Insider Knowledge From a Diabet

Dr. Ahmet Ergin

THE ULTIMATE DIABETES BOOK

This book is dedicated to the millions of people who are struggling with diabetes, my faithful followers, and my loyal patients. Thank you all for your continued support.

Foreword/Introduction

You are now reading the only guide you will ever need to support you on your diabetes journey. These pages are not just filled with tips and advice from a diet guru or general practitioner. As an endocrinologist and diabetes educator, I've spent my entire career as a physician working with diabetic patients. On a daily basis, I saw firsthand the problems my diabetic patients were facing and the many challenges they had to overcome which became the inspiration for this book.

Whether you have diabetes or know someone with diabetes, the diagnosis can be overwhelming. But it doesn't have to be. Since the discovery of diabetes in 1899 many advancements have been made to help improve the lives of those living with the disease. As an endocrinologist, my job is to help those inflicted with the disease control, manage, and overcome it with the help of new technologies, lifestyle changes or medications. In these pages you will find insightful guidance and advice on some of the topics my patients ask me about most.

My personal journey into diabetes world began when I was only 18 years old in medical school. I quickly gained an interest in diabetes and after my fellowship at Cleveland Clinic in Ohio, it became my passion. This passion stemmed from not only a medical interest but an interest of the heart. My mother has been living with type 2 diabetes for years. I watched her suffer from debilitating and uncontrollable lows for too long. But it's not just her. Over 425 million people worldwide suffer from diabetes so I live each day with the hope to change patient lives… hopefully one of them will be yours. Regardless if you are a patient of one of my clinics, YouTube follower or simply a reader, I want to make a difference in your life and in the way you see and treat your diabetes. Diabetes is a lifelong disease but it's not a lifelong burden. It simply depends on the way you view and treat it.

This book was written to serve as a beacon of light, a ray of hope and a trusted guide to help you manage and overcome your diabetes. No matter what type of diabetes you may have, you will find invaluable knowledge and expertise on every page.

The answers to your many questions about your diabetes care, treatment and management can all be found in one place…***The Ultimate Diabetes Guide.***

Acknowledgments

I want to take a moment to give thanks to the following who filled me with inspiration, motivation, and love.

My patients who may not even be aware, have given me both inspiration and motivation to fill these pages with knowledge. From the very beginning, my patients provided me with the experience I needed to grow as a physician.

I want to send my love and give a special thanks to my wife, Jacqueline A. Ergin, who provided endless support and love during the SugarMD journey. Thank you for standing by me during all the late nights and weekends worked.

And of course, God who made all of this possible. I'm truly humbled by God's everlasting grace.

Table Of Contents

CHAPTER 1: WHAT IS DIABETES AND WHAT CAUSES IT? 20

- What Is Blood Sugar? 21
- Where Does Glucose Come From? 22
- How Does Your Blood Sugar Get Regulated When You Don'T Have Diabetes? 24
- How Is Diabetes Defined? 25
  - Can I Test And Diagnose Myself With Diabetes Via Fingerstick? 27
- Who Needs Testing For Diabetes? 30
- What Causes Diabetes? 31
- Is Diabetes A Progressive Disease Or Can It Be Cured? ... 32
- Can Bariatric Surgery/Gastric Bypass Surgery Cure Diabetes? 33
  - Who Is Eligible For Bariatric Surgery? 35
  - Can Bariatric Surgery Prevent Diabetes In Obese People? Will It Last? 36
- Defects In The Body That Lead To Diabetes 37
- The Root Cause Of Other Types Of Diabetes 39
- Miscellaneous Factors That Can Cause Diabetes 40
- Medications That Contribute To Developing Diabetes 40
- Final Thoughts 42

CHAPTER 2: TYPES OF DIABETES 44

Insulin Resistance, Metabolic Syndrome And Prediabetes 46
Who Is More Likely To Develop Insulin Resistance? 49
What Diseases Are Linked To Being Insulin Resistant? 56
Prediabetes 58
Metabolic Syndrome 61
A Brief Review Of What To Do 62
Summary Of Insulin Resistance And Its Complications 64
Type 1 Versus Type 2 Diabetes 65
Risk Factors For Diabetic Ketoacidosis 71
Are Type 1 Diabetics Guaranteed To Have Thyroid Disease Or Adrenal Insufficiency? 71
LADA (Latent Autoimmune Diabetes Of Adults) 72
A Rare Kind Of Diabetes That Runs In Families: MODY (Maturity-Onset Diabetes Of The Young) 73
Final Thoughts 74

CHAPTER 3: DIABETES BASICS 76

Risk Factors For Diabetes 79
How To Prevent Diabetes 81
Lifestyle Modifications 82
Medications Or Supplements That Can Help Prevent Diabetes 83
Signs And Symptoms Of High Blood Sugar Due To Diabetes 83
What Is A High Blood Sugar Level? 89

    When Should You Seek Medical Attention?.. 91

    Why Are Your Blood Sugars High In The Mornings?.........................92

The Dawn Phenomenon And Somogyi Effect....................93

    Why Are My Blood Sugars So Up And Down In The Mornings?.....94

    The Bottom Line: How Does Insulin Resistance
Cause High Blood Sugar In The Morning? 96

    Do I Have To Worry About My Sugar Spiking After Eating?........... 98

What Is Low Blood Sugar/Hypoglycemia And How Can You Prevent Or Correct It? 99

    Factors That Contribute To Low Blood Sugar....................................101

    What Can You Do To Manage Low Blood Sugars? 104

    Low Blood Sugars Without Symptoms.. 105

    How Can You Avoid Low Blood Sugars In The First Place?...........106

    Why Do The Symptoms Of Low Blood Sugar
Differ Between Individuals?... 107

    Insulin And Sulfonylurea Drugs Increase The Risk
Of Low Blood Sugar!... 109

    Continuous Glucose Monitoring Systems Help A Lot 109

    Diabetic Drugs That Don'T Cause Low Blood Sugar 110

    What Other Measures You Can You Take To Prevent
And Control Low Blood Sugar?..110

    Fear Of Hypoglycemia (Low Blood Sugar)..111

What Causes Blood Sugar Fluctuations? 112

The Bottom Line On Blood Sugar Fluctuations 116

What Is HbA1C?..117

    What Is A Good A1c Goal? 119

    Using The A1c Level To Help Manage Your Diabetes.....................120

    Advantages And Disadvantages Of The A1c Test............................ 121

    What Are Some Alternatives To A1c Measurements? 123

Why Is My A1c Not Coming Down Below 7%? 124
A1c Testing During Pregnancy.. 125
Final Thoughts On The A1c Level.. 125

Individualized Blood Sugar Goals **126**
What Is A Normal Goal For The HbA1c?... 126

Final Thoughts **127**

CHAPTER 4: DIABETES MANAGEMENT......... 128

6 Pillars Of Diabetes Control: What You Need To Know To Be Fully Prepared To Manage Your Diabetes Easily ... 130

1. Eat Healthy.. 130
Should I Lose Weight, And If So, How Much? 134
What Is The Best Diabetic Diet?.. 134
Specific Diabetic Diets... 135
    Keto Diet..135
    What Types Of Fats Are In The Keto Diet?..138
    What Are The Effects Of A Ketogenic Diet On Blood Sugar?.............138
    Is There A Downside To The Keto Diet? 138
    What Not To Eat On A Ketogenic Diet...139
    Monitoring Your Diabetes On A Keto Diet...140
    Is There Any Evidence To Back Up The Benefits Of A Keto Diet?........141
    The Final Word On The Keto Diet… 141
Intermittent Fasting 143
    What Is The Difference Between Reducing Calorie Diet Versus Intermittent Fasting? 144
    Will I Lose Muscle While Intermittent Fasting?..................................145
    What Changes Happen In Your Body When You Fast? 145
    What Are The Benefits Of Using Ketones As A Source Of Energy?....146
    How Do I Deal With The Side Effects Of Intermittent Fasting? 148

    Can I Exercise During Intermittent Fasting? 149

    Important Points For Diabetics Trying Intermittent Fasting…..............149

Mediterranean Diet 151

Diabetic Diet Basics 152

    What Are The Different Food Groups, And How Do They
    Affect Your Blood Sugar?..152

    How Does Protein Affect Blood Sugar?...152

    What Are Carbohydrates?..153

    Are All Carbohydrates The Same? 154

    How Do Carbohydrates Metabolize In The Body? 154

    What Do Carbohydrates Do? 155

    What Are Complex And Simple Carbohydrates? 156

    Complex Carbohydrates 156

    Examples Of Complex Carbohydrates 157

    Simple Carbohydrates..158

    What Are The Glycemic Index And Glycemic Load?
    And How To Use The Glycemic Index To Your Advantage? 159

    The Essential Role Of Fiber In Carbohydrates...161

    Recommendations On Fiber Intake 162

    Why Does The Body Absorb Refined Carbohydrates
    Very Quickly And Raise Blood Sugars? 163

    The Role Of Your Diabetes Coach And Endocrinologist......................164

    In Summary...165

    How Many Carbs Should A Diabetic Have? 166

    What Does "Counting Carbs" Mean?..166

    How Do I Count Carbs?... 167

    Do I Have To Count Carbs For Diabetes Or Are There Any
    Other Alternative Ways To Manage My Diet?..168

    Do I Have To Eat At The Same Time Every Day? 168

    How Do I Determine The Number Of Carbs I Need? 169

    Do Men And Women Have Different Carbohydrate Goals? 170

    How Many Carbs Should A Diabetic Person Eat Later In Life? 171

Can I Go With No Carbs To Cure My Diabetes?..172
Are Artificial Sweeteners Safe For Diabetics To Take? 172
Do Artificial Sweeteners Help With Weight Loss? 173
Do Artificial Sweeteners Cause Cancer? 174
What Are The Disadvantages Of Artificial Sweeteners?................................174
What About Sugar Alcohols?...174
How Much Pasta Can A Diabetic Have? Are There Any
Pasta Alternatives Diabetics Can Eat?...175
How Much Rice Can A Diabetic Eat And Is There A Rice
Alternative For Diabetics?...176
Can Diabetics Eat A Potato? Is Sweet Potato Better
Than A Regular Potato?...177
Can Diabetics Eat Oatmeal Or Cereal? 178
Are Oatmeals A Low Glycemic Index Food?..179
Can Diabetics Eat Bread? What Types Of Bread Are
Good For Diabetics?...180
Calories And Calorie Distribution On A Diabetic Diet....................................182
But I Only Had A Salad...183
What Are The Other Important Things Besides Carbs
In Anyone'S Diet Living With Diabetes?..184

2. Being Active 186

How To Exercise For Diabetes.. 187

Activity Tips To Help Control Your Diabetes:..188
How Do I Transition From Being Sedentary To Active? 188
Developing A Structured Diabetes Exercise Program 189
Types Of Exercises That Are Helpful For People With Diabetes 190
Safety Precautions For Diabetics Deciding To Undertake Exercise: 191
Determining The Intensity Of Exercise For Diabetes 191
The Rating Of Perceived Exertion (RPE)..192
How Long Should I Exercise To Benefit My Diabetes? 193
In Summary..194
Avoid Exercise-Induced Low Blood Sugar 196

3. Checking Blood Sugars (Monitoring)..................................196

What Can Frequent Monitoring Glucose Do For You? 198

How To Make Glucose Testing Easy With Fingersticks And Get The Most Out Of Limited Data...202

Which Factors Affect Blood Glucose Levels? 203

Which Factors Affect Blood Sugar The Most?..204

Do You Really Have To Check Your Blood Sugar 7-10 Times A Day To Know Your Blood Sugar Is Controlled? 205

How Many Times Do You Need To Check Your Blood Sugars At The Early Stages Of Diabetes? 207

Can I Stop Taking My Blood Sugars If They Are Consistently Normal?..208

How Many Times A Day Should I Check My Blood Sugars On Insulin?..208

How To Check Your Blood Sugar Accurately With Minimal Pain And Effort 210

Which Glucose Meter To Choose From? 211

How To Record Blood Sugars Accurately And Quickly 211

Common Factors Affecting The Accuracy Of Blood Glucose Results...212

Blood Sugar Monitoring Tips To Help Control Your Diabetes:..............213

Trending Now: CGM (Continuous Glucose Monitoring Systems) 214

Are Fingersticks Necessary On Dexcom G6 Or Freestyle Libre CGM?..215

Is CGM The Right Option For Me? 216

The Benefits Of CGM Systems...217

4. Taking Medications 217

Tips You'Ll Need To Optimize Your Medication Management: 218

Medications That Affect Blood Sugars...219

Generic Drugs For Diabetes 220

Sulfonylureas And Meglitinides: Why You Shouldn'T Use Them As First-Line Agents 221

How Do The Sulfonylureas Work? 221
Why Do Sulfonylureas Have Such A Bad Reputation? 222
Sulfonylureas And Low Blood Sugars 222

Metformin: Advantages And Disadvantages 223
When Should Metformin Be Avoided? 225
Metformin Side Effects 226
Metformin And Weight Loss 228
Metformin And Diarrhea 228
The Bottom Line On Metformin 229

Pioglitazone - Good Or Bad? 230
Most Common Adverse Reactions From Pioglitazone (Actos) 231
Is Pioglitazone Effective And Are There Risks To Worry About? 232
The Bottom Line 233

Name-Brand Drugs For Diabetes 233

DPP-IV Inhibitors (Januvia, Tradjenta, Saxagliptin, Alogliptin, And Others) 233
What Are The Side Effects Of DPP-4 Inhibitors? 234
DPP-4 Inhibitors And Pancreatic Disease 235
The Bottom Line 235

GLP-1-Smart Insulin Secretion- Why Are They So Popular Now? 236
Common GLP-1 Medications: Ozempic, Rybelsus, Victoza, Trulicity, Bydureon, And Byetta 236
GLP-1 Agonists Effects 237
Rarely Reported Problems With GLP-1 Agonists 237
Avoiding Side Effects With GLP-Agonists 238
Who Should Not Take A GLP-1 Agonist Drug? 239
About Thyroid Cancer And GLP-1 Agonists 239
Disorders Which Might Impact Side Effects From A GLP-1 Agonist . 240
How To Take A GLP-1 Agonist Drug 241
Using A GLP-1 Agonist During Pregnancy And Breastfeeding 241

- Positive Effects Of Taking A GLP-1 Agonist Drug 242
- Summary Of GLP-1 Agonist Pros And Cons 242

SGLT2 Inhibitors: Jardiance, Farxiga, Invokana, And Steglatro. 242
- Pros And Cons Of SGLT2 Inhibitors 243
- Avoid SGLT2 Inhibitors Under These Circumstances: 245

Insulins 246
- The Type And Duration Of Diabetes Determine Whether You Need Insulin Or Not! 246
- What Types Of Insulins Are Available? 248
- Pay Attention To These 3 Important Features: 248
- Common Insulins On The Market And Their Features: 249
- How Do I Take Insulin? 250
- Insulin Pen Priming 251
- Injecting Insulin 251
- More About Long-Acting Insulins 253
- What Happens If You Have Low Blood Sugar On Long-Acting Insulin? 254
- Practical Information On Taking A Long-Acting Insulin 255

Diabetic Medications And Alcohol Use 256
- Diabetic Medications, Alcohol Use, And Lactic Acidosis 257
- What Are The Symptoms Of Lactic Acidosis When Taking Your Diabetic Medications And Alcohol? 257
- If You Drink Alcohol, Should You Stop Taking Metformin Or Other Diabetic Medications? 257

Diabetes Drugs That Cause Weight Gain Or Weight Loss 258
- Common Reasons For Weight Gain In Diabetes: 258
- Diabetes Medications That Cause Weight Loss 260
- Metformin 260
- Ozempic, Trulicity, Rybelsus, And Bydureon 260
- What About An SGLT2 Inhibitor Like Invokana, Farxiga, Or Steglatro And Weight Loss? 261
- The Bottom Line 262

5. Problem-Solving And Healthy Coping 262

    Stress And Depression 264

    Depression "Stats" In Diabetes And How To Seek Help 265

    Alarming Symptoms Of Depression In Diabetic Patients 265

    What You Can Do About Diabetes And Depression 266

    Your Social Life With Diabetes.. 269

    Common Financial Problems With Diabetes................................ 270

    Sick Day Management Of Diabetes 271

    Follow These Additional Steps When You're Sick Even If Your Blood Sugar Is Within Good Range: 272

    Eating Out 272

    Vacations And Holidays 273

    Traveling For Diabetics..274

    Playing Sports With Diabetes 276

6. Reducing Your Risk Of Complications 278

    The Legacy Effect...279

    How Do You Know If Your Diabetes Is Under Control In The First Ten Years?..280

    Reducing Your Risks Of Heart Disease And Stroke....................... 282

    Diabetes Is The Most Common Reason For Heart Attacks And Strokes. 282

    The Biggest Risk: Heart Disease And Stroke 282

    Is Diabetes-Related Heart Disease Preventable? 284

    What Does It Mean To Have Each Of These Risk Factors Controlled In A Diabetic? 286

    How Can I Stop Insulin Resistance, Prevent The Progression Of Diabetes, And Lessen The Chances Of Developing Heart Attacks And Strokes? 287

    Diabetic Neuropathy 287

        Signs Of Diabetic Neuropathy 288

- Different Types Of Diabetic Neuropathy 288
- Detecting Diabetic Neuropathy 291
- Some Diabetic Foot Ulcers Are Due To Diabetic Neuropathy 292
- Risk Factors/Causes Of Diabetic Neuropathy 293
- Treatment Of Diabetic Neuropathy 293
- Diabetic Foot Care 296
- Preventing Diabetic Neuropathy 297

Peripheral Vascular Disease 298
- How Do Diabetic Foot Ulcers And Gangrene Begin? 298

Kidney Disease 300
- How Does Diabetic Kidney Disease Develop? 301
- What Are The Risk Factors For Diabetic Kidney Disease? 303
- Signs And Symptoms Of Chronic Kidney Disease 304
- How Is Diabetic Kidney Disease Prevented And Managed? 304

Diabetic Retinopathy 306
- Symptoms Of Diabetic Retinopathy 308
- Testing For Diabetic Retinopathy 309
- Preventing Diabetic Retinopathy 309
- Treating Diabetic Retinopathy 310
- In Summary 311

Gastroparesis 311
- Medications That Can Cause Or Worsen Gastroparesis 312
- How Do We Diagnose Diabetic Gastroparesis? 312
- How To Treat Diabetic Gastroparesis 312

Erectile Dysfunction 313
- Could Erectile Dysfunction (ED) Be A Symptom Of Diabetes? 314
- Risk Factors For Erectile Dysfunction In Diabetics 314
- Other Types Of Sexual Problems Seen In Men 314
- Types Of Sexual Problems In Women 316
- Management And Treatment 317

Final Thoughts 318

CHAPTER 5: DIABETES TECHNOLOGY.......... 320

Insulin Pumps 321
What Is An Insulin Pump And How Does It Work?............................322
Who Is A Good Candidate For An Insulin Pump?............................323
Is An Insulin Pump Right For Me?..324
Advantages Of Using An Insulin Pump 325
Disadvantages Of The Insulin Pump 325
Components Of An Insulin Pump 326
Various Kinds Of Infusion Sets Are Available 327
Various Types Of Insulin Pumps 327
Choosing An Insulin Pump.. 328
Tandem Pumps..329
Medtronic Insulin Pumps 330
How An Insulin Pump Works... 333
Checking Sugars On The Insulin Pump 333
Wearing An Insulin Pump.. 334
Maintaining And Troubleshooting Your Insulin Pump 334
Final Thoughts 336

Continuous Glucose Monitoring Systems 336
Dexcom G6 System- Soon To Be G7... 336
Is CGM The Right Option For Me? 337
The Benefits Of CGM Systems 338
How To Choose The Right CGM? 339
Using CGM Systems And Troubleshooting Them 340
Using Your CGM System To Make Treatment Decisions 342
Interpreting Your CGM Numbers 342

If You See An Arrow That Is Diagonal Up Or Diagonal Down: 343
If You See A Straight Up Or Straight Down Arrow On Your Dexcom G6: 343
Making Treatment Decisions Between Meals Or When Fasting Using A CGM Device..344
CGMCost And Coverage Issues 346
Final Thoughts 347

A Modern Concept: What Are The Benefits Of Telemedicine And Remote Patient Monitoring? 348
How Does Remote Patient Monitoring Work? 349
How Remote Patient Monitoring And CGM Work Together In SugarMDs Center? 350
The Future Of Telemedicine 351
CONCLUSION 352

CHAPTER 1
WHAT IS DIABETES AND WHAT CAUSES IT?

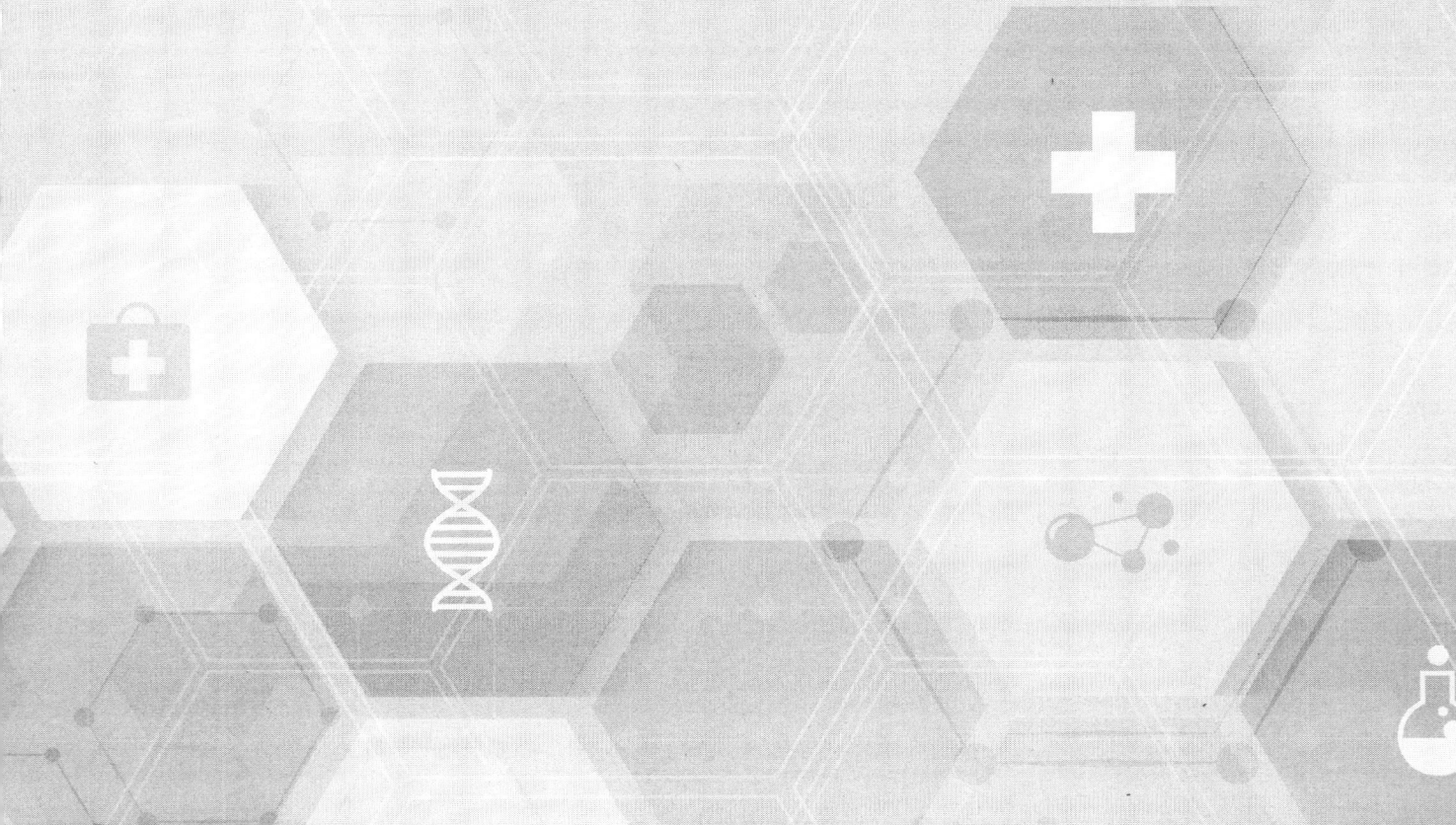

CHAPTER 1
WHAT IS DIABETES AND WHAT CAUSES IT?

Unless you've really not paid attention to the world around you, you probably already know that diabetes has something to do with blood sugar. You would be right about this fact to a point, but you will find out that diabetes is more than just "high blood sugar" as you read this book. This is because there are many reasons a person's blood sugar might be too high.

At the end of this first chapter, I hope you will feel informed, educated, and empowered because knowledge is power. And power will help you succeed against diabetes. Let's take a brief look at diabetes and what it means to have it. To understand diabetes, you have to understand what blood sugar is first.

What Is Blood Sugar?

When you have your blood sugar measured at home or the doctor's office, what the test is actually measuring is your blood "glucose" level. Glucose is just one type of sugar, but for the cells in your body, it is the only one that really counts when it comes to giving your cells the fuel it needs.

Every cell in your body needs fuel so you can make the energy you need to drive all of the chemical reactions your cells must have so they can function. Glucose is the simplest fuel for most of your cells. You could survive without much sugar in your diet if you had to, but it would be harder on your cells without any glucose to use as fuel. In order to use other types of nutrients besides glucose for fuel, your cells have unique biochemical pathways to take just about anything you eat and funnel these into making glucose before going on to make the energy for your cell.

Most cells in your body can use things like fats and proteins for energy (usually after turning these nutrients into glucose first). Your brain cells, however, are not as flexible and only run best on pure glucose aka sugar.

Even if your body can use ketones, if your blood sugar becomes really low, you will not be able to survive unless the blood sugar is corrected. To see just how it feels to have a low blood sugar, I gave myself 30 units of fast-acting insulin. Do NOT try this at home, ever. My wife was on standby with a glucagon injection and I had my camera rolling. I figured that was the only way to have empathy with my patients. And yes, my blood sugar went down to 50 mg/dL (2.775 mmol/l), and no, it wasn't a pleasant feeling.

So, what does the body do with the glucose, anyway? Well, the final end-product of consuming glucose aka sugar from a cellular standpoint is that glucose gets broken down into carbon dioxide and water. This is the same carbon dioxide you exhale with every breath. While carbon dioxide or CO_2 is a waste product of your cells' metabolism, its production has a big bonus: you make tons of energy. Your body then uses this energy for bodily functions such as breathing, digesting, walking, etc.

Where Does Glucose Come From?

You can't survive long without food. The food you eat is where your glucose comes from. Hardly ever would you eat pure glucose, however. Instead, you eat food which is composed of major macronutrients: carbohydrates, fats, and proteins.

When you eat, your digestive system releases a cocktail of different chemicals and enzymes that break large, complex molecules like carbohydrates, fats, and proteins into their simplest components. These essential building block molecules (like glucose) are small enough to be absorbed by your gastrointestinal tract (GI tract), so they can pass into your bloodstream to be distributed to all the cells in your body.

✈ Fast Fact

Are carbohydrates, sugars, and glucose the same thing? Not really. Carbohydrates or carbs can mean sugar or glucose, but they can also mean much bigger chains of simple sugar molecules linked together. The starch in the potato you ate for dinner has glucose in it but not in its simplest form. This long chain of glucose molecules must be broken down in your gut into glucose molecules so you can absorb them. Also, "sugar" can mean carbs, glucose, or something else. For example, table sugar is a combination of glucose and fructose (fruit sugar) linked together. You can also call milk sugar (lactose) a kind of sugar, even though it is a combination molecule made of glucose and galactose (another simple sugar). Usually, when I say the term "sugar," I mean simple sugars made from one or two simple sugar molecules. If I say "carbohydrates," I probably mean the long-chain version that needs to be broken down in the gut.

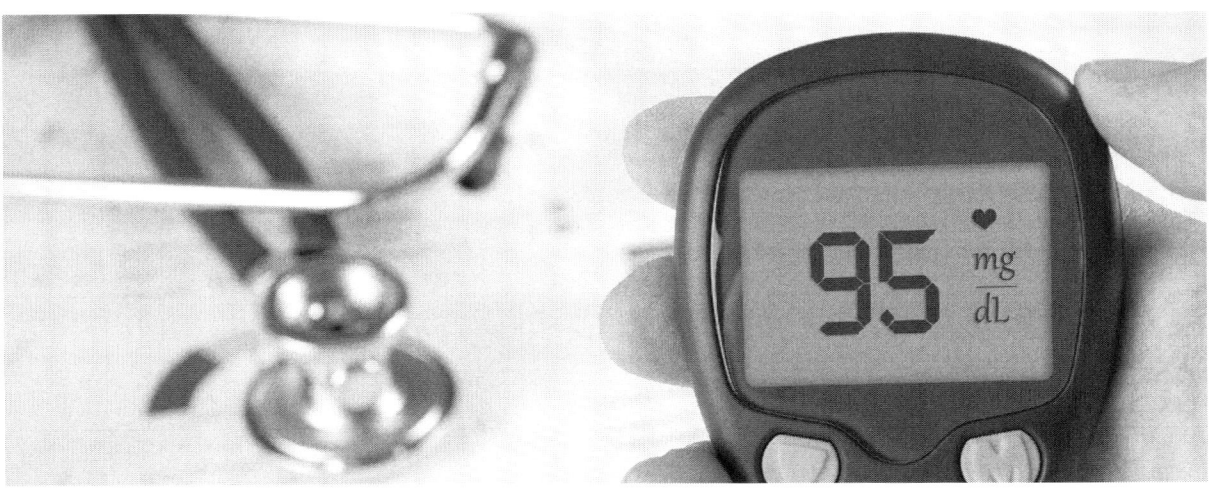

How Does Your Blood Sugar Get Regulated When You Don't Have Diabetes?

Insulin serves to coordinate the use of fuels (glucose, free fatty acids, and amino acids) to meet your body's energy demands during cycles of feeding and fasting and in response to exercise.

To put it simply, when you eat, your insulin levels go up. It increases the most when you eat carbohydrates. It can also go up when you eat protein and fat (but not as much). Although insulin responds to the protein and fat you eat, it is much less responsive to them than it is to the carbohydrates you eat. As a result, I concentrate most on carbohydrate consumption when treating my diabetic patients while letting them know that a lot of animal fat in the diet can increase insulin requirements.

Insulin allows glucose to enter into the cells so it can be utilized as an energy source. Insulin also helps store unused glucose in the form of glycogen stores. Glycogen is a long chain of glucose molecules in a row. When the glycogen stores are full, insulin will help make fat from the same glucose cells. That explains why carbohydrates cause weight gain.

Exercise uses up a lot of glycogen at once. When you do not exercise enough, the glycogen stores in the body remain full. Unless the carbohydrates (which turn into glucose in the intestinal system before absorption) are used as an immediate energy source, insulin will help turn this glucose into fat.

When you are fasting, your insulin levels go down. In turn, glucagon (made in the pancreas' alpha cells) goes up to help convert glycogen into glucose. Glucose is then readily available for energy for the cells. This tradeoff of insulin and glucagon keeps your blood sugars regulated day and night, whether you are fasting or not.

How Is Diabetes Defined?

The simplest definition of diabetes is that it involves a persistent state of high blood sugar. The reasons for this vary from person to person. I like this definition because it avoids calling a person "diabetic" if they have a high blood sugar level after getting a cortisone shot, for example. If the blood sugar rises after you get one of these steroid shots but is normal all other times, it doesn't mean you don't have any trouble handling sugar in your body. In fact, you probably do have some difficulty with this. It also doesn't necessarily mean you have diabetes, however.

The concept of "diabetes" is mostly a numbers issue. It means you have inappropriately high blood glucose levels, but the reasons behind it vary according to the type of diabetes you have. I will talk much more about the different kinds of diabetes we know about. Regardless of the kind you have, it is diagnosed by your blood sugar numbers more than anything else.

About the numbers: you can have several tests in your doctor's office or have some other screening test that will tell you whether or not you have diabetes. Based on what the numbers say, your doctor can tell you whether or not you have the disease. Let's look at the different tests used to make the official diagnosis of diabetes. You will need 2 of 3 tests positive to confirm your diabetes. Let us review what these tests are:

1. *Fasting blood sugar:* This is a common screening test for diabetes. It involves having an overnight fast (nothing but water and most medications for at least 8 hours). You will have your blood tested once for this test. These are the current rules for what this test means:

    » Normal blood sugar—less than 100 milligrams per deciliter (mg/dL) (5.55 mmol/l)

    » Prediabetes—between 100 and 125 mg/dL (5.55 mmol/l – 6.9375 mmol/l)

- » Diabetes—above 125 mg/dL (6.9375 mmol/l)
- » Normal range for known diabetics—80 to 130 mg/dL (4.44 mmol/l – 7.215 mmol/l)

If the number falls close to the dividing line between two levels, it is usually a simple matter to recheck it or to confirm the diagnosis with another test.

2. *Glycosylated hemoglobin (HbA1c):* I will talk more about this test in a little bit but essentially it is a measure of how "sugar-coated" your red blood cells have been lately. Because red blood cells live in your body for about 120 days, this test can be done any time of the day without any fasting and will tell you how high your average blood sugar was over the previous three months. This is because glucose sticks to your red blood cells for their entire lifetime. We use this number to make these diagnoses:

- » Normal—less than 5.7%
- » Prediabetes—between 5.7% and 6.4%
- » Diabetes—6.5% or above

This is an excellent test for several reasons. 1) It requires no fasting. 2) It ignores isolated highs and lows in order to give a nice "average" blood sugar number. 3) It is a good way to see if anything you've done to treat your diabetes has been effective. For this reason, it can be repeated as often as every three months among known diabetics.

3. *Glucose Tolerance Testing or GTT:* This is a test done in the doctor's office. You need to fast overnight and then drink a glucose-containing syrup with exactly 75 grams of glucose in it. Your blood sugar is tested two hours later. These are the results:

- » Normal—less than 140 mg/dL (7.77 mmol/l)
- » Prediabetes—140 to 199 mg/dL (7.77 mmol/l – 11.04 mmol/l)

» Diabetes—200 mg/dL or more (11.1 mmol/l)

Note: 200 mg/dl (11.1 mmol/l) at any time during the test also confirms diabetes.

Can I Test And Diagnose Myself With Diabetes Via Fingerstick?

The fasting blood sugar, 2-hour post-meal blood sugar, and HbA1C tests are essential to screen and diagnose diabetes. But, if you think you have diabetes and do not have a normal blood sugar level, it's important to avoid diagnosing yourself by doing a fingerstick with a home blood glucose meter. There are standards that laboratories use for diagnosing diabetes you won't get with a fingerstick.

For this reason, you should ask your doctor's office to test you at a laboratory. Although, if you checked your blood sugar with another person's meter and found a high blood sugar level such as 200 mg/dL or more (11.1 mmol/l), it can indicate you may have diabetes. In that case, I would strongly recommend seeing your doctor as soon as possible.

It's also important to talk with your Endocrinologist to ensure you know how often you should check blood sugars, such as fasting blood sugar or HbA1C test. Also, understand what your results mean and what your blood sugar and HbA1C targets are.

If you have not been previously diagnosed with diabetes, prediabetes, or insulin resistance and your results are above "normal," your endocrinologist may recommend other tests.

Treatment may include lifestyle changes such as weight loss, a healthy diabetic eating plan, and regular exercise. You may need to start taking diabetes medications when lifestyle changes fail, including insulin, although that is usually the last resort in most cases.

If you are diagnosed with diabetes, I recommend getting a proper education on checking your blood sugars with a meter or a CGM such as a Dexcom or Freestyle Libre system. Also, work with your doctor to collaborate on a treatment plan that will work for you.

Miscellaneous sugar-related tests: A random blood sugar test done any time of day without regard to eating can also be helpful. Any random blood sugar level greater than 200 mg/dL (11.1 mmol/l) is also considered to be diabetes, especially if there are symptoms of the disease. Some people will learn they have "sugar in their urine," but this is a flawed test for diabetes. Still, having this finding might indicate that further testing is needed.

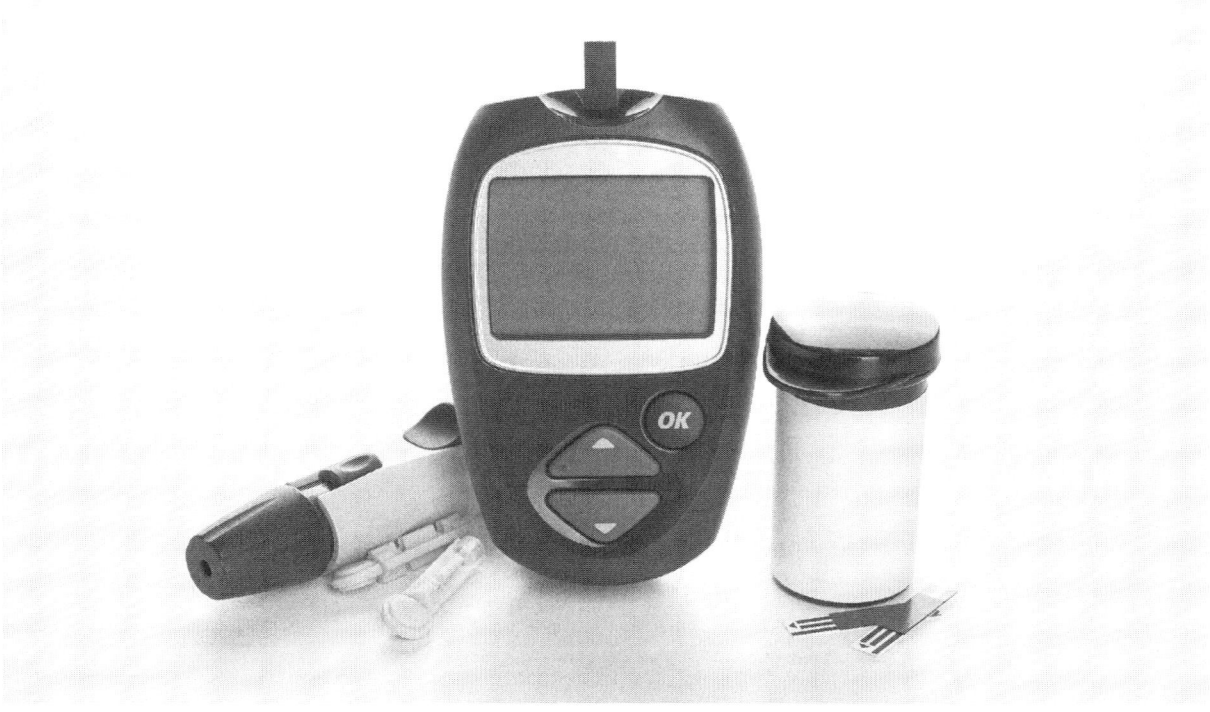

Tests to determine the diabetes type: Some testing can be done to see what type of diabetes you have. Not everyone needs these tests, but they are sometimes helpful. One test, called the C-peptide test, is done to see if you are making insulin. C-peptide is a small chunk of protein that breaks off after insulin is made by the pancreas, and before the insulin can be "activated." If this test is low, you probably have type 1 diabetes. If this test is high or even normal, you probably have type 2 diabetes.

The normal range for C-peptide is between 0.5 and 2.0 nanograms per milliliter, although reference ranges may differ from laboratory to laboratory. In addition to that, C-peptide test levels should be interpreted knowing what the blood glucose levels are at the time of the test. I would highly recommend an Endocrinologist interpret your C-peptide test levels.

Antibody screening is another possible test for certain types of diabetes. Some of these include the following:

- Islet cell cytoplasmic antibodies (for type 1 diabetes or latent autoimmune diabetes, also called LADA)
- Glutamic acid decarboxylase antibodies
- IA-2 alpha antibodies
- IA-2 beta antibodies

As you will learn, type 1 diabetes and type 1.5 diabetes (LADA) are truly immune-related disorders where your immune system makes antibodies that destroy insulin-making cells (beta cells). Other types, like type 2 diabetes, don't involve these types of immune molecules. This is why antibody testing can be helpful, especially at the time of the diagnosis.

On the other hand, antibody testing is not necessarily done for every diabetic patient. Patients who are candidates for these antibody tests are younger individuals or patients who are not necessarily overweight. For example, a 45-year-old male who is 5'10" and 170 pounds (not overweight) with high blood sugars may have type 1.5 diabetes with positive antibodies in his blood.

On the other hand, a 10-year-old-year-old girl with obesity may have type 2 diabetes instead of type 1. Because of her young age, I would order antibody testing to rule out type 1 diabetes.

I see patients almost every day who have been misdiagnosed previously. The most common misdiagnosis is type 2 diabetes, while in reality, the patient has type 1.5 diabetes.

Fast Fact

So, is diabetes a matter of having too much insulin or too little? This is a trick question because, as you've probably figured out, diabetes isn't defined by the amount of insulin you have. Some people with diabetes have little or no insulin, so it makes sense they have diabetes. Others have a great deal of this hormone, but because they can't use it properly (a problem also known as insulin resistance), they also have diabetes. I will talk more about how this works in a later section.

Who Needs Testing For Diabetes?

The whole reason to test for diabetes in most cases is to find out as soon as possible if someone has diabetes or is at risk for it. This often means being able to make a difference in whether or not there are long-term complications of the disease. It is beneficial for people with prediabetes because they can make lifestyle changes to avoid ever getting actual diabetes.

These are the people who would benefit most from getting screened for high blood sugar:

- » Everyone aged 40 to 70 years who are overweight or obese should be screened at least once for diabetes according to recommendations made by the US Preventive Services Task Force.

- » Everyone at the age of 45 years, even without risk factors, should be screened for diabetes according to recommendations made by the American Diabetes Association (ADA).

» The American Association of Clinical Endocrinologists has more complex recommendations for screening, including those 45 years or older, those who have a skin disease called acanthosis nigricans, those taking certain antipsychotic drugs, those with other risk factors for heart disease, women with polycystic ovarian disease, and people with parents or siblings who have type 2 diabetes.

» Children aged 10 or older with a strong family history of type 2 diabetes, obesity, or evidence they might have diabetes should be screened according to ADA recommendations.

» All pregnant women are screened for gestational diabetes at about 24 to 28 weeks' gestation.

» The ADA has an online diabetes risk calculator at this link: https://www.diabetes.org/risk-test. If you take the written test, and it shows you are at risk, your doctor might decide to screen you based on this test result.

Most screening tests will be definitive and will indicate if you have or don't have diabetes. People who are at risk because they have prediabetes are often screened every few years for the rest of their lives.

What Causes Diabetes?

Diabetes has a lot to do with supply and demand. The supply side is the insulin you make, and the demand side is usually your body weight. The more you weigh, the more insulin you need. If you can shift the supply and demand in specific ways, you can determine whether or not you develop diabetes.

Let's use an analogy: The definition of being wealthy versus poor all depends on how much money you make and how much money you spend. You could be making $1 million a year and can still be in debt or go bankrupt because of uncontrolled expenses. On the other hand, you could be making $50,000 a year yet be very cautious about your spending, which will lead to a significant amount of savings over time. So the person making $1 million a year may end up with millions of dollars of debt, and the person making $50,000 a year can accumulate millions of dollars by retirement time with a good savings and investment strategy.

The capacity to make insulin is usually genetically determined. This is your supply side and is something you can't change. You can, however, adjust your demand for insulin by remaining in a healthy weight range. If you never become overweight, even if you don't make a lot of insulin, you have a good chance of avoiding diabetes altogether. On the other hand, if you are overweight or obese, you may still develop diabetes even if you genetically make decent amounts of insulin.

Is Diabetes A Progressive Disease Or Can It Be Cured?

Before we dive into how diabetes progresses over time, I want to emphasize that the idea of a "diabetes cure" is a relative one. If you consider having an A1c level of less than 5.7% a cure, this is certainly possible in almost every case. On the other hand, if you consider having an A1c less than 5.7% forever in any diabetic, this is virtually impossible.

If you already have type 2 diabetes and lose a significant amount of weight (which can change depending on the person and the duration of diabetes), you can be "cured" from diabetes. The most common example of a diabetes cure can be seen in people who have had gastric bypass surgery. Very soon after the surgery, these individuals stop taking medications and literally become diabetes-free. We will talk more about bariatric surgery later.

Since diabetes is a supply and demand disease, just because you are cured of diabetes at one time does not mean that diabetes will not come back. From a medical standpoint, we call that "remission." For example, just because you had pneumonia or a common cold and were cured with antibiotics, this does not mean that you will not have another episode of pneumonia or common cold if you have the same risk factors.

This means that managing your risk factors is the most important part of "curing" diabetes. The reason we were able to eradicate a lot of viral or bacterial infections seen throughout history is that we have implemented risk-reduction measures in the entire population, such as vaccines, hygiene, preservative agents in the water, etc. With diabetes, you are mostly on your own in controlling your personal risk of developing diabetes again.

And yes, the ugly truth we accept or not is that diabetes is a pervasive hormonal glandular disease caused by permanent damage to the beta cells in your pancreas. Through various mechanisms, when you reduce the demand on the pancreas through diet and exercise and/or you increase the potential insulin production by taking certain medications, diabetes can be put into remission.

Remember that your maximum insulin production capacity is also genetically determined. With diabetes, the amount of insulin you can maximally make is not enough to overcome the insulin resistance you have. In addition to that, by the time you are diagnosed with diabetes, you have lost almost 80% of your insulin-making beta cells. Still, most people have plenty of insulin, but it is mostly ineffective in helping glucose enter the cells. This process happens faster when you are already genetically inclined to have diabetes. As a result, you may not be able to keep up with your insulin needs, especially when you gain weight.

Can Bariatric Surgery/Gastric Bypass Surgery Cure Diabetes?

Bariatric surgery can be an excellent alternative when dietary and medication approaches fail for type 2 diabetes. Bariatric surgery has been a popular treatment for obesity for this reason.

Can bariatric surgery cure diabetes? Sometimes, but in not all cases. People who have a milder form of diabetes (controlled with diet) for less than five years and who achieve greater weight loss after surgery are more likely to achieve complete resolution of diabetes mellitus.

When it comes to "curing" diabetes or putting it into remission, the Roux-en-Y gastric bypass is the gold standard for bariatric surgery. Surgeons reroute the food to skip part of the stomach and the beginning of the small intestine. There are other options for bariatric surgery, but these are less effective in producing prolonged weight loss.

Bariatric surgery can definitely help improve diabetes, high blood pressure, severe joint pains, infertility, and numerous other disorders. Bariatric surgery changes the anatomy of your intestinal tract, so you naturally lose weight.

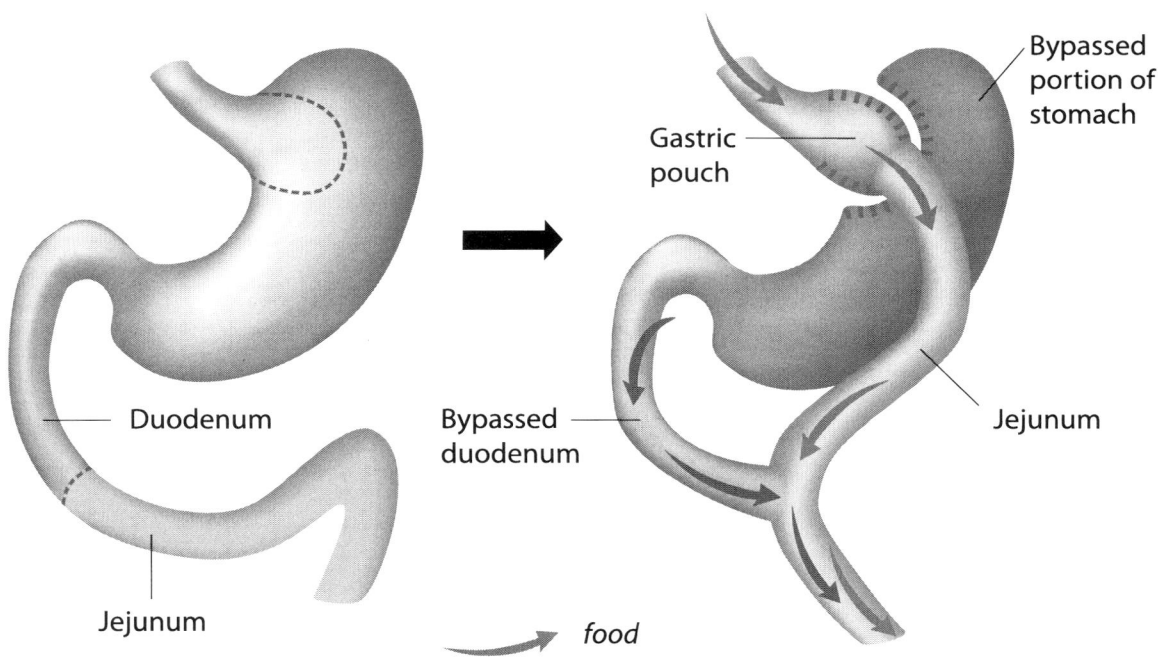

Weight loss surgery typically results in more significant and sustained weight loss than traditional treatment like exercise and diet for weight loss. Bariatric surgery also leads to improvements in quality of life and obesity-related complications such as diabetes, hypertension, sleep apnea and, orthopedic problems.

Who Is Eligible For Bariatric Surgery?

Before you can become eligible for bariatric surgery, you must meet certain criteria. These include the following:

- » You must understand the risks during and following the surgical operation.

- » You need to have a Body mass index (BMI) of 40 or more, which is about 45 kg (100 pounds) overweight for men and 35 kg (80 pounds) for women.

- » You can also possibly qualify for it if you have a BMI between 35 and 39.9 and a serious obesity-related health problem such as type 2 diabetes, heart disease, or severe sleep apnea.

As you know, the majority of individuals with type 2 diabetes tend to be obese. For obese diabetic people who fail lifestyle management and the available medical treatments, bariatric surgery may be an effective treatment alternative. I see long-term diabetes remission in 23 to 60 percent of patients, depending on the baseline severity and duration of their diabetes.

A recent study on over 20,000 patients showed that 84 percent who underwent Roux-en Y gastric bypass (RYGB) experienced a complete reversal of their type 2 diabetes, at least in the short term. In the long term(>7 years), weight gain is common if strict dietary guidelines are not followed.

The effects of bariatric surgery on blood sugars following the operation can be visible within a few days. Some theories explained are with a significant increase in incretin hormone release from the gastrointestinal system.

Can Bariatric Surgery Prevent Diabetes In Obese People? Will It Last?

An international survey was done in France on the effects of bariatric surgery. They looked at 300,000 very obese patients who had this type of surgery. A third of those who underwent bariatric surgery were up to 6 times less likely to develop type 2 diabetes. They were also much less likely to develop type 2 diabetes complications.

Having bariatric surgery decreased the HbA1c by 2-3.5 percent in those who had surgery compared to 1-1.5 percent in those who chose regular medical treatment. Most of these medical studies also showed that surgery was better than standard nonsurgical treatment in causing weight loss and eliminating metabolic syndrome.

Almost all of these studies also included only people who were obese. They showed that people who were less obese also benefited from the surgery—just as much as people who had a very high BMI above 40.

Many of the research studies followed people for one to three years after surgery. They showed there was continued diabetes remission in about 78 percent of these patients. Overall, there was an improvement in blood sugars in 87 percent of people who had type 2 diabetes.

Most people want to know if bariatric surgery lasts. How long diabetes remission lasts after bariatric procedures has been a subject of debate. In one large study, the diabetes remission rate after seven years was 60.2 percent. This is a lot of people who are no longer diabetic for so many years.

As you know, heart attacks and strokes are the major causes of death in people who have type 2 diabetes. Bariatric surgery seems to help reduce the chances of getting these complications too. Many research studies have shown that there may be up to a 50% reduction in the risk of heart attacks in the years after bariatric surgery.

As you can imagine, the chances of having diabetes complications such as kidney disease, diabetic eye disease, and neuropathy were also reduced. The people who had bariatric surgery were 2-3 times less likely to have these complications compared to those who didn't have bariatric surgery.

There are many complications of Roux-en-Y gastric bypass surgery.. These include gastric distension, narrowing of the stomach opening, ulcer formation, gallstone formation, hernias, small bowel obstructions, low blood sugar if on insulin or sulfonylurea drugs (glipizide, glyburide, glimepiride), dumping syndrome, metabolic and nutritional deficiencies, and weight regain.

Some bariatric surgery complications are seen soon after surgery, while others may present weeks to months, even years following the surgery. You need to know these risks before you consider having this type of surgery.

Defects In The Body That Lead To Diabetes

There are several possible defects your body can have that could lead to diabetes. I call this the "octet" because there are eight of them. Let's review the different reasons why your blood sugar might be persistently high enough to say you have diabetes:

Defect:	What this means:	Diabetic Type Involved:
Defect in the pancreatic beta cells	Beta cells in the pancreas start to fail due to predetermined genetic weakness or because of metabolic stress from excessive nutrition, too many fat cells, and inflammation from excessive fat buildup.	Insulin resistance Type 2 diabetes Prediabetes Type 1 diabetes and LADA (from antibodies against the beta cells)
Defect in pancreatic alpha cells	Insulin normally blocks the pancreatic alpha cells from producing glucagon after meals. Some types of diabetes involve alpha cell resistance to insulin. If insulin levels are also low, there will be too much glucagon and high blood sugar levels.	Insulin resistance Type 2 diabetes Prediabetes
Defect in fat cell glucose utilization and resistance to insulin	When excessive amounts of fat are packed in your fat cells, it causes inflammation. This is why many people with insulin resistance feel tired and why we call obesity an inflammatory disease state. The same inflammation also stresses the beta cells and alpha cells in the pancreas. When fat cells get too full, fatty acids start circulating in the blood causing all cells to be resistant to insulin.	Insulin resistance Type 2 diabetes Prediabetes
Defect in the gut hormones	You have gut hormones called "incretins". These hormones communicate with the beta cells in the pancreas. When you eat, these hormones tell the pancreas to make insulin. In diabetics, cells making incretins are defective. As a result, insulin is not produced enough after consuming a meal.	Insulin resistance Type 2 diabetes Prediabetes
Defect in the kidney's glucose regulation	Normal kidneys reabsorb all the glucose they filter from the blood so it isn't wasted. When blood sugars go above 180 mg/dL (9.99 mmol/l), the kidneys spill glucose into the urine. Kidneys also make glucose themselves. When the kidney is resistant to insulin, glucose production increases too and the threshold to spill glucose goes above 220 mg/dL (12.21 mmol/l), making it harder to control the blood sugar.	Insulin resistance Type 2 diabetes Prediabetes

The Root Cause Of Other Types Of Diabetes

We have the entirety of chapter 2 to talk about types of diabetes. Here I will briefly explain a few more causes of diabetes. In case you do not want to drill into the next chapter, here is a brief summary ahead of time.

Autoimmune destruction of the beta cells of the pancreas is the cause of type 1 diabetes. There is probably both a genetic and environmental reason for this. The destruction of beta cells starts happening at a very early age. The process is often very fast, but in other cases, it can take a while. When the process is fast, it is called type 1 diabetes; it usually happens at a very early age (often in the first five years of life).

When the process happens more slowly, diabetes doesn't present until the individual is between 20 and 40 years old. This is sometimes called type 1.5 diabetes or latent autoimmune diabetes in adults (LADA). The reason behind this kind of diabetes is the same; both of these disorders happen because the individual makes antibodies against the beta cells of the pancreas. They just differ in when it occurs in a person's lifetime.

Lastly, there is an entirely genetic type of diabetes that has nothing to do with insulin resistance or environmental factors. It is called MODY (maturity-onset diabetes of the young). This is an inherited condition, usually involving a single defective gene that leads to diabetes. Most cases of MODY are mild and do not cause the same complications of diabetes seen in other causes of high blood sugar.

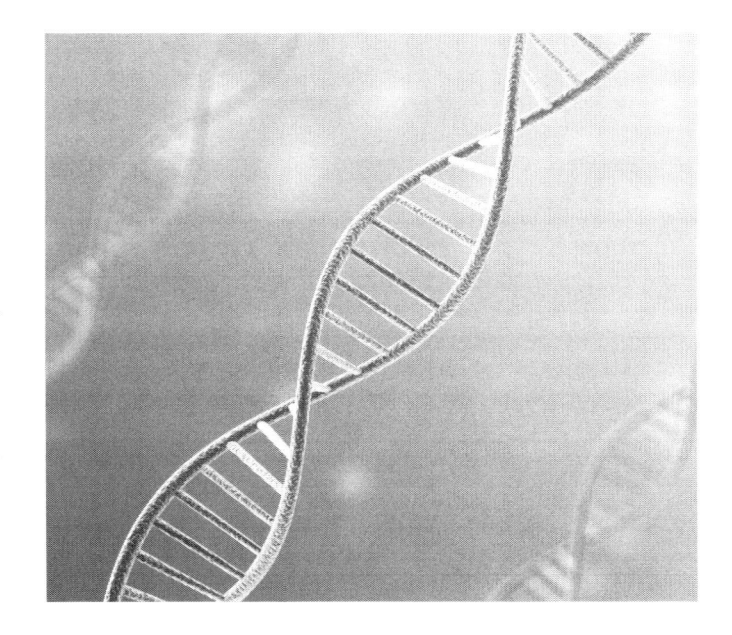

MODY has six different types. The most common types are MODY–2 and MODY–3. I test patients for MODY if they are young, have a strong family history of diabetes, and do not have positive antibody levels. Common types of MODY (MODY-2 and MODY-3) can be treated very easily so it is essential to test for it when it is clinically indicated.

Miscellaneous Factors That Can Cause Diabetes

Many studies indicate that both low birth weight and high birth weight can factor into the development of insulin resistance and diabetes. So if you came into this world underweight and later turned out to be overweight, your diabetes risk is very high.

Even among infants of average birth weight, if they grow too slowly in the first three months of life, these babies have a higher chance of diabetes in the future. Also, having a high birth weight can be a cause of later developing diabetes.

Sometimes a high birth weight is related to being born to a mother who had gestational diabetes or high blood sugar during pregnancy. This increases the risk of diabetes in later life. Prematurity at birth also can be a cause of diabetes.

Medications That Contribute To Developing Diabetes

Many medications can contribute to the development of diabetes. I am going to tell you about the medications that can potentially contribute to the development of this disorder; however, these medications are often essential, and I do not recommend you stop taking any of these drugs before you discuss with your physician regarding a potential alternative medication. Some of these include the following:

- » Steroids like prednisone or dexamethasone if taken orally or injected into the body. I see a lot of patients in my clinic who are diagnosed with diabetes after steroid treatments. Some of these patients never go back to having normal blood sugar levels after such treatments.

- » Antipsychotic drugs used for schizophrenia or bipolar disorder. These include clozapine, iloperidone, olanzapine, paliperidone, quetiapine, risperidone, which cause diabetes by increasing insulin resistance. In my clinic, I get regular referrals for uncontrolled diabetes due to the use of antipsychotic medications.

- » Beta-blocker drugs commonly used for heart problems such as atenolol, metoprolol, and propranolol can also reduce insulin sensitivity and are a potential cause for diabetes.

- » Niacin (nicotinic acid) increases the glucose release from the liver, while statins used for high cholesterol also increase the risk of diabetes through unknown mechanisms.

- » Blood pressure medications such as hydrochlorothiazide, chlorthalidone, chlorothiazide, and indapamide cause diabetes by decreasing insulin secretion and increasing insulin resistance.

- » Combination estrogen-progestin oral contraceptives and progestin-only contraceptives can also increase insulin resistance and cause diabetes.

- » Immunosuppressive agents used for organ transplants such as cyclosporine (cyclosporin), sirolimus, tacrolimus can cause diabetes by reducing insulin secretion.

When it comes to medications that cause or contribute to diabetes, it is usually a matter of the risks versus benefits of taking the drug. If your doctor prescribed any of these medications for other reasons, ask your physician if there is an alternative. Do not stop any medications you are on because you are afraid of becoming diabetic. Consult with your doctor. Not taking these medications may have more severe consequences than taking them.

Final Thoughts

The simple answer to "what is diabetes?" is that it means your blood sugars are regularly too high. As you have learned, there are many reasons why you can develop the disorder. Regardless of the reason, the result is the same: your blood sugars will be too high. Later on, I will talk about why it is important to have normal blood sugars and the complications of not keeping your blood sugars under reasonable control.

I am also an avid supporter of diagnosing diabetes very early on, even at the insulin resistance and prediabetes stage, to prevent progression to diabetes. This is because many of the complications settle in even before the diagnosis of diabetes or very early on, right after the diagnosis is made.

Most cases of diabetes are due to lifestyle factors that lead to obesity and derangements of the body's glucose regulation mechanisms that come with being overweight. Heredity has a lot to do with who gets diabetes and who doesn't but this doesn't mean you can't do anything about your genetic lottery ticket. You can do many things that might lead to the remission of certain types of diabetes and a sharp reduction in diabetic complications later in life, even if you can't "cure" your own diabetic state completely.

If, instead of type 2 diabetes, you have type 1 diabetes (where obesity is not nearly as important in developing it), you can do many things to prevent complications and improve your quality of life (and even your longevity).

Actually, most of my type 1 diabetic patients are my best patients because many of them get diagnosed at an early age and learn how to live with it successfully. A type 1 diabetic who can control their blood sugars in a reasonably controlled range will never develop complications.

I will talk a lot more on ways to manage your blood sugars so you can have the best possible outcome, even if you are technically still a "diabetic." A "cure" is definitely possible if you put your mind to it or if you choose the right medications or a combination of both.

CHAPTER 2
TYPES OF DIABETES

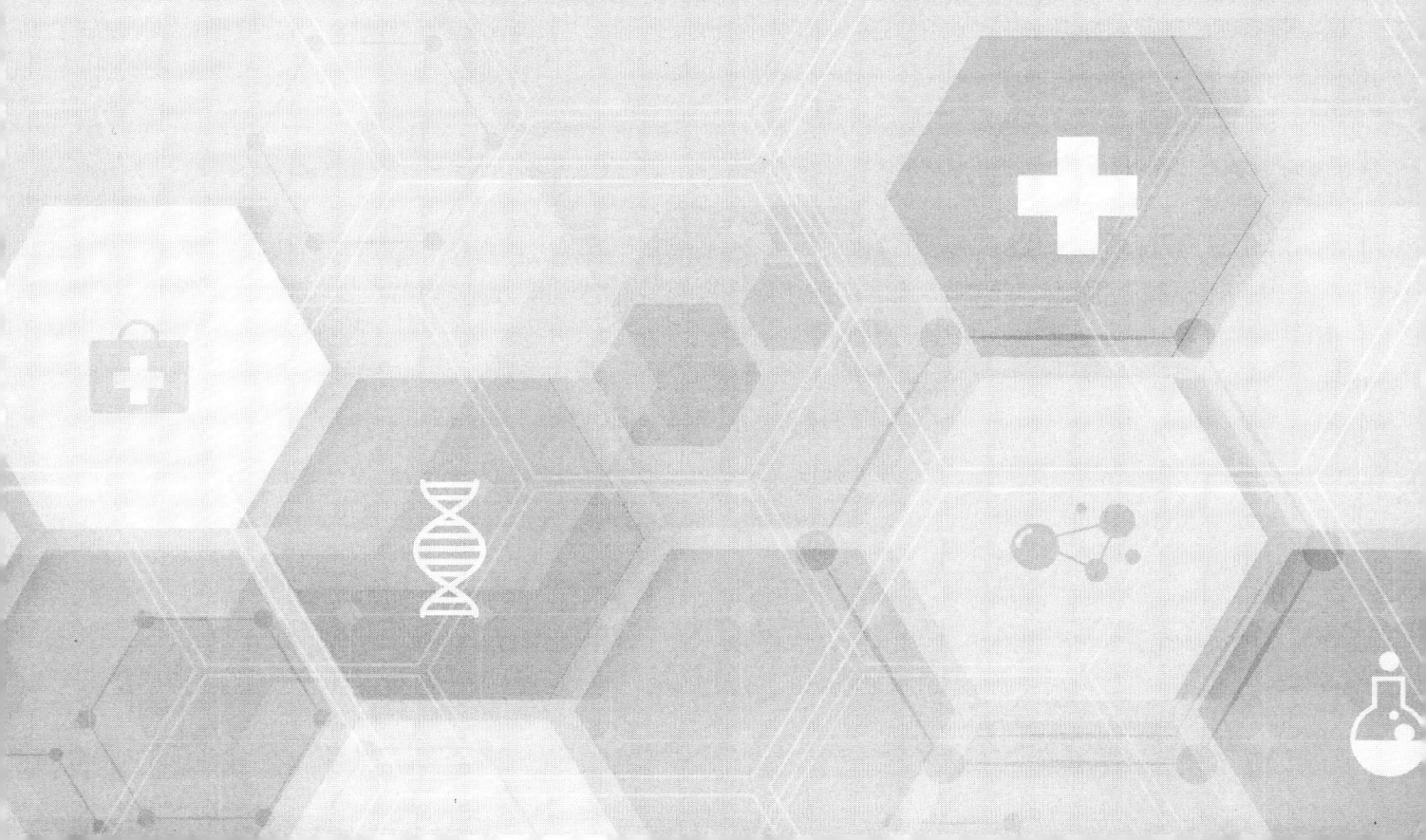

CHAPTER 2
TYPES OF DIABETES

You likely already know that there are several kinds of diabetes. I talked briefly about the different types in the first chapter of this book so you could see how diabetes can develop. I want to talk now about the different kinds of diabetes in more detail so you can see what they might look like in your own situation. We will also discuss how to prevent and possibly cure your type 2 diabetes or some related conditions, especially if detected in its earliest stages.

Even though all cases of diabetes involve high blood sugar, they differ significantly in what causes them and the ways they are treated. Even the type and timing of complications of the different types of diabetes will vary based on which type you are talking about.

Because type 2 diabetes is so much more common than any other kind of high blood sugar disease, I will focus more on what it looks like and how it develops. It is an interesting disorder, mostly because it is a "spectrum disease" and not an "all-or-none" condition.

I talked earlier about numbers being important in the diagnosis of diabetes but with type 2 disease, it really starts along a spectrum of insulin resistance to blood sugar dysregulation--progressing over time to more severe disease if not managed early enough. The key here is "manage". This is the one type of diabetes where the advantage of knowing you are at risk is the greatest.

Insulin Resistance, Metabolic Syndrome And Prediabetes

The terms insulin resistance, prediabetes, diabetes, and metabolic syndrome are all related to one another in some way, so it can be confusing to figure out which of these you might have. I will try to explain what they mean and tell you more about how they are related.

Insulin resistance is often the first sign you might be at risk for diabetes. It is defined as having a less than usual response to normal insulin concentrations. In fact, insulin resistance is the most common environmental trigger in causing type 2 diabetes in the setting of genetic predisposition. The genetic predisposition part is not something you have control over; it's what you do with having this predisposition that counts.

If you have insulin resistance, it might be hard to diagnose. It's common to have a normal fasting blood sugar with insulin resistance. Most individuals with insulin resistance actually seem to have perfectly normal glucose levels at first. Some people, as they progress towards prediabetes, should they have a glucose tolerance test (75-gram glucose challenge), they would see that they may not handle glucose very well.

Insulin resistance is also not just about glucose regulation. People with insulin resistance may have completely normal glucose levels. However, they may still have other signs of insulin resistance such as low HDL, high triglycerides, high blood pressure, and difficulty in losing weight. Insulin resistance is the most common reason for cardiovascular mortality in the USA and all around the world. We will talk more about these signs in a later section.

In the initial stages, such as when you have metabolic syndrome or prediabetes, insulin resistance is the main problem. At this point, your glucose levels are still normal, although the insulin levels are very high in your body. The pancreatic beta cells put out more and more insulin, depending on your needs.

CHAPTER 2 - TYPES OF DIABETES

Moderate Insulin Lowering

Insulin

Adiposity

Insulin Resistance

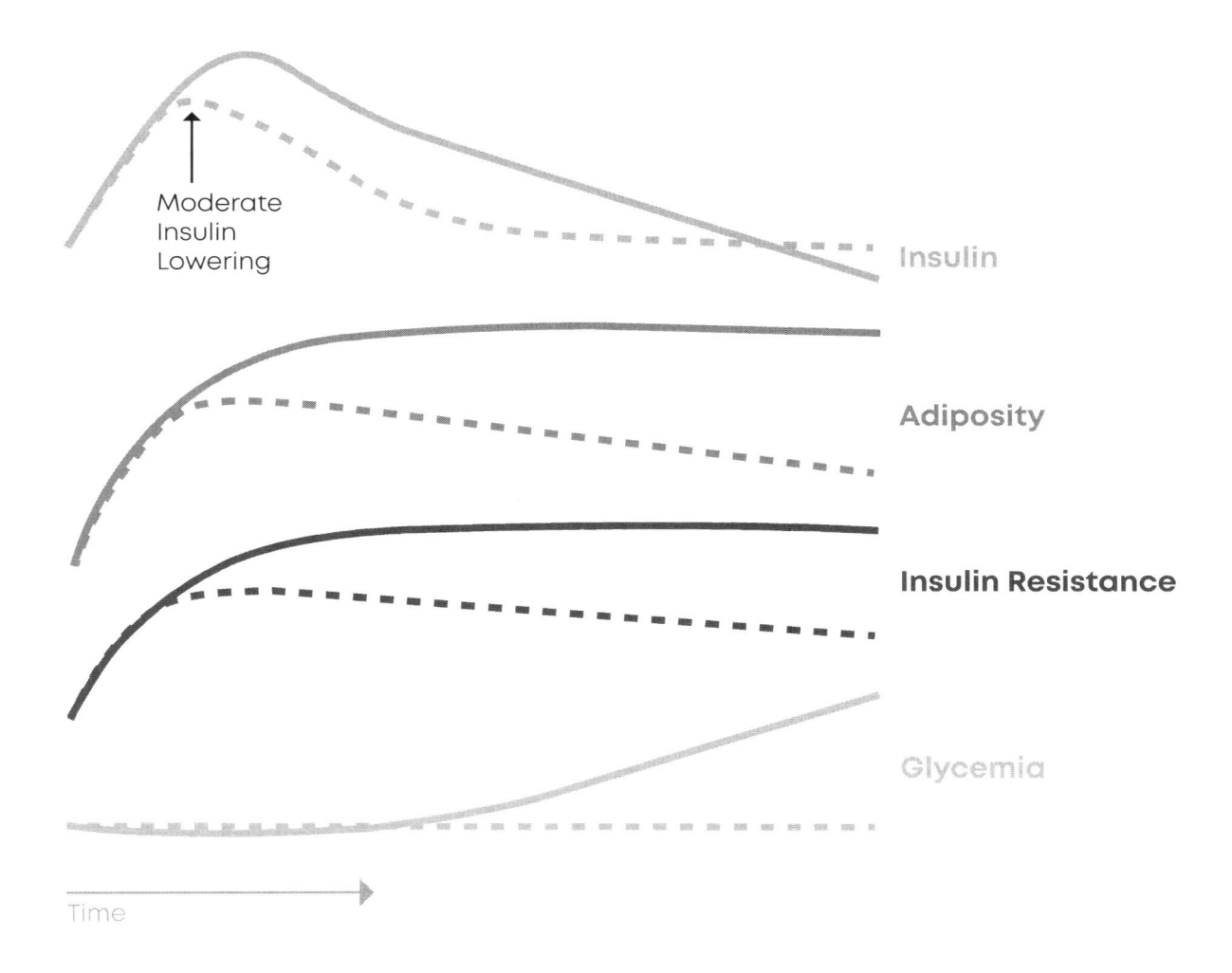

Glycemia

Time

At some point, the beta cells start to die off because of the excessive metabolic stress on them; as a result, they will not be able to make as much insulin; the insulin levels will begin to drop off. This combination of insulin resistance and a reduction in insulin production leads to uncontrolled high blood sugars. Uncontrolled blood sugar above 130 mg/dL (7.215 mmol/l) on average, is defined as diabetes. Unfortunately, damage to other organs can start even before this threshold is achieved.

Patients with diabetes generally start with one single oral diabetes medication. Most of the time, doctors who treat diabetes will continue to add medications even if their patients try their best to change their lifestyle.

You need more and more medications because the beta cells that produce insulin continue to die slowly over time. This is inevitable. You need to know that this process can be slowed down if you control your diabetes as early as possible. This requires aggressive management at the beginning of the disease process. We call this the "legacy effect," which I will talk about shortly.

One distressing impact of type 2 diabetes is that primary care doctors often wait too long to start any treatment. When people do not change their lifestyle and let their blood sugars stay high for too long, this is what causes even further damage to their beta cells. It is like keeping a damaged engine running in your car and not fixing the problem, which may cause further damage down the road.

On the bright side, it is a lot easier to manage diabetes and keep it under control early in the course of this progressive problem rather than later on. You need to get treatment before severe damage to your organs and pancreas occurs.

When severe damage happens, and you lose most of your insulin-producing cells, then you become insulin-dependent. To prevent being insulin-dependent, using the right diabetes medication and instituting a diabetes care plan is important. Remember, lifestyle changes are the best "medication," even though lifestyle changes alone may not be enough to control progressive diabetes.

I have created Dr. Ergin's SugarMD Advanced Glucose Support for my patients who insist on avoiding medications for various reasons such as cost, side effects, etc. It is available on Amazon.com and some health stores. However, if my patients need more medications even after lifestyle changes and SugarMD diabetes supplements, I always advise them not to defer the treatment because doing so could cause further damage to pancreatic beta cells.

Who Is More Likely To Develop Insulin Resistance?

This is what to look out for in terms of risk factors:

- Abdominal obesity
- Increased stress hormones (cortisol, growth hormone, catecholamines like adrenaline, glucagon)
- Medications (glucocorticoids, HIV drugs, contraceptives)
- Pregnancy (placental hormones)
- Genetic predisposition
- Physical inactivity
- Aging

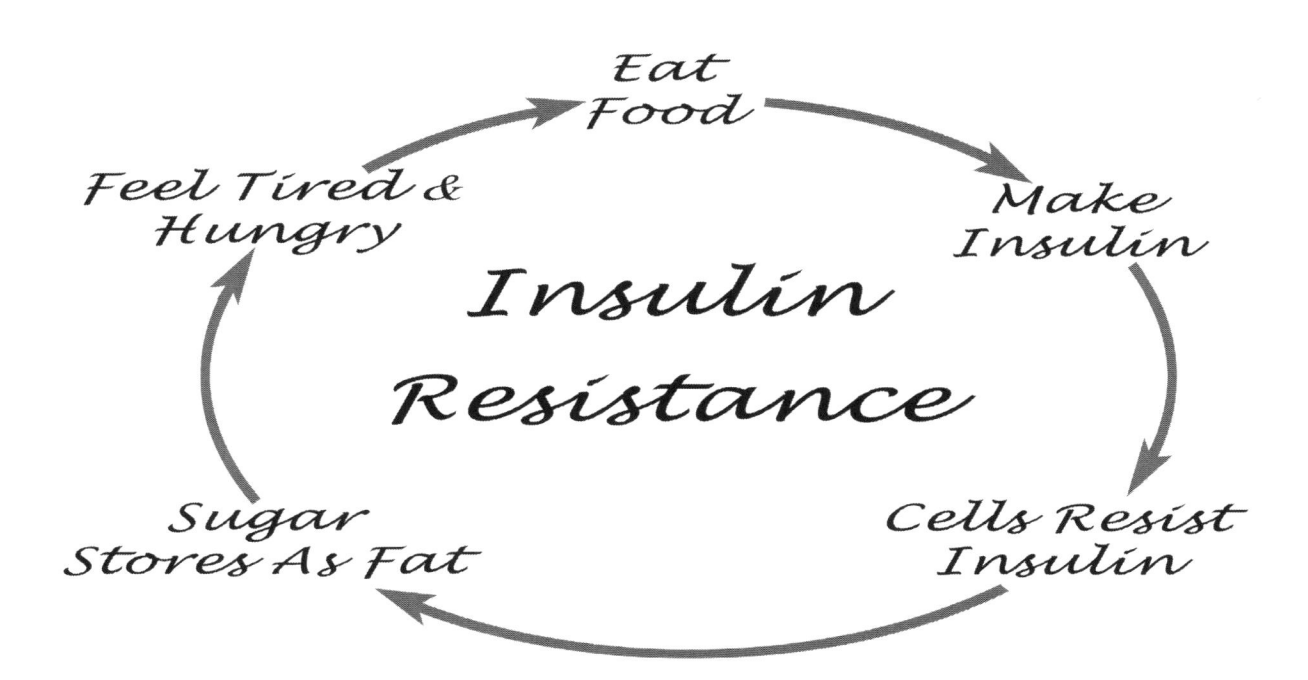

<u>If you have one or more of the factors below, you should be evaluated for insulin resistance or diabetes.</u> These factors can cause diabetes or can simply be linked to insulin resistance; this insulin resistance eventually leads to diabetes and cardiovascular mortality (heart attacks, stroke).

- HDL below 50 mg/dL in women and below 40 mg/dL in men
- Elevated blood pressure (above 120/70)
- Elevated triglyceride levels above 150
- Acanthosis nigricans, which is the darkening of the skin at the back of the neck and under her arms, also has a velvety texture
- Body mass index more than 27 for Americans, 23–24 for Asians and Indians.
- Waist circumference over 40 inches/102 cm (men) or 35 inches/89 cm (women)
- Polycystic ovarian syndrome
- Gestational diabetes history
- Delivering a large baby

There is a huge genetic component in developing insulin resistance and diabetes. As insulin resistance gets worse with age, becoming more obese, or more sedentary, your insulin resistance will progress and will eventually lead to a defect in insulin production. When the body cannot produce enough insulin to accommodate the body's needs due to insulin resistance, diabetes will develop.

For example, a person who has inherited diabetes genes from their family would never develop type 2 diabetes if they did not develop insulin resistance first due to the risk factors we discussed above. In other words, it's hard to have type 2 diabetes without first being insulin resistant.

This makes it so important to know if you have it. It's like the canary in the coal mine; it warns you of impending disaster ahead if you don't do something about it. Let's dig deeper into how it develops.

- ***Chemicals/hormones as a possible cause for insulin resistance and diabetes:*** Insulin resistance occurs due to certain chemicals/hormones that overly-filled fat cells secrete in the body. Some of them are leptin, interleukin and tumor necrosis factor-alpha. These cytokines are called "pro-inflammatory cytokines." That is why many people with insulin resistance tend to feel tired and exhausted all the time. The inflammation in their body makes them feel like they have the flu all the time.

- ***Insulin resistance often starts many years before high blood sugars appear.*** Eventually, you might begin to see mildly elevated blood sugar levels. We call this prediabetes. When blood sugars are very high, we call it diabetes.

  One of the early signs that your body is trying to keep up with the insulin it needs is that your proinsulin levels increase. Proinsulin is the molecule your beta cells produce first that is later cleaved to turn into insulin (leaving behind the C peptide I talked about before). Elevated insulin or proinsulin levels can be a clue indicating the development of diabetes in the future.

- ***Lifestyle factors as a cause for diabetes and insulin resistance:*** The most common risk factors for diabetes and insulin resistance are weight gain, obesity, and inactivity. With excessive weight gain and obesity, stress develops in your fat cells. It's this stress that causes inflammatory markers to rise. These inflammatory markers in your blood are often toxic to your pancreatic beta cells (the insulin-producing cells in the pancreas).

  It can become a vicious cycle, as you can see.

INSULIN RESISTANCE

Other Health Problems

High Carb Diet

Constant High Glucose In Blood

Constant High Insulin Demand

Pancreas

Insulin
Cells
Glucose

Insulin Receptors Become Resistant

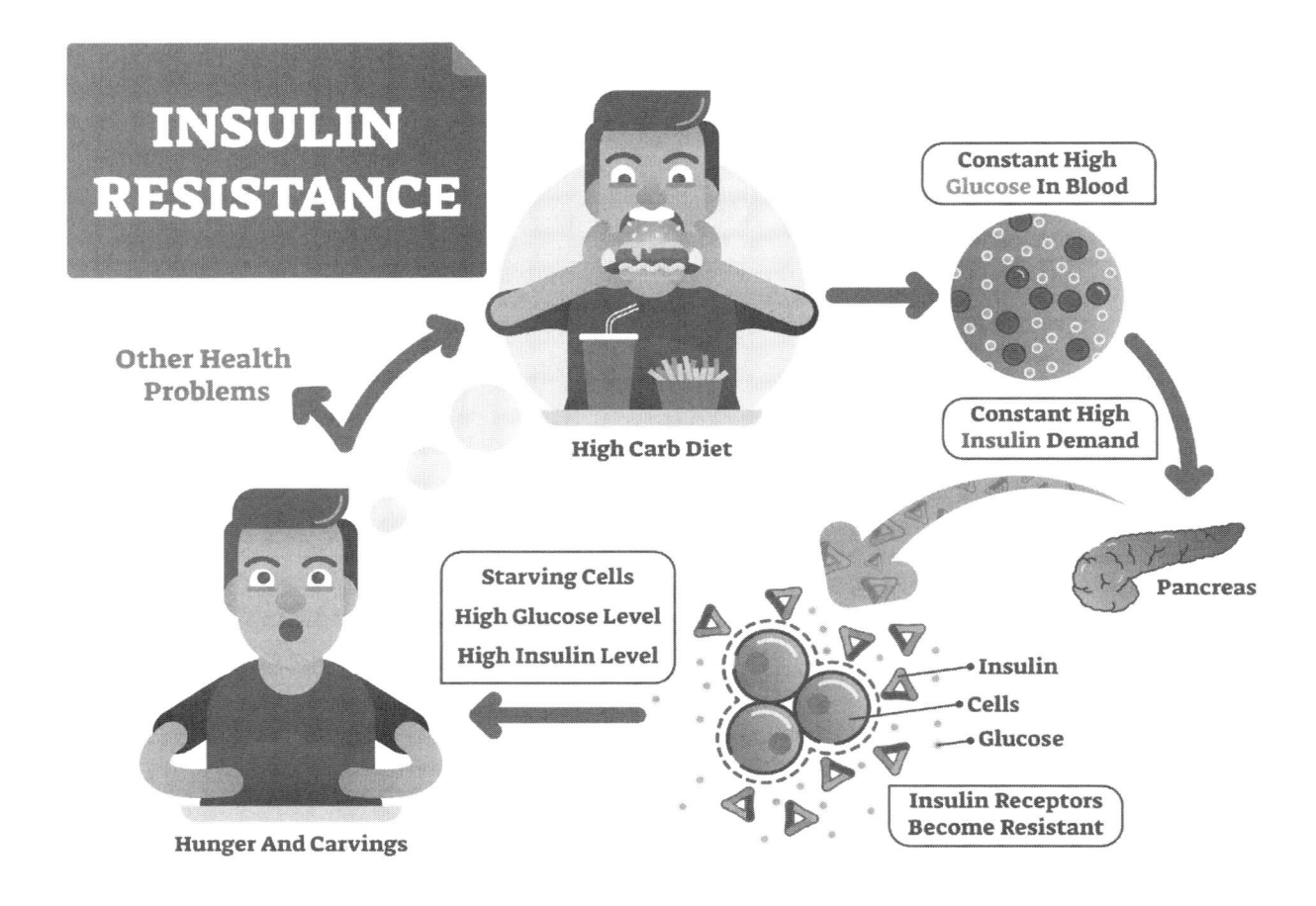

Starving Cells
High Glucose Level
High Insulin Level

Hunger And Carvings

- ***Cytokines as the cause of insulin resistance and diabetes:*** Cytokines are hormones that help your cells communicate with one another. Some of these cytokines are messengers that lead to inflammation in the body. They can be released from stressed fat cells that are stressed, simply because they are too filled with stored dietary fat. These cytokines can also disable the insulin receptors on your cells that normally recognize the insulin in the bloodstream.

   You need these receptors to allow insulin to put glucose into the cells. When there is a problem in the receptor, the body cannot use insulin appropriately, and you will need more insulin to stimulate the receptors. This is the reason for insulin resistance most of the time.

Due to the presence of these inflammatory substances in your body, you will often feel tired and run down most of the time. This problem leads to more inactivity. As a result, obesity and insulin resistance worsen in another type of vicious cycle.

Factors that lead to Insulin Resistance

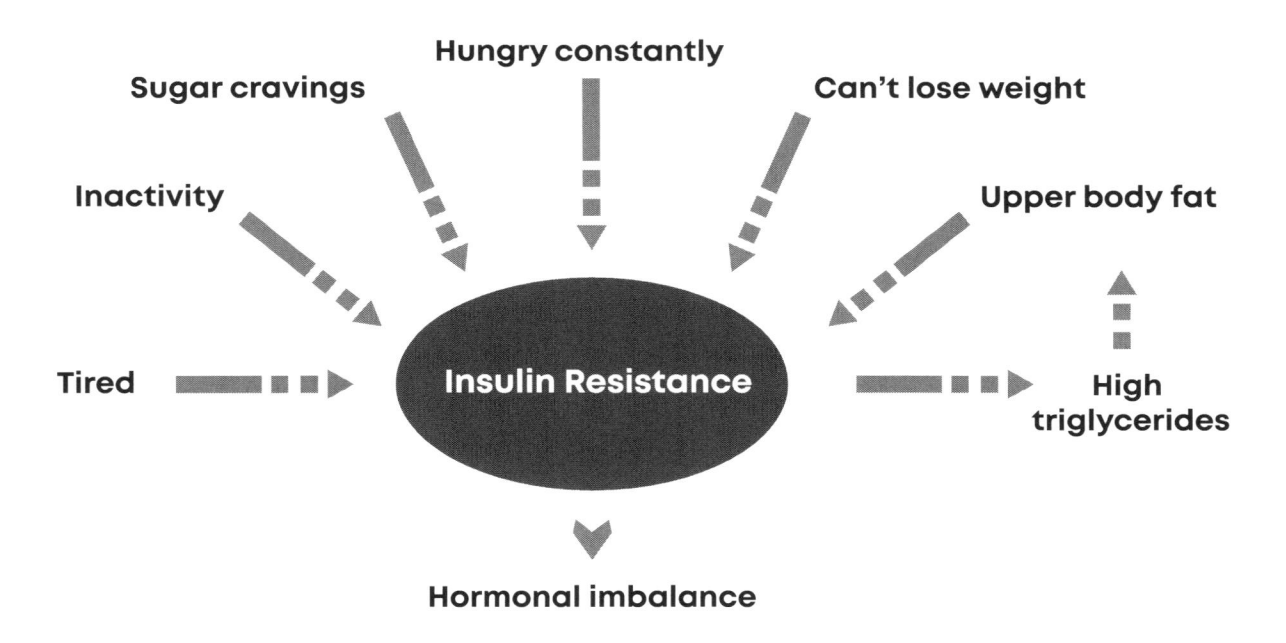

- Sugar cravings
- Hungry constantly
- Can't lose weight
- Inactivity
- Upper body fat
- Tired
- High triglycerides
- Hormonal imbalance

→ Insulin Resistance

- ***Fatty acids as a cause for diabetes:*** When there is too much fat in the fat cells because you are overweight or obese, the fatty acids inside them also start to escape into the bloodstream. Fatty acids are just like cytokines and disable the function of insulin receptors. Fatty acids also reduce the pancreas's ability to make insulin.

- ***The type of obesity matters:*** The type of obesity also makes a difference in whether or not you develop insulin resistance. The fat in the abdominal area is more likely to cause insulin resistance and diabetes than the fat in the buttocks and thighs.

> ## ✈ Fast Fact
>
> *When it comes to abdominal fat or "belly fat," it's safe to say that "fat doesn't make you fat." It's mostly sugar that contributes to belly fat (although trans fats are also big culprits). Foods that increase belly fat include sugary sodas, flavored coffee drinks, high fructose corn syrup, and excess alcohol intake. Just remember this link: Sugar spikes ▸ insulin spikes ▸ fat deposition in your fat cells. Avoid triggering this link to reduce abdominal fat.*

Leptin is a hormone related to the number of fat stores in your body. This is because it is made by your fat cells. In "normal" people, it tells the hypothalamus (in the brain) that you don't need to be hungry because the fat stores are full. Leptin deficiency and resistance to leptin are both possible causes of diabetes, partly because the signal to stop eating isn't present or your hypothalamus doesn't respond to it.

Leptin deficiency is very rare and can be a genetic disorder. While increasing leptin sounds like a cure for obesity and diabetes, many studies and medications have failed to address this problem. Unfortunately, there is no medical approach at this time to address leptin resistance or leptin deficiency.

Adiponectin is a hormone that reduces insulin resistance. It is an anti-inflammatory hormone. A deficiency of adiponectin also correlates with insulin resistance and diabetes. Healthy fat cells release adiponectin. As we discussed, excessive fat storage within fat cells will lead to stress. In turn, your adiponectin levels will go down.

Too many people in Western societies have general obesity and/or abdominal obesity. They have high free fatty acid levels in the circulation and/or excess fat deposition in muscle or liver. This is what can lead to insulin resistance and prediabetes.

Free fatty acids come from enlarged adipose or fat cells. When the storage capacity of your fat cells overflows, fatty acids start circulating in the blood. The body's defense system (immune cells) tends to be attracted to the areas where there is a fat deposition.

When your body's defense systems meet fat cells, a clash happens. Immune cells start eating up fat cells, which leads to inflammation. Inflammation creates a state of fatigue. This is why most people with obesity or excessive fat deposition complain of excessive tiredness. They aren't lazy; they act much like you'd act if your body were infiltrated with the flu, and they don't feel well enough to get up and exercise.

The interaction between Obesity, Leptin and Adiponectin

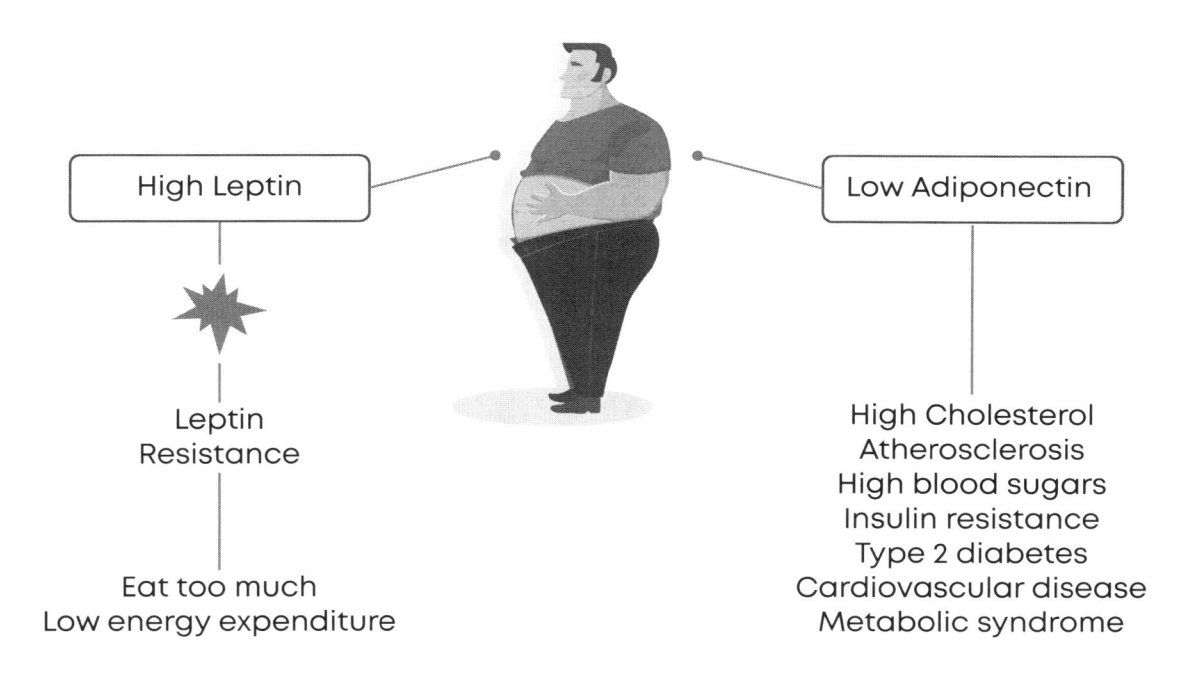

High Leptin

Leptin Resistance

Eat too much
Low energy expenditure

Low Adiponectin

High Cholesterol
Atherosclerosis
High blood sugars
Insulin resistance
Type 2 diabetes
Cardiovascular disease
Metabolic syndrome

What Diseases Are Linked To Being Insulin Resistant?

People with insulin resistance and prediabetes are at an increased risk of many other health problems. These are the different disorders we know are associated with prediabetes and insulin resistance:

- Coronary Artery Disease
- Metabolic Syndrome
- Polycystic Ovary Syndrome (PCOS)
- Nonalcoholic Fatty Liver Disease
- Certain obesity-related cancers (especially colon, breast, and endometrial cancers)

In most cases, we do not know the precise basis for the link between insulin resistance and clinical findings such as heart disease. We believe that elevated insulin levels from insulin resistance can over-stimulate other organs in the body. This can lead to disturbances in many different organ systems.

Abdominal obesity also reduces the good chemicals that prevent heart disease. Remember that healthy fat cells make adiponectin, which is good to have in reducing inflammation. Adiponectin levels go down when you have a lot of belly fat but increase when you have healthy dietary patterns and exercise regularly.

Low adiponectin levels are associated with high circulating levels of insulin and other inflammatory chemicals. Inflammation leads to inflamed blood vessels that are more likely to be narrowed from atherosclerosis. When you get too many narrowed blood vessels in the heart, brain, and blood vessels supplying the limbs, you can easily develop heart attacks, stroke, and peripheral vascular disease, respectively. Now you can see why diabetes is such a big risk factor for heart disease.

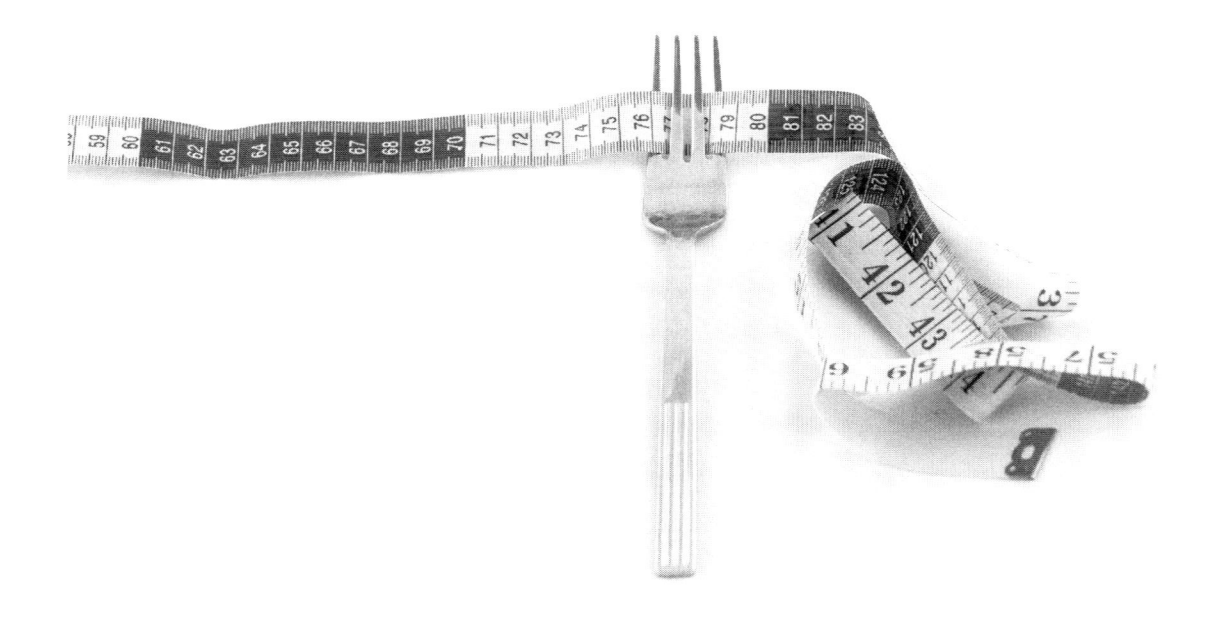

Quick tip

It's a good idea to know if you have too much belly/abdominal/visceral fat. Get a cloth measuring tape like those used in sewing. Stand with a bare belly and find a spot about the level of your belly button. Wrap the tape around snuggly, but don't cinch it tight, and don't suck your stomach in. Relax and exhale before getting a measurement. If the total circumference you measure (all the way around) is more than 35 inches (89 centimeters) for women or 40 inches (102 centimeters) for men, this is too high and puts you at risk for health complications, like type 2 diabetes, heart disease, sleep apnea, high blood pressure, and some types of cancer. It isn't a given though, because you can reverse your risk by eating healthy, exercising, and avoiding alcohol.

Prediabetes

Prediabetes is just one step further along a path toward developing type 2 diabetes. Again, it starts with having insulin resistance in the first place. You have prediabetes when even an elevated amount of insulin cannot keep your blood sugar levels within the normal range. A fasting blood sugar level between 100 mg/dL and 125 mg/dL (5.6 to 7.0 mmol/L) indicates you can no longer use the insulin you have to control your blood sugars.

Obesity (particularly abdominal obesity) causes this derangement in the effectiveness of insulin in the body. Prediabetes naturally follows insulin resistance. Later, having prediabetes leads to developing type 2 diabetes mellitus provided you remain obese or gain even more weight. This is especially problematic when you realize how hard it can be to lose weight when your body is too inflamed and you are too tired or sluggish to exercise.

Many people with obesity-related insulin resistance initially have normal or only slightly high blood glucose concentrations. Eventually, however, the pancreatic beta cells (insulin-making cells) fail to compensate for the fact that the cells in your body are insulin resistant and you develop high blood sugar levels.

It's also possible to have elevated blood glucose levels after meals before developing overt type 2 diabetes or even without having a high fasting blood sugar. High blood sugars after meals may be the first sign you are developing diabetes because you can't handle the carbohydrate loads you get with meals.

> ## Quick Tip:
>
> *"If you know someone with diabetes, use their glucose meter and try to check your own blood sugar 1 hour after a carb-heavy meal. If your glucose spikes above 160 mg/dL (8.88mmol/L) after one hour, chances are you have insulin resistance and are likely to develop diabetes soon. Also, get tested for a 2-hour glucose tolerance test and HbA1c. It is a good idea to improve your lifestyle now, rather than waiting until diabetes diagnosis".*

Moreover, every person's response to obesity can be different. Some patients start developing elevated glucose levels with only slight insulin resistance. Other people may have all the signs of insulin resistance without any glucose changes until the very late stages of the disease process. This is all mostly determined by your genetics.

So you can see how abdominal obesity causes insulin resistance. Insulin resistance then causes high insulin levels as your pancreas keeps trying to catch up. When it can't, you will have high blood sugars. Your excess fatty tissue creates inflammation due to an immune attack on your body.

Multiple Factors in Diabetes Leading to Blood Vessel Disease

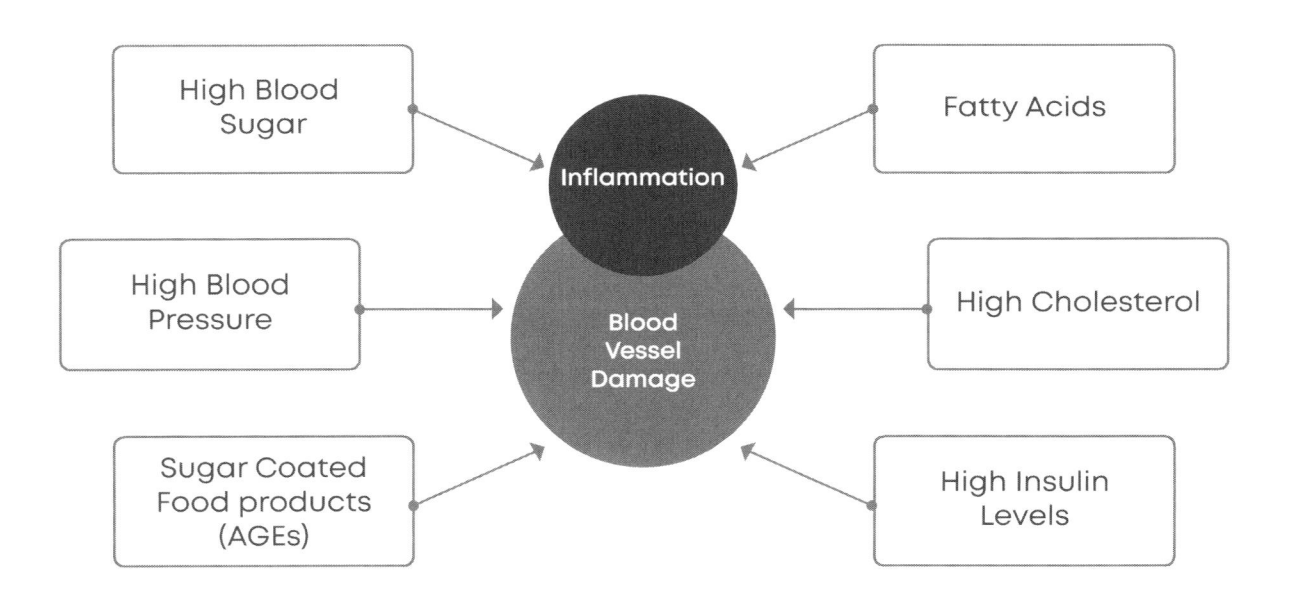

- High Blood Sugar → Inflammation
- Fatty Acids → Inflammation
- High Blood Pressure → Blood Vessel Damage
- High Cholesterol → Blood Vessel Damage
- Sugar Coated Food products (AGEs) → Blood Vessel Damage
- High Insulin Levels → Blood Vessel Damage

All of this inflammation plus high insulin levels often combine to cause vascular destruction. It's these same factors that lead to high cholesterol, hypertension, and vascular inflammation. In the end, you have an increased risk of developing cardiovascular disease (CVD).

🖅 Fast fact

Acanthosis nigricans as a sign of insulin resistance. It looks like a brown/darker color soft/velvety skin on the neck or under the armpits. Skin tags and acanthosis nigricans are common with insulin resistance. The lesions are usually found on the back of the neck, the axilla, the groin, and over the elbows, but they may cover the entire surface of the skin, sparing only the palms and soles of the feet.

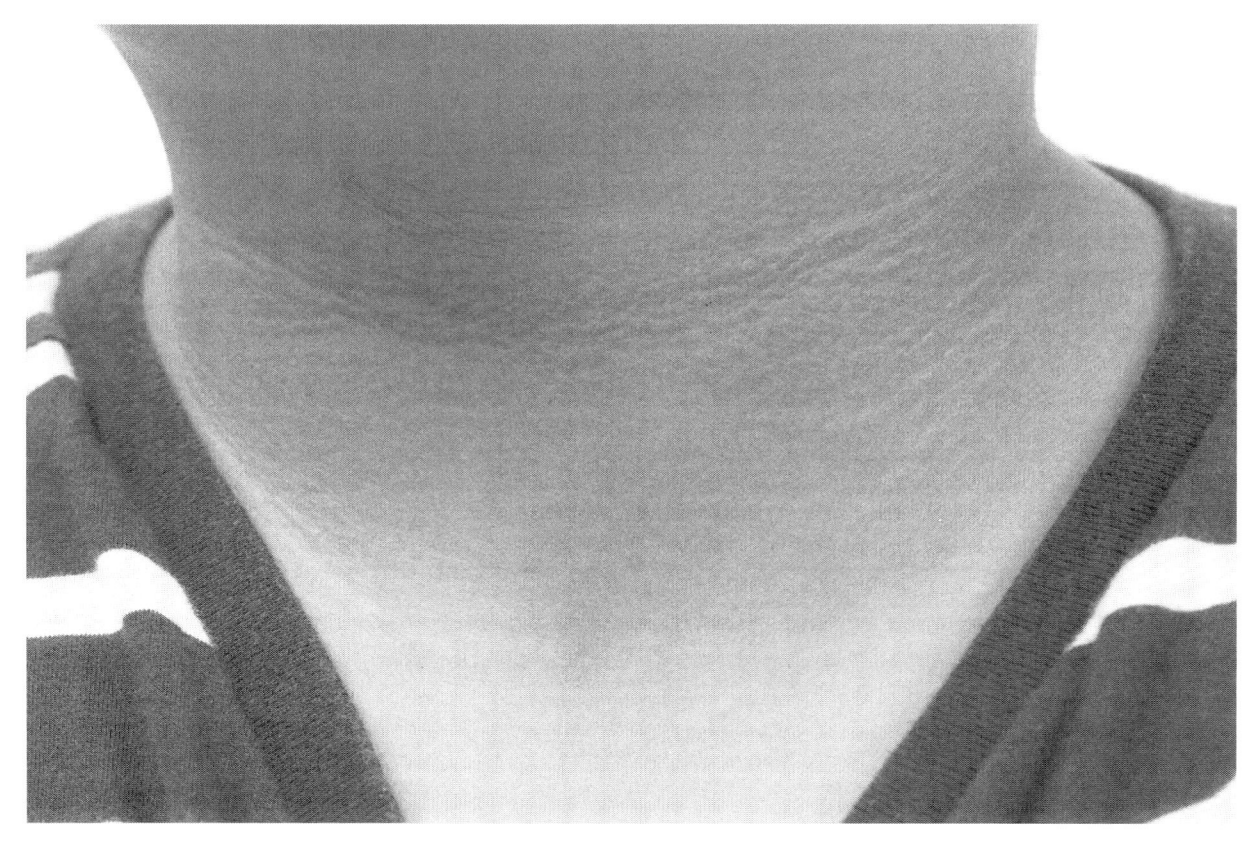

The common denominator in all cases of acanthosis nigricans, with the possible exception of tumor-induced lesions, is insulin resistance.

Metabolic Syndrome

Metabolic syndrome is a combination of metabolic derangements such as high blood pressure and high cholesterol. Metabolic syndrome is the end-stage syndrome caused by insulin resistance and its many effects on the body. It develops when you have insulin resistance for so long that you develop high glucose, high blood pressure, and abnormal cholesterol or triglycerides.

The person with this disorder has the co-occurrence of metabolic risk factors for both type 2 diabetes and heart disease. You probably recognize the cardiovascular disease risk factors: abdominal obesity, hyperglycemia (high blood sugar), dyslipidemia (high lipid levels), and hypertension. All of these factors go hand in hand to contribute to cardiovascular disease. Insulin resistance is the common denominator of all of these things.

When I see these high-risk patients, I find it useful to quantify how much insulin resistance they have. In nondiabetic overweight individuals, I measure the serum triglyceride level, the ratio of triglyceride to high-density lipoprotein (HDL) cholesterol, and fasting insulin concentration for identifying insulin resistance. Optimal cutoff points are triglyceride levels less than 130 mg/dL, 3.0 for triglyceride to HDL ratio, and 15.7 microU/mL for insulin level.

Also, the American Heart Association suggests having three of these or more means you have metabolic syndrome:

- » Abdominal obesity
- » Triglyceride level of 150 mg/dL of blood (mg/dL) or greater
- » HDL cholesterol of less than 40 mg/dL in men or less than 50 mg/dL in women
- » Systolic blood pressure of 130 millimeters of mercury (mm Hg) or greater, or diastolic blood pressure of 85 mm Hg or greater
- » Fasting blood sugar of 100 mg/dL (5.55 mmol/l) or greater

A Brief Review Of What To Do

II will talk more in the next chapter about the specifics of what you should do if you think you are at risk for the complications of insulin resistance, but these are the basics:

If you have pre-diabetes, metabolic syndrome, or insulin resistance, make lifestyle changes. If you do these things, you will reduce the chance that you will get full-blown diabetes and its complications.

Here are a few things you can do.

- *Lose weight* – Losing 5 to 10 percent of your body weight can lower your risk a lot. If you weigh 180 pounds, that means you should lose 9 to 18 pounds. If you weigh 160 pounds, that means you should lose 8 to 16 pounds.

- *Eat right* – Choose a diet rich in fruits, vegetables, and low-fat dairy products but low in meats, sweets, and refined sugar. Pay attention to portion size. Eat small portions. Stay far away from sweet drinks, like soda and juice.

- *Exercise for 30 minutes a day* – You don't have to go to the gym or break a sweat to get a benefit. Walking, gardening, and dancing are all activities that can help.

- *Quit smoking* – If you smoke, ask your doctor or nurse for advice on how to quit. People are much more likely to succeed if they have help and get medicines to help them quit.

- If your doctor or nurse prescribes any **medicines**, take them every day as directed. The most common medications that help prevent diabetes are metformin and pioglitazone. I also recommend "SugarMD's diabetic support formula," that I have created from totally natural ingredients. It is a good alternative for those patients who are not ready to start taking medication or are afraid of side effects from regular medications such as metformin. There are others you can take to lower your blood pressure or cholesterol. People with pre-diabetes have a higher-than-average risk of heart attacks, strokes, and other problems, so taking those medicines are important to reduce the risk of these serious complications when lifestyle adjustment is not enough.

Your diet will be one of the most important things you can do to prevent diabetes. The Mediterranean diet is the best choice, so I will cover that in detail later. Carbohydrates raise your blood sugar level the most. This is why your doctor, nurse, or dietitian will teach you how many carbohydrates you should eat at each meal or snack. Most prediabetics should limit total carbs to less than 30-45 grams per meal.

Foods that have carbohydrates include these:

> » Bread, pasta, and rice
> » Vegetables and fruits
> » Dairy foods
> » Foods with added sugar

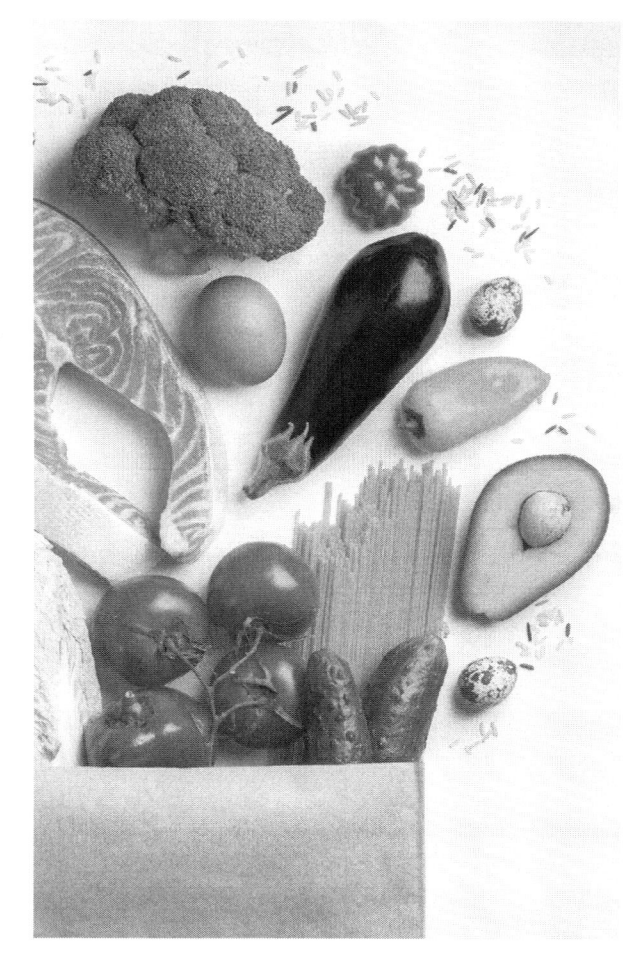

It's best to get your carbohydrates from fruits, vegetables, whole grains, and low-fat milk, as you'll see when I talk more about diabetes nutrition. Also, talk to your doctor or dietician about how much protein you should eat each day. I generally recommend 50-75 grams of total protein daily. It is best to eat lean meats, fish, eggs, beans, peas, soy products, nuts, and seeds as your main protein sources.

You need fat too, but I usually recommend avoiding "saturated" and "trans" fats because these can increase your risk for heart problems, such as heart attacks. Foods that have saturated fats include red meat, butter, cheese, and ice cream. Avoid them. Foods that have trans fats include processed food with "partially hydrogenated oils" on the ingredient list. This may include fried foods, store-bought cookies, muffins, pies, and cakes. Avoid these as well. "Monounsaturated" and "polyunsaturated" fats are better for you. Foods with these types of fat include oily fish, avocado, olive oil, and nuts.

Summary Of Insulin Resistance And Its Complications

Insulin resistance is a state in which a given insulin concentration is not enough for a normal response to glucose in the diet. Important long-term consequences of insulin resistance you need to remember include prediabetes, type 2 diabetes, cardiovascular disease (CVD), and certain cancers associated with obesity.

Insulin resistance is associated with a variety of clinical presentations, depending on how severe it is. For those who are obese, the diagnosis of insulin resistance is mostly based on clinical findings and not necessarily on lab testing. These clinical factors include high blood sugars, high cholesterol, abdominal obesity, and hypertension.

So if you are overweight, having problems losing weight, feeling fatigued, or do not have the energy to do anything, you are likely to have insulin resistance. You will often see low HDL levels, high triglyceride levels, and high total cholesterol in your blood work. Your blood sugars may start to go up over time, and your doctor may tell you that you have prediabetes (or diabetes in a worst-case scenario).

High blood pressure generally follows insulin resistance and abnormal cholesterol levels. As a result, most people start developing cardiovascular disease and can even have heart attacks before being diagnosed with diabetes. Most heart attacks actually happen to people in the prediabetes stage.

This is why you need to take action as soon as you can. If you think you are at risk for any of these abnormal blood sugar states (insulin resistance, prediabetes, diabetes, or metabolic syndrome), seeing an endocrinologist early on will save you many headaches and trouble in the future.

Type 1 Versus Type 2 Diabetes

While both of the main types of diabetes involve high blood sugars, they are caused by completely different things. Most of the time, it is relatively easy to tell the difference between the two from a clinical perspective, but this isn't always true. I sometimes have to do some specialized testing to be able to tell the difference.

People with type 1 diabetes don't make enough insulin because their own immune system has destroyed their pancreatic beta cells. For reasons we don't yet understand completely, those with type 1 diabetes have immune systems that don't recognize their own beta cells as part of their body but rather as something foreign.

After all the beta cells are gone, the person with type 1 diabetes can't make any insulin at all. Beta cells can't regenerate themselves, and if they could, the immune system would still be active and destroy any that developed.

Without insulin, glucose can't enter the cells, so the cells instead start using mostly fats as an alternative fuel source. Using fat for energy creates waste chemicals called ketones and, when ketones build up in the blood, they make it more acidic. If ketone levels get too high, it can lead to a life-threatening condition called diabetic ketoacidosis or DKA.

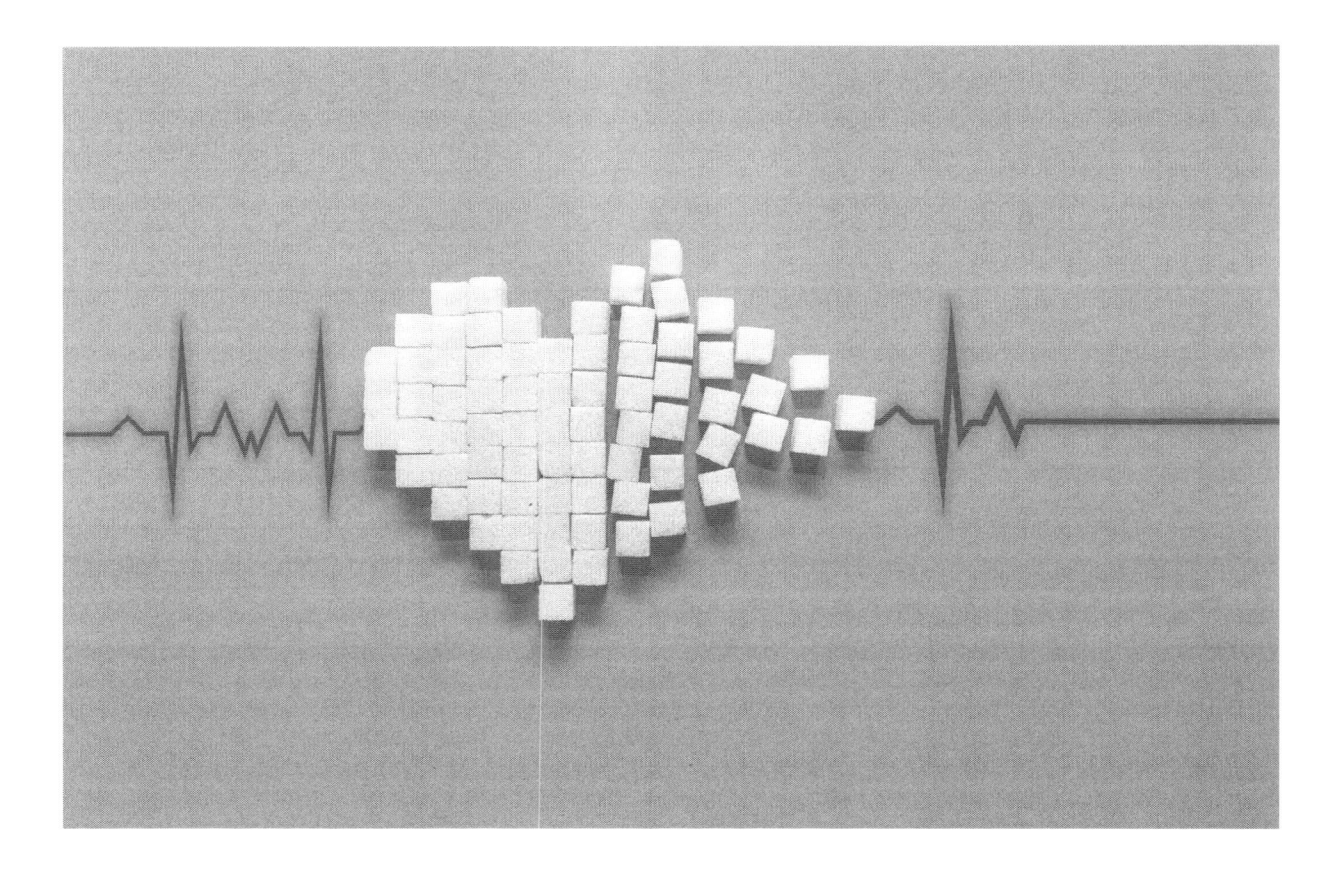

Unfortunately, most people with type 1 diabetes find out they have it only after being hospitalized with DKA. Type 1 diabetics are insulin-dependent, meaning they have to take insulin to survive. There really is no other good treatment for it other than insulin replacement in almost every case.

Type 2 diabetes is a combination of insulin resistance, reduced insulin production, and elevated blood sugars. Genetic factors and environmental factors are the two main contributors that cause type 2 diabetes. We have already covered how things like obesity and lifestyle play an important role in getting it, but I haven't yet said how much genetics plays a role in this disorder.

When we talk about a person's genetic risk factors, we are talking about the genes you inherit from your mother and father that affect your risk of diabetes. Some races are more prone to have diabetes than others. African Americans,

Alaska Natives, American Indians, Asian Americans, Hispanic/Latinos, Native Hawaiians, and Pacific Islanders are generally at a higher risk of diabetes because of their genetic makeup.

Beta cells, which are the only insulin-producing cells in your body, are located in the pancreas. How much insulin they make is genetically determined, so you can produce only so much insulin based on your inheritance of certain genes. Just like your height is mostly genetically determined, your insulin production capacity is also genetically determined. First degree relatives have a higher risk of developing T1D than unrelated individuals from the general population (approximately 6% vs. <1%, respectively). On the other hand, studies estimate that the heritability of T2DM is anywhere between 20%-80%.

In addition to that, when environmental factors put stress on the beta cells to make more and more insulin, they will eventually fail. Your genes determine how resilient your beta cells are to these kinds of stressors. The most significant environmental stress impacting the risk of type 2 diabetes is whether or not you have insulin resistance.

Sometimes a single genetic mutation can lead to diabetes independent of any environmental factors. This type of diabetes is called maturity-onset diabetes of the young (MODY).

◢ Fast Fact

> *You may have figured out now why you would still feel starved with so much blood sugar (fuel) in your body. It's because your cells are really starving without the ability of insulin to help them use the glucose you have. It would be like being stranded on a deserted island with a huge pile of canned food but no can opener. The fuel is there; it's just hard to have access to it.*

The Differences Between Type 1 and Type 2 Diabetes

Type 1 Diabetes	Type 2 Diabetes
Caused by the destruction of beta cells	A combination of insulin resistance and destruction of beta cells
Patients are positive for autoantibodies against the beta cells	There are no associated autoimmune markers
insulin deficiency is absolute	Insulin deficiency is relative
Patients are totally dependent on insulin	Total insulin dependency happens at the later stages of the disease
Patients can only use insulin, glucagon, and Symlin (pramlintide)	There are more than 80 different diabetic medications to treat it
DKA (diabetic ketoacidosis) happens fairly frequently	DKA is very rare
Patients are not overweight or obese most of the time	Patients tend to be overweight or obese
Patients may have associated autoimmune disorders such as Hashimoto's thyroiditis, celiac disease, or adrenal insufficiency	There is no association with other autoimmune disorders
The hypoglycemia risk is much higher	Low blood sugar (hypoglycemia) is not commonly seen unless on insulin.

Whether you've had diabetes for a long time or are newly diagnosed, you may still not be sure what type of diabetes you have. Unfortunately, many doctors also cannot give you a clear answer most of the time. So, how do you know you have type 1 versus type 2 diabetes? Are there any other types of diabetes? Does it even matter what kind of diabetes you have? I think it does.

In fact, knowing whether you have type 2 diabetes versus type 1 diabetes makes all the difference, especially in the treatments that work best. When you have type 1 diabetes, you know that you are totally insulin-dependent. You know that your beta cells that make insulin are almost completely destroyed. You understand that you may end up with diabetic ketoacidosis or DKA if you do not take your insulin.

Diabetic ketoacidosis is a very dangerous and potentially deadly problem that those with type 1 diabetes face. Even so, having type 2 diabetes doesn't mean you are free of any danger. Type 2 diabetics can get very sick if their blood sugars are high with a complication called hyperosmolar hyperglycemic state or HHS.

If you develop HHS from type 2 diabetes and very high blood sugars, statistics say you have an 8 percent chance of dying from the complication. If instead, you have type 1 diabetes and develop DKA, your risk of dying is only 5 percent. Part of the difference in mortality is that type 2 diabetics with HHS tend to be sicker and older before they develop the complication, so they don't do as well as the younger diabetic with DKA.

Also, when you have type 2 diabetes, you have more time to work on your lifestyle, eat better, and exercise. This isn't true for type 1 diabetes. Type 2 diabetics can start taking maybe one pill at first and then try to keep the number of medications limited by changing their lifestyle at the same time.

Some type 2 diabetics will eventually need insulin. It doesn't mean they suddenly have type 1 diabetes. Like any other organ, your pancreas makes insulin less when you age. As a result, insulin production capacity becomes lower and lower over time. Even if insulin resistance did not change at all, when the insulin production drops, diabetes will still progress. This may not happen within a few years, but it will happen in decades in most cases. I typically see this pattern in my diabetes clinic myself on a daily basis.

Eventually, if a person with diabetes lives long enough, he or she will become insulin-dependent. Exactly when it is that someone with type 2 diabetes becomes insulin-dependent depends on many different factors. Diet, exercise habits, medications, and genetics will all determine the outcome. When a type 2 diabetic needs insulin, it will often be in much larger amounts than are required by type 1 diabetics.

Remember that type 2 diabetes is a progressive disease. Remission for diabetes is definitely possible by reducing the demand for insulin. By now, you know the factors determining the demand, such as dietary sugar intake and body weight. Most people can achieve diabetes remission if they can reduce the carbohydrates in their diet significantly or totally. On the other hand, your genetic ability to produce enough insulin determines whether or not your diabetes comes back in the long run.

You probably already know that people with type 2 diabetes have dozens of different medication choices unavailable to those with type 1 diabetes. Why is this true? This is a good question and fundamental to the differences between these two diabetes classes. The answer to this relies on knowing the pathology behind the different types of diabetes. Most medications that we use for type 2 diabetes work on helping the beta cells work better.

Since most beta cells are dead in type 1 diabetes, the medications designed for type 2 diabetes may not be appropriate for these individuals. On the other hand, your endocrinologist may choose to use some medicines normally used for type 2 diabetes off-label for type 1 diabetes if they determine that a type 1 diabetic patient has developed insulin resistance.

Why does DKA affect type 1 diabetics but not type 2 diabetics as much? Again, when we talk about type I versus type 2 diabetes, we are talking about a fundamental difference in the amount of insulin present. When there is no insulin in the body, your body starts making ketone bodies as byproducts of alternative fuel metabolism. Type 2 diabetics have insulin, so ketone bodies specific to produce DKA don't get made.

People with type 1 diabetes start making too many ketone bodies because of a prolonged lack of insulin. This lack of insulin might only be hours—not usually days. The ketone bodies are acidic. They change the body's pH level. The pH of your body is very tightly regulated for good reasons. Any minor changes in the pH can cause devastating consequences. This is why it is imperative for people with type 1 diabetes to continue to take their insulin as instructed.

Risk Factors For Diabetic Ketoacidosis

If the person with type 1 diabetes gets sick for any reason, their insulin requirements may change while they are sick. During those times, type I diabetics are at a higher risk for developing DKA. Sickness is a time when blood sugars need special attention and insulin needs adjusting.

Are Type 1 Diabetics Guaranteed To Have Thyroid Disease Or Adrenal Insufficiency?

There is no guarantee that this will happen. Still, there is definitely an increased risk of Hashimoto's thyroiditis, adrenal insufficiency, and celiac disease (all autoimmune diseases) in patients with type 1 diabetes but not type 2 diabetes. This is because the tendency to develop any autoimmune disease (including type 1 diabetes) is largely inherited.

As a result of this heightened risk, many endocrinologists will perform yearly screenings for these disorders to make sure they are diagnosed before they become severe. Type 2 diabetics, on the other hand, are not at high risk for autoimmune diseases, so they usually don't need these routine screening tests.

Another big difference between type 1 and type 2 diabetes is the number of times the blood sugar becomes too low. The risk of low blood glucose is far higher in type 1 diabetes. Remember that people with type 1 diabetes are on insulin only. They take insulin injections 3-6 times a day. Taking long-acting insulin such as Tresiba, Toujeo, Levemir, or Lantus, and short-acting insulin such as NovoLog, Humalog, or Fiasp together increases the risk of low blood sugars.

On most occasions, patients with type 2 diabetes are on one or just a few basal insulin injections daily. Others only take oral agents such as metformin. Even when type 2 diabetics are on multiple daily injections, the chances of low blood sugar are still reduced because they also have insulin resistance. Insulin resistance definitely reduces the risk of low blood sugar.

LADA (Latent Autoimmune Diabetes Of Adults)

LADA, or what we call type 1.5 diabetes, is exactly how it sounds. It is something in between the two types of diabetes. It has the same underlying cause as type 1 diabetes (autoimmune dysfunction), but it happens in adulthood and not in childhood. It can be hard to diagnose easily in the beginning because we sometimes initially expect it to be type 2 disease; the patient is too old for it to logically be type 1 diabetes. It's only when they quickly become insulin-dependent or if antibody testing is done early that it becomes clear that it is instead of type 1.5 diabetes.

Here is a good question: Are all type 2 diabetics overweight and are all type 1 diabetics very thin? Absolutely not. These are all general features we see when we study diabetic patients. There are always exceptions to this rule. I see many patients with type 1 diabetes who, in time, start gaining weight due to excess calories and the effects of insulin, which eventually leads to insulin resistance.

Similarly, some patients with type 2 diabetes are not overweight; however, their insulin production capacity is much lower in general than other diabetics. As a result, their insulin resistance is of a lesser magnitude as a factor in developing diabetes. Remember, type 2 diabetes is a state of *relative* insulin deficiency.

Sometimes we refer to this unique and uncommon situation as LADA, especially If the patient has the same antibodies type 1 diabetics have. This is because they are not as insulin deficient as type 1 diabetics, but they are also not as insulin resistant as type 2 diabetics. They might have autoantibodies plus low insulin production so they are in between type 1 and type 2 diabetes.

A Rare Kind Of Diabetes That Runs In Families: MODY (Maturity-Onset Diabetes Of The Young)

It is important to know if you have MODY because, if you know that you have one of the more common types of MODY, it is likely that all you need to manage your diabetes is dietary management or very simple treatments such as a sulfonylurea drug during your entire life with this type of diabetes.

These are some clues to know if you might have MODY:

» If you have diabetes diagnosed at a young age (often in the late teenage years) but your blood sugars are only mild to moderately elevated.

» You have a strong family history of people in your family with a type of diabetes that does not progress or cause complications (most people in your family either use no medication or a single oral pill for decades).

» They think you may have type 1 diabetes because you are young, but antibodies such as GAD-65 and IA-2 antibodies are negative in blood testing.

If you or your doctor think you have MODY, there are tests you can have to see what gene is defective in your body. This will say what type of MODY you have. Because this is highly hereditary, you may wish to see a geneticist, so your children and siblings can also be tested to see if they have inherited the disorder.

Final Thoughts

While testing for diabetes will show if you have pre-diabetes or diabetes, it won't necessarily say which kind you have. The two main types of diabetes I see most often are type 1 and type 2 diabetes. While both types can be managed with treatments I will outline later, the person with type 2 disease, insulin resistance, or prediabetes has the best chance of curing their problems with regulating blood sugars using things like diet and exercise, especially when it is caught early enough.

You can see how insulin resistance is the root of type 2 diabetes. It is not easy to diagnose this before the blood sugars are elevated, but if you have the risk factors we discussed previously or meet the criteria for metabolic syndrome, you should start taking measures to keep it from progressing any further. The consequences of failing to do this can be catastrophic, especially if you develop severe type 2 diabetes.

You need to keep going back to the idea of supply and demand. If you don't make enough insulin for any reason, OR if you don't make enough to suit your body's needs, you will develop diabetes. If you are overweight or obese, your insulin needs are greater (the demand goes up). It means that, if you are genetically predisposed to making less insulin than normal, it isn't hard for you to have a relative insulin deficiency simply because the demands for insulin in obesity are higher than they should be.

The other types of diabetes: type 1 diabetes, LADA, and MODY, are less common but still need careful management. Both type 1 diabetes and sometimes LADA at later stages are managed with insulin. However, things like eating correctly and consuming healthy foods that aren't so high in simple sugars are still important no matter what type of diabetes you have.

CHAPTER 2 - TYPES OF DIABETES

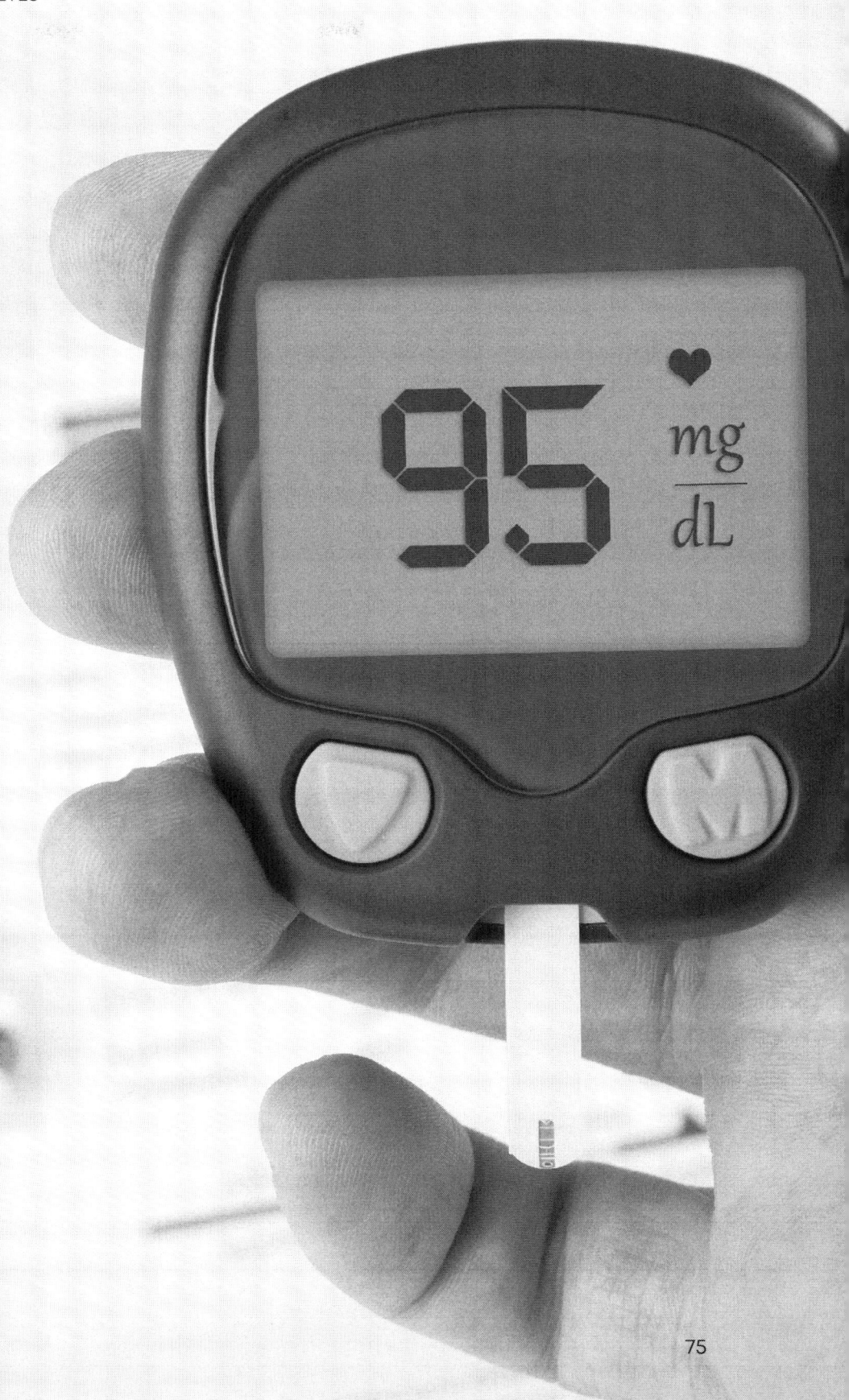

CHAPTER 3
DIABETES BASICS

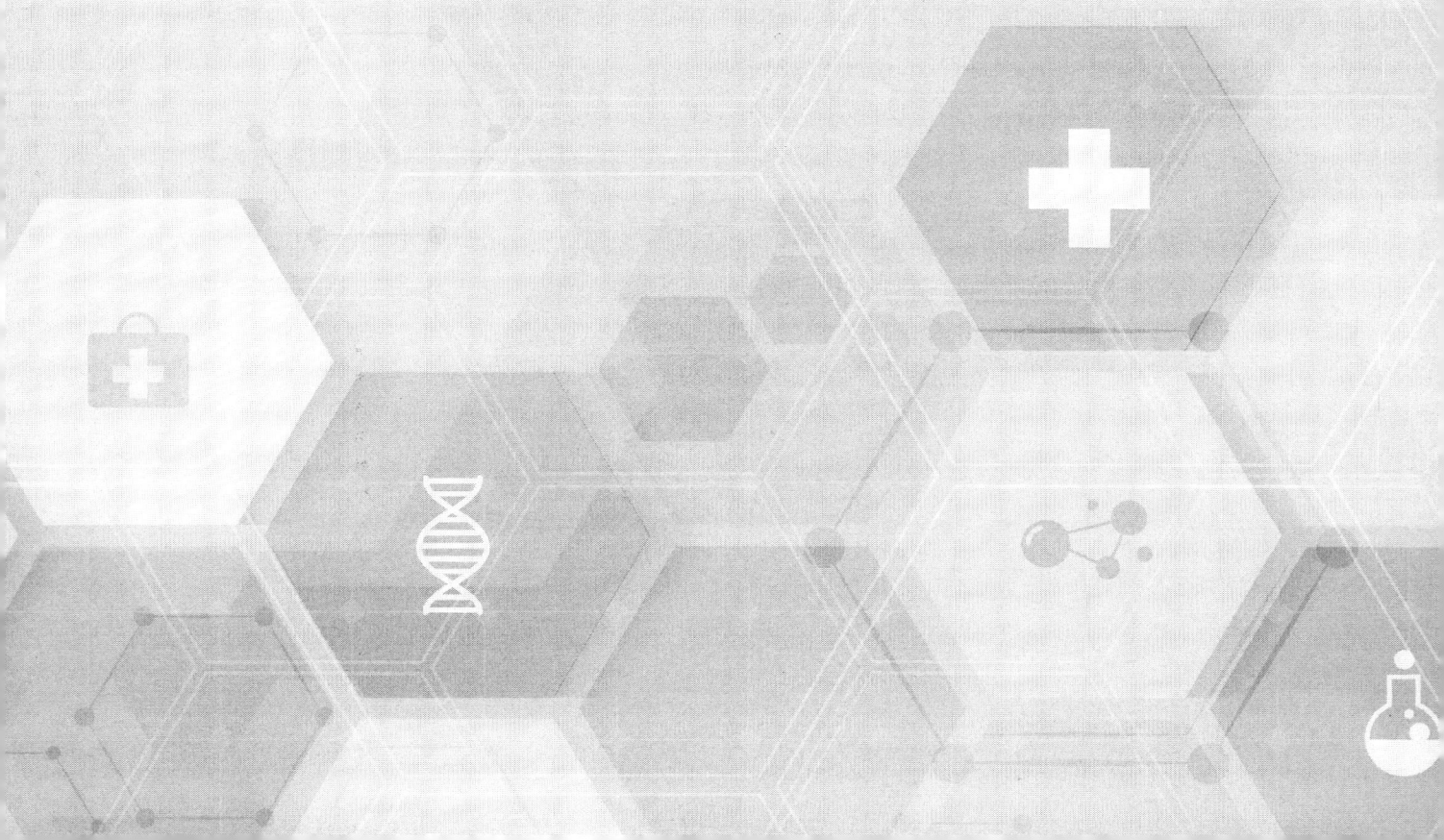

CHAPTER 3
DIABETES BASICS

I want to talk now about the things you most need to know if you are diabetic. There are some basics that every person with diabetes should be completely familiar with, such as the signs of diabetes, how to check your blood sugars, and what to do if the blood sugar reading is too high or too low. Like anything in life, if you know your basics, you should stay safe in most cases.

One thing you need to remember is diabetes is not a death sentence. It is another chronic condition like high blood pressure or high cholesterol. It can be a little more demanding than just taking a pill for cholesterol, for example, but you will realize it is not a big deal once you get the hang of it. I hope that you will be able to improve your self-confidence you'll need to manage this disorder. When you do this, not only will you feel comfortable managing your diabetes, but you will also learn to control it or even put it into remission.

Regardless, anytime you are dealing with a chronic condition (especially if it's new to you), it can feel very overwhelming at first. You might feel as though there is just too much to absorb at one time, especially in the beginning. I recommend you keep coming back to this chapter as a guide for practicing the skills it takes to manage your symptoms and blood sugars successfully; there are ways you can do this that will not only make having the disorder more tolerable but will help you have mastery over its management. The goal is to improve your quality of life.

Having diabetes is often a wake-up call telling you that major changes are in order. Don't feel like you have to cram it all into one day. Change happens slowly and involves a lot of practice in finding what works best. As long as you remain committed to improving your health for the better in small ways every day, you will be successful in seeing large and meaningful changes over the long-term.

With these things in mind, use this chapter to familiarize yourself with the particulars of what it is like to live with diabetes using the skill and empowerment you'll need to succeed. Yes, you can gain control over your blood sugars and your health.

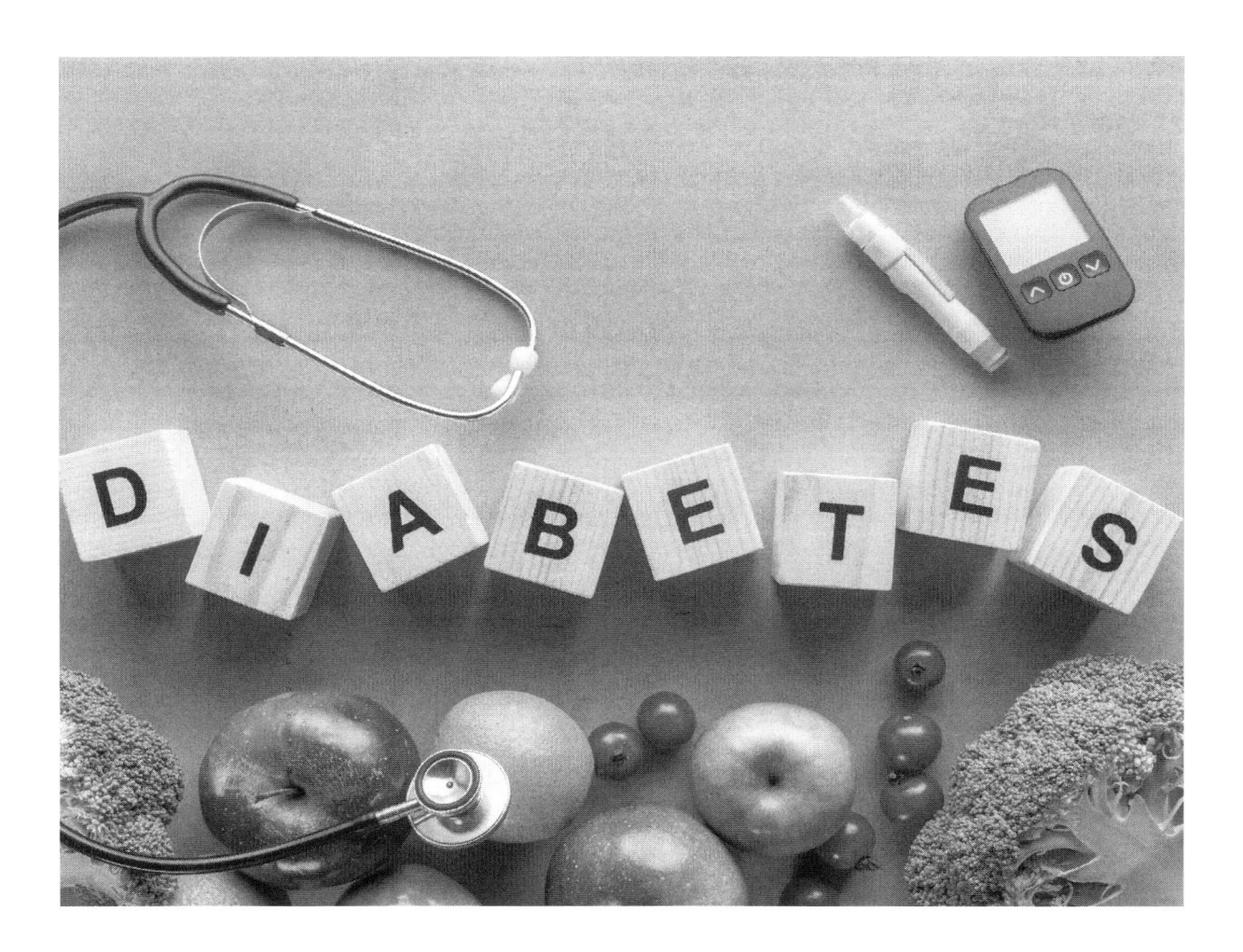

Risk Factors For Diabetes

When you understand the risk factors for diabetes, you'll have a better idea about how and why you developed the disease yourself. Knowing your risk factors is less about beating yourself up over things you did or didn't do years before and more about looking at each risk factor carefully and deciding how you can tackle each one now. Yes, it is not too late yet. If you do something to change those risk factors, you will be able to prevent a possible progression to insulin injections and will reduce your chances of developing complications.

The goal is to reduce your risk of having your diabetes worsen over time and maybe, if you are very successful at changing your lifestyle, to cure yourself of the disease altogether. Of course, you can't change some things, like your genetic background and ethnicity. These are things you can use instead to tell your children and grandchildren of their own potential risk long before they develop diabetes themselves.

These are the main risk factors for type 2 diabetes:

- *Being overweight or obese:* This is the main risk factor for type 2 diabetes. While it is possible to develop diabetes without being overweight, remember that this happens when you have the genetic tendency to make less insulin than most others. You can improve your outcomes with diabetes or prevent getting it at all if you maintain a normal weight for your height. Your first goal should be to lose only 5-10% of your body weight within a few months. Ideally, 1-2 pounds per week on average will be enough. We will talk more about this later.

- *Having most of your fat around your midsection:* As I mentioned, having belly fat or abdominal fat is linked more to type 2 diabetes than is true of fat that builds up in the thighs and buttocks. There are many environmental factors related to having too much abdominal fat, including eating a high-sugar diet, being inactive, and suffering from chronic stress. Stress releases a major stress-related hormone called cortisol. High cortisol levels predispose you to put more fat into your fatty abdominal areas. What helps? Avoiding high sugar and a high saturated fat diet (in my opinion and based on studies, the Mediterranean diet is the best) as well as incorporating 150 minutes of aerobic exercise and some strength training into your week.

- *Being physically inactive or sedentary:* Part of maintaining a healthy weight is regular exercise. This makes a lot of sense but it's not all about simply not burning enough calories. When your muscle cells aren't active enough, they become less sensitive to insulin. Also, remember "use it or lose it." If you are not engaged in aerobic exercise and strength training, you will lose a lot of muscle. This only gets worse as you get older. When you have less muscle overall, your basal metabolic rate will slow down, and you will gain fat a lot easier. As we discussed earlier, this development of fat is one of the main reasons you get the kind of inflammation that triggers diabetes.

- *Genetic background:* With certain types of diabetes (like MODY), you might be able to predict that your child has a high chance of developing the same type of diabetes you have. With other diabetes types, the genetic linkage is not as clear-cut, while inheriting type 2 diabetes risk is much higher than inheriting type 1 diabetes.

- *Race or ethnicity:* This may have something to do with genetics and which genes for diabetes might be higher in certain ethnic groups compared to others. As I mentioned earlier, those with the highest risk of developing type 2 diabetes include people of Hispanic descent, American Indians, Alaskan natives, Asian-Americans, African-Americans, and those whose ancestors came from the Polynesian Islands, including native Hawaiians.

- *Older age:* There is an increased risk of type 2 diabetes in older individuals, with the risk being particularly significant after the age of 45 years. Being sedentary and having a higher proportion of fat to muscle increases with age, which might be part of why the risk increases in older people.

- ***Having gestational diabetes:*** The risk of type 2 diabetes increases in women who have had an episode of gestational diabetes in pregnancy. This could be because pregnancy increases the demand for insulin, so it might indicate a woman who has a genetic tendency toward having a decreased natural ability to put out enough insulin under the stress of pregnancy maximally. If you have gestational diabetes, it isn't guaranteed that you'll later develop type 2 diabetes, but your risk becomes higher, so you should test for diabetes more frequently later in life.

- ***Polycystic Ovarian Syndrome:*** Women with polycystic ovarian syndrome (PCOS) have similar metabolic derangements affecting their reproductive system and the ability to regulate their blood sugars simultaneously. Insulin resistance is a major part of having PCOS. As you know, being insulin resistant is essential for later developing type 2 diabetes.

As I mentioned, you can't do much about age, ethnicity, family history, and whether or not you've had PCOS or gestational diabetes. This means you need to focus more on what we call "modifiable risk factors" like diet, weight, and exercise. These are things you have the most control over; I will talk more in the next chapter about exactly how you manage these lifestyle issues.

How To Prevent Diabetes

Although diabetes type 2 is genetically inherited, there are ways to prevent it early in life, so it doesn't happen as you age. Even if you have family members with diabetes, there are certain things you can pay attention to so you can avoid developing diabetes yourself. Some measures you can take will help delay the development of diabetes, while others will totally cancel the risk of getting the disease.

To prevent diabetes, you need to understand your own risk factors. As I discussed earlier, if you have these risk factors, you should take measures to prevent diabetes now.

- » A first-degree family member with diabetes
- » If you are of African American, Latina, Asian, or Native American descent
- » High blood pressure or abnormal cholesterol levels
- » Sedentary lifestyle
- » History of cardiovascular heart disease or PCOS

It is better to start prevention efforts knowing that you have risk factors even if you have no blood sugar abnormalities now at all. On the other hand, if your fasting blood sugar is between 100 and 126 mg/dL (5.55-7.0 mmol/l) and your A1c is between 5.7 and 6.5, you are considered to have prediabetes. In this situation, you have to hurry up and do something to prevent progression to diabetes as soon as possible.

Lifestyle Modifications

The most important aspect of lifestyle modification in diabetes prevention is behavior modification plus dietary changes and increased physical activity. Smoking cessation is also extremely important. The goal is, of course, to return to a normal healthy weight. For people who want to use a strict diet, I would recommend following the Newcastle diet or the Mediterranean keto diet to achieve rapid weight loss. Following that, you may gradually increase your calories; however, you need to continue to weigh yourself every day and make sure you do not start gaining the weight back while introducing the calories.

Exercising daily will help you keep the weight off. Discipline and perseverance are extremely important when it comes to exercise. You need to have a routine. You will learn more about diet and exercise in the following chapter of this book.

In a nutshell, your motto should be to have a low-carbohydrate, mostly Mediterranean, and portion-controlled diet. If you can embrace this type of diet and add 30 minutes of daily exercise, you will have your exit ticket to the development of diabetes.

It is sometimes better to work with a diabetes coach or life coach to help you achieve your goals if you do not have enough self-motivation by yourself. Our YouTube channel, called SugarMD, is another good source that can help you stay motivated while learning about diabetes and diet.

Medications Or Supplements That Can Help Prevent Diabetes

Some individuals may need medications or some natural herbal remedies. The only two proven medications that can help prevent diabetes are metformin and pioglitazone. For patients who have side effects of these agents or are afraid to take them, I have developed a "SugarMD Advanced Glucose Support" supplement, which will also help you prevent diabetes. In my experience, this supplement not only helps prevent the progression of diabetes but also helps patients reduce the number of medications and insulin they take.

In addition to supplements, you will have to develop strategies to help you stay motivated, manage stress, and solve the problems coming your way; these could derail you when it comes to sticking with your goals.

Signs And Symptoms Of High Blood Sugar Due To Diabetes

The majority of people with type 2 diabetes had no idea they had the disease at the time of their confirmatory test. Only the presence of a high blood sugar reading or abnormal response to a sugar load may have led to the diagnosis. This is because most symptoms don't develop unless the numbers are much higher than the cutoff values indicating diabetes.

Still, there are several symptoms of high blood sugar you'll start seeing if the blood sugar is above 180 to 200 mg/dL (10.0 to 11.1 mmol/L). Let's review what these are:

- *Excessive thirst and urination:* This is seen because the kidneys start to excrete excessive blood sugar above a certain threshold; this threshold is typically when the blood sugar is above 180 mg/dL (10.0 mmol/l). In individuals with long-standing uncontrolled diabetes, that threshold can be higher (above 220 mg/dL or 12.2 mmol/l). When the body urinates glucose (a process called glucosuria), it also attracts the water with it.

  Because water is also excreted along with glucose in the urine, dehydration and thirst are two of the most common symptoms of diabetes. There are other causes of excessive thirst and urination, such as diabetes insipidus, which give similar symptoms but aren't the same as diabetes mellitus at all. This is why you need to see an endocrinologist who can make the correct diagnosis.

- *Excessive hunger:* Because the body excretes excessive glucose, a calorie deficit starts to happen, which leads to excessive hunger. Hunger also happens because of insulin resistance and the inability to utilize glucose by the cells. Due to this excessive hunger, many people start eating a lot more to compensate for the energy loss. Eventually, this becomes habitual, and when the diabetes is finally treated, the person may start gaining weight, especially if they are on insulin.

  Excessive hunger can be from other hormonal disorders such as hyperthyroidism or Cushing syndrome. In my clinic, we always do the proper workup to differentiate between these hormonal disorders that can give similar symptoms as diabetes. You should make sure your doctor does the same.

- *Fatigue:* Since the body cannot utilize glucose, which is the primary energy source under most circumstances, fatigue sets in. The fatigue is generally chronic and persistent, even when the person is apparently rested. The individual may wake up feeling unrefreshed. They may also start feeling extremely exhausted by the afternoon and fall asleep very early in the evening. Fatigue is the most nonspecific symptom of diabetes so, in the absence of other symptoms related to diabetes, having only fatigue may not mean you have diabetes.

- *Weight loss:* Because of excessive glucose loss in the urine and the body's inability to utilize the glucose properly, these lead to excessive weight loss. Some people think that weight loss results from their minor efforts to lose weight; however, most of the time, unless the person was on a very strict diet, weight loss is generally an indicator of significant health problems. If you are experiencing weight loss, obtain an endocrinologist's opinion for further insight into why it could be happening.

- *Nausea:* Excessive blood sugars can lead to a sluggish stomach that doesn't empty well. This is called gastroparesis, which is often complicated by nausea. Certain medications that are taken for diabetes also can lead to nausea. Food allergies and certain other medications taken for other reasons also contribute to nausea.

Abdominal obesity, often seen in people with type 2 diabetes, contributes to gastrointestinal reflux disease or GERD. One of the major signs of this is nausea, which is usually worse in the morning, especially if the blood sugar is also high, causing acute gastroparesis (discussed later). Monitoring blood sugars and keeping them stable will help prevent nausea during diabetes care as well.

Fast Fact:

Nausea and vomiting can be a sign of something more serious, especially in type 1 diabetes. These are symptoms among type 1 diabetics who have ketoacidosis or DKA. As the body starts to burn fat, the cells will produce ketones as a waste product. Ketones can make you feel sick to your stomach. In severe cases of DKA, nausea and vomiting contribute to the dehydration seen in the disorder.

- *Dry mouth:* Due to the dehydration from high glucose and water excretion in the urine, dry mouth is a common presentation of diabetes. Unfortunately, some individuals continue to drink sugary beverages that fuel the fire and make the dehydration worse. Remember, dry mouth can also be a symptom of rheumatologic disorders such as Sjogren's syndrome, psychiatric disorders, and many other disorders unrelated to diabetes.

- *Itching:* When dehydration happens, it directly affects the skin, leading to diffuse itching. In essence, the skin is dehydrated along with the rest of the body, so it becomes very dry and itchy. Instead of taking over-the-counter supplements or creams for itching, people who have diabetes should consider the possibility of dehydration and the likely prospect of also having significant health problems from this diabetic complication. Glucose monitoring and diabetes care are very important, but avoiding hot showers, baths, and drying soaps will also help. Also, using moisturizers regularly is an important part of diabetes care. These will prevent fluid loss from the skin surface.

- *Dizziness:* Dehydration in diabetes happens from excessive glucose and water excretion in the urine. When the fluid is not replaced with appropriate hydration, dizziness can occur from excessive volume loss and a reduction in blood pressure. Dizziness typically happens when the individual first stands up. If this happens to you, you need to be careful and get up slowly. Along with hydration with a non-caffeinated beverage, using compression stockings on the legs can help older people with diabetes.

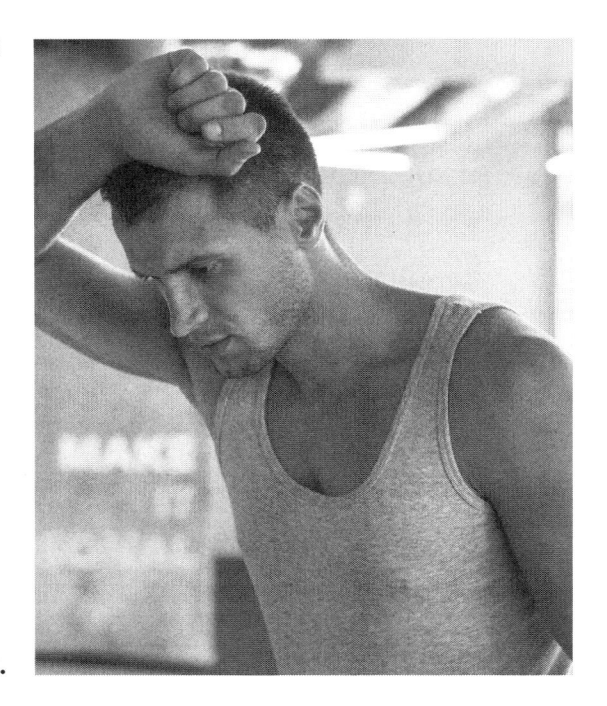

- *Frequent infections:* Because of excessive urination of glucose, people with diabetes become especially susceptible to urinary tract infections. Bacteria and fungi like the sweeter environment in the urine from the glucose in it, so they grow faster. Also, individuals with diabetes are typically prone to infections because the disorder suppresses the immune system. Strict diabetes control with an appropriate diabetes care plan should help improve the ability to fight infections. Of course, the doctor in charge of your diabetes care may also prescribe antibiotics or antifungals to treat the infection, depending on what is causing it.

- *Decreased or blurry vision:* This happens because high blood sugars in the lens of the eye cause the lens to swell with fluid, changing its shape. Rapid changes in blood sugars also will change the thickness of the lens, which can also lead to blurry vision. Early retinal disease from diabetes (called diabetic retinopathy) is also possible, leading to vision loss. It may not be a bad idea to see an ophthalmologist along with seeing an endocrinologist. Once appropriate diabetes care is given, your symptoms should resolve unless there is a significant underlying problem with the eyes themselves.

- *Dark, velvety skin:* This is due to acanthosis nigricans, as I mentioned earlier. Most people will see patches of it behind the neck and under the armpits that are darker and softer than the rest of their skin. This usually means there is insulin resistance, which typically leads to diabetes. It isn't dangerous by itself, but it is still something you do not want to ignore. Insulin resistance is the initial stage of diabetes and cardiovascular disease so, if you see the typical skin changes of acanthosis nigricans but don't think you have diabetes, you should still seek medical care. Talking to an endocrinologist will reduce your chances of progressing to diabetes or dealing with the complications of diabetes that can happen very early, even if you are still prediabetic.

- *Numbness, tingling, or pain in the feet:* Neuropathy is one of the earliest complications of diabetes types 1 and 2. The only symptoms of neuropathy can be numbness or tingling on both feet. There can also be pain that is typically worse at night. Cramps in the calves are also not uncommon. It is very important to protect the feet against cuts, corns, or calluses. Unnoticed problems such as these can lead to more serious issues, such as foot ulcers.

- *Foot ulcers:* Sometimes, neuropathy is silent and only presents itself as the inability to feel the ground, which leads to corns and calluses, and eventually to foot ulcers. If not noticed and treated promptly, foot ulcers can be infected, and these infected ulcers can lead to gangrene and amputation. Foot ulcers can be extremely complicated to treat. The reason is that people with diabetes generally have underlying vascular disease (poor circulation). They are also immunosuppressed (poor immune functioning). These factors contribute to delayed healing or progression of the infection into the underlying soft tissue and bone.

  Because diabetic foot ulcers are both hard to treat and very serious, aggressive diabetes care using a multidisciplinary approach is needed. This care often involves consultations with an endocrinologist, podiatrist, and a vascular surgeon who work together to treat this complex problem before gangrene and an amputation are necessary.

- *Erectile dysfunction or impotence:* This symptom is also very common. It results from neuropathy and vascular dysfunction together, which affects the ability to have a male erection. Unfortunately, this complication can happen very early and can lead to significant interpersonal family problems. This can lead to a reduction in self-confidence and feelings of rejection. Aggressive diabetes care will help prevent the occurrence or progression of this problem. The most common treatment for erectile dysfunction is medications like Viagra or Cialis. There are also penile injectable medications or penile implants that can be used as a last resort.

- *Chest pain, heart attack, and stroke:* Although most people believe that uncontrolled long-standing high blood sugars are what causes a heart attack or stroke in diabetes, the truth is that cardiovascular disease establishes itself very early in the disease process. As a result, aggressive diabetes care as soon as you know, you are at risk is crucial in preventing these complications. <u>Your endocrinologist will treat not only your blood sugars but also the high cholesterol and high blood pressure that often coexist in diabetics. Control of these things will be of equal value to prevent these common cardiovascular complications of diabetes.</u>

- *Slow healing sores or cuts:* This is a well-known diabetic sign or symptom. High blood sugars over time cause decreased blood flow to the skin and nerve endings. The problem is worse in the feet because of their distance from the heart and poorer blood supply. The combination of poor circulation and poor immunity makes it much harder for your body to heal any wounds.

- *Yeast infections:* Both men and women can get yeast infections with diabetes. It is more common in women due to anatomical differences in the reproductive system. As a result, diabetic women often get vaginal yeast infections or similar infections under the breasts. Yeast organisms thrive best in warm and sweet environments. Now it is easier to see how diabetics are at a higher risk for these infections when the blood sugars are poorly controlled.

Again, you need a healthy immune system to fight yeast infections, which is a problem for diabetics. Yeast (mycotic) infections tend to be seen most in moist, warm skin folds, such as between the fingers, around sex organs, or under the breasts. Although treatment is not difficult or complicated, recurrent yeast infections can be quite annoying and disturbing for people with diabetes. They can also be a sign that the individual's diabetes needs to be better managed.

What Is A High Blood Sugar Level?

Normal blood sugar in a healthy individual is between 70-90 mg/dl (3.9-5 mmol/L) before meals and to 90-140 mg/dl (5-7.8 mmol/L) after a mixed meal composed of carbs, protein, and fat. When you have diabetes, keeping blood sugar within a completely normal range can be difficult for some, especially at later stages of diabetes.

We prefer to keep blood sugar below 120mg/dl (6.7 mmol/L) before meals, and below 160 mg/dl (8.9 mmol/L) You don't usually see symptoms unless the blood sugar is regularly above 180 mg/dL (10 mmol/l). What's true, though, is that optimizing blood sugar in diabetes isn't just about eliminating these symptoms or keeping the blood sugar below this level.

Some signs of diabetes and its complications happen when the blood sugars are less than 180 mg/dL (10 mmol/l), but you will still see things like yeast infections and erectile dysfunction even when the blood sugars are somewhat better than that. That is why we try to keep blood sugar as close to normal as possible without causing harm to the patient.

There is one complication of type 2 diabetes you'll want to remember the symptoms of before it becomes too life-threatening or unmanageable:

This complication is called a ***diabetic coma*** or ***hyperosmolar hyperglycemic nonketotic syndrome (HHNS)***. This is a consequence of diabetes nobody wants to have. It happens when the pancreas essentially goes bankrupt. When there is almost no insulin coming out of the pancreas, the result can be a diabetic coma, especially in the setting of severe dehydration.

HHNS is a serious complication that can lead to death in both type 1 and type 2 diabetes; It is more common among type 2 diabetics. Common symptoms include:

» Blood sugar levels over 600mg/dL (33.3 mmol/l)

» Warm, dry skin that doesn't produce sweat

» Extreme thirst

» Fever over 101 degrees Fahrenheit

» Vision loss

» Hallucinations

- » Sleepiness and or confusion
- » Weakness on one side of your body
- » Dry mouth

If you see any of these symptoms in yourself or a loved one with diabetes, check the blood sugar immediately and be prepared to seek emergency medical help as soon as possible. This isn't something you can simply treat at home.

When Should You Seek Medical Attention?

Whether you know you have diabetes or just think you might, there are some symptoms of high blood sugar that you should not avoid. If you have access to a glucose meter in the home, you can check your blood sugar when you have symptoms to see if they correlate with high blood sugar levels. If you aren't sure what's going on, you need to seek help anyway.

These are the symptoms you should be aware of, and that should prompt you to make an appointment with your doctor as soon as possible. You may need to go to the emergency room if your symptoms are significant, such as:

- » Urinate a lot more than usual
- » Feel weak or tired
- » Sick to your stomach
- » Have sweet-smelling breath
- » Breathe faster or more deeply than normal

These symptoms can mean your blood sugars are much higher than they should be. These symptoms listed can also be a sign of diabetic ketoacidodic coma. If you have nausea, vomiting, abdominal pain, or heavy breathing, please do not wait; go to the emergency department. As I mentioned, once you have symptoms like this, you shouldn't try to ignore them or manage them on your own.

Why Are Your Blood Sugars High In The Mornings?

Have you ever wondered, "why is my blood sugar or my glucose always so high in the morning"? High blood sugars in the morning are a fairly common problem that many diabetics face daily, and I get this question from newly diagnosed diabetics all the time in my clinic.

In the morning, almost everyone experiences a slight increase in blood sugar levels. A person without diabetes will not necessarily realize this as a problem because their body can adjust to this phenomenon. However, for a person with diabetes, high blood sugar/glucose in the mornings can be problematic. It may even need to be something your endocrinologist wants to treat.

On the other hand, high blood sugar in the morning is not always a problem for every person with diabetes. This is because, if you are on medications like metformin or long-acting insulins, like Toujeo, Tresiba, Levemir, or Lantus, your blood sugar may end up being okay in the morning or even too low if taken in excess. This complication can happen because some of these medications work at night to help regulate your blood sugars. Like any medication for diabetes, too much of these may increase the risk of low blood sugars in the morning.

With regard to high blood sugars in the morning, these are the key issues to remember:

» In most people with diabetes, insulin resistance is the primary reason for elevated blood sugars in the morning.

» Two factors, the dawn phenomenon and the Somogyi effect, can also play a role (these will be discussed separately next).

» Depending on the circumstances, things like insufficient insulin intake, incorrect medication dosage, and sweet snacks before bed are common causes for high blood sugars the following morning.

The Dawn Phenomenon And Somogyi Effect

Morning hyperglycemia in diabetics may occur due to the dawn phenomenon. The dawn phenomenon occurs when the diabetic's insulin secretion decreases or because the medications they take for diabetes (including insulin) wears off during the night. This is combined with a physiological increase in insulin-opposing hormones.

The most common hormones that lead to this problem are growth hormone and cortisol. The increases in these hormones as part of the dawn phenomenon are normal physiological events and cannot be prevented. On the other hand, your endocrinologist can help you manage the condition.

The Somogyi effect is present in diabetics taking an excessive amount of insulin or insulin-secreting oral diabetic medications. Due to excess insulin levels, the blood sugars can go too low when the body is the most sensitive to the action of insulin. This time is between midnight and 3 AM.

The Somogyi effect happens if blood sugars go too low during these nighttime hours, which results in a rebound increase or spike in blood sugar levels. Low blood sugar events will trigger cortisol, growth hormone, and adrenaline increases. This hormonal response will trigger a rebound in the blood sugar levels.

The dawn phenomenon is more common than the Somogyi effect. To diagnose these phenomena, it is useful to measure plasma glucose levels for several nights between 3 am and 5 am. You can also use a continuous glucose monitoring system.

If the blood sugar is low at 3 am (in the range of 60 mg/dL or 3.3 mmol/l) and high (in the range of 200 mg/dL or 11.1 mmol/l) at 8 am, this can be explained by the Somogyi effect. In this case, the endocrinologist will adjust your medications to avoid this late night or early morning low blood sugar. If instead, the blood sugars are somewhat high (in the range of 150 mg/dL or 8.3 mmol/L) at 3 am, this is easily recognized as morning high blood sugar. Although the treatment differs, the best way to prevent both the dawn phenomenon and the Somogyi effect is to find optimal diabetic control using insulin therapy.

Why Are My Blood Sugars So Up And Down In The Mornings?

You will never wake up with the same blood sugar every morning. So forget about trying to keep your blood sugars the same every day. That simply doesn't happen. Everything in your body is constantly changing, and many things will affect your blood sugar levels. A normal person wakes up with blood sugar values between 80-90 mg/dL (4.4-5.0 mmol/l). When you are diabetic, you might not have a tight range of blood sugars each day; there are too many factors that play into that morning blood sugar number. If you wake up with a blood sugar less than 120 mg/dL (6.7 mmol/l), that's great.

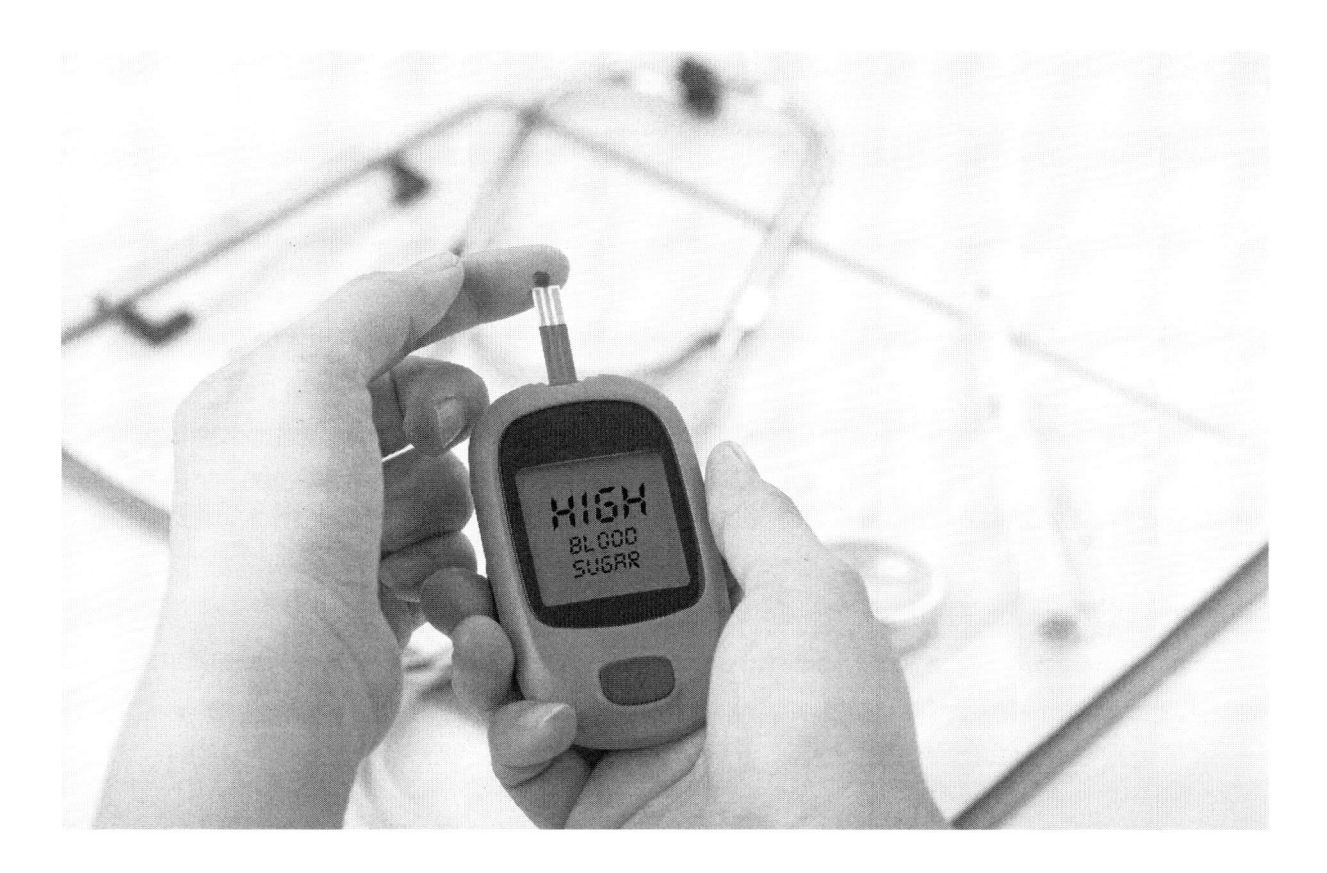

On the other hand, you don't want to go to be at 200 mg/dL (11.1 mmol/l) at nighttime and wake up at 120 mg/dL (6.66 mmol/l) if you're on insulin. This could be a dangerous sign that your blood sugars may go too low in your sleep. You want to make sure that your blood sugar is similar overnight and in the morning if you are taking a basal insulin injection each day.

What a lot of people do wrong is that they try to give too much basal insulin so they can control higher morning blood sugar values. That can be a problem because you will probably have blood sugar levels that become too low during the night. This can be very dangerous. For this reason, if you want to keep your blood sugar very stable in your sleep, you want to keep it as steady as possible. If there is a 20-30 mg/dL (1.1-1.7 mmol/l difference in your blood sugar between morning and night, this difference is very acceptable. It's not going to put you into any danger zone.

Let's do an example: If you consistently go to bed with a blood sugar of about 120 mg/dL (6.7 mmol/l) and wake up with blood sugars around 90 mg/dL (5mmol/l), that isn't a big deal. If your blood sugars are typically dropping 100 points overnight instead, this is possibly because of the insulin or sulfonylurea drug you're taking. In this case, you are putting yourself at a significant risk of becoming dangerously low during the night. The main goal of taking basal insulin is to keep the blood sugar stable overnight, but in this case, that's not happening.

You can see why I recommend checking your blood sugar at night before bed and again in the morning. Once you're stable and know nothing is really changing in your life, you don't have to keep repeating that testing pattern. You can instead just check your blood sugar at bedtime to make sure it's not too low before you go to bed.

Many people are really afraid of using insulin because they have been prescribed too much insulin or because they do their own thing, not thinking about the consequences of taking too much of it. For example, they might just increase their insulin dose, thinking that it will result in better overall blood sugar values. While that might be true, you have to be respectful of the power of insulin in your body and instead consult with your endocrinologist.

The Bottom Line:

The dawn phenomenon is simply an exaggeration of insulin resistance affected by cortisol and growth hormone. When the blood sugar is already high, these hormones will have a more noticeable effect on morning blood sugar.

I tell my patients to avoid carbohydrates at bedtime, which often helps. I also sometimes adjust their insulin or other medications to avoid morning highs and lows. Patients who are on insulin pumps are easier to manage when it comes to the dawn phenomenon. This is because insulin pumps allow for hour-by-hour insulin delivery adjustments.

Also, some insulins are better than others. When it comes to long-acting insulin, I sometimes switch my patients to Tresiba or Toujeo because these have a more long-lasting effect than Lantus or Levemir. Occasionally I will tell the patient to change the time they take their insulin. Levemir, for example, may not last for an entire 24 hours. In patients on this drug, I often advise taking it in the evening to control the high blood sugars seen in the dawn phenomenon.

How Does Insulin Resistance Cause High Blood Sugar In The Morning?

The liver produces glucose during overnight fasting when you sleep. Insulin is the main hormone that regulates glucose production in the liver. As you know, when insulin levels go down, the production of glucose in the liver increases. In the same way, when insulin levels go up, the production of glucose decreases.

If you are insulin resistant or diabetic, this is the same as not having enough insulin. The liver is also resistant to the effects of the insulin you are producing. When it can't recognize your insulin, the liver makes more glucose than it should. The result is that you have higher blood sugars in the morning.

Your blood sugars might still be high when you are taking diabetic medications. Most medications for diabetes are taken in the morning in order to force your body to make insulin. This prepares your body for the food you will eat that day. Medications like glipizide, for example, produce insulin that helps with your meals. But over the course of a day, its effects wear off. At night, your body still needs insulin it doesn't have, so your blood sugars increase.

🖅 Fast fact

> *You need to remember that insulin is not just needed for the meals you eat; your body also needs insulin during times of fasting.*

This means that, even if you're eating no carbs whatsoever, you still need insulin. In cases of relative deficiency or resistance to insulin, many diabetics will end up waking up in the morning with high blood sugars. Much of the time, this is because the medications they take for diabetes have worn off.

The good news is that there are things you can do to regulate your morning blood sugar effectively. The best options are intermittent fasting, eating with portion control, and exercising daily for at least 30 minutes. If lifestyle changes are very difficult or not effective enough to keep the blood sugars better regulated, then we start discussing diabetes medications. Metformin or pioglitazone are two commonly prescribed medications that act specifically to combat insulin resistance.

The "SugarMD Advanced Glucose Support" is a diabetic supplement as an alternative natural solution if you are not a big fan of using medications. I still do not want you to undermine the need for medications. You should never stop medications prematurely, hoping a diabetes supplement will work instead. On the other hand, while trying SugarMD Advanced Glucose Support supplement, many of my patients were able to reduce the number of medications they were taking while using this supplement. It primarily includes natural ayurvedic herbs that have been used for hundreds of years to treat diabetes safely.

Your diet is crucial in helping you reduce insulin resistance and high blood sugars. As I mentioned, among the different diets out there, only the Mediterranean diet has been found to contribute to lasting weight loss and improvement in longevity. In fact, this diet has been studied multiple times and has been proven repeatedly to reduce heart attacks, decrease stroke risk, and improve diabetic blood sugar numbers.

Ketogenic diets have not proven to be superior to other diets in terms of cardiovascular risk reduction. Yet, these diets can also help prevent type 2 diabetes. You should discuss your lifestyle changes and medications with an endocrinologist. He or she may refer you to a nutritional specialist who can make specific recommendations for your particular situation.

Do I Have To Worry About My Sugar Spiking After Eating?

Your blood sugar will usually rise after eating, but high spikes after meals can be damaging. What I typically ask my patients is not only what their fasting blood sugars have been like but also what their blood sugars are like after meals. I tell them to check their blood sugars one day after breakfast, one day after lunch, and one day after dinner (using the staggered method). The idea is to get a range of numbers without having to do too many finger sticks.

I ask them to check these numbers, so I see whether the blood sugar spikes to more than 180-200 mg/dL (10-11 mmol/l) after certain meals. That's a red flag I want to know about. I try to adjust the diet, of course, reducing the carbohydrate intake; I might ask them to exercise more, etc. If they can do these things and they help, that's great. If they can't do it or it doesn't help much, I know we have to use medications.

There are a lot of great medications that help control blood sugar spikes after meals. Again, not everyone is the same. Some people do great with diet and exercise, but these things might not be enough depending on their disease state status. Type 1 diabetics, for example, have to take insulin with meals no matter what their diet and exercise patterns are like. Others, like those with LADA, have to take insulin by the time they reach the later stages of their disease. You might think that your diabetes will be cured if you stop eating sugar. Avoiding sugar will help many people but not those who don't make insulin at all. It helps the most in individuals in the beginning stages of type 2 diabetes.

In my practice, I see a lot of complicated cases. You might hear about the diabetic with simple disease in the earliest stages. They will say that they just stopped eating carbs, and now they are fixed for good. But diabetes is not a disease like that. It's a very complex, diverse, and philosophical disease. Most people don't understand how complicated it is and all the different complex aspects of it. You know now that it isn't just a sugar problem, and it isn't something you can cure by just avoiding carbs, nor is it maintainable by the majority of people.

If you're on basal insulin, check it once a day at night and again in the morning to make sure the numbers are stable. When your fasting blood sugars are stable, you should then look at your blood sugars after meals. Keep post-meal blood sugars below 180 mg/dL (98.9 mmol/L) and if possible below 160 mg/dl (10 mmol/L) at all times. The idea of monitoring is to get useful information that will guide your treatment strategy.

What Is Low Blood Sugar/Hypoglycemia And How Can You Prevent Or Correct It?

Low blood sugar or ***hypoglycemia*** happens when blood sugars are below a certain level. Everybody feels hypoglycemia/low blood sugar at different blood sugar levels depending on their baseline blood sugar. We will talk about this later. Medically, hypoglycemia/low blood sugar is defined as a blood sugar less than 70 mg/dL (3.9 mmol/L). Clinically significant hypoglycemia/low blood sugar is defined as a blood sugar less than 55 mg/dL (3.05 mmol/L).

The most common symptoms of hypoglycemia involve feeling shaky, sweating, anxious, having a racing heart, feeling hot, or feeling nervous. These symptoms start early and are seen with mild to moderate hypoglycemia/low blood sugar. When there is severely low blood sugar, the diabetic may experience neurological symptoms such as severe dizziness, confusion, inability to talk, hearing loss, and being unable to move. If you reach this point, you may be too confused to help yourself and may need help from someone else to correct the hypoglycemic symptoms. I tell my diabetic patients at risk for this problem to teach their loved ones the signs of hypoglycemia, check blood sugars, and help manage low blood sugars.

Some people who do not have diabetes and who engage in prolonged fasting can have hypoglycemia/low blood sugar after this type of fasting. Normally the liver generates glucose for 8 to 10 hours during fasting. After that, the body starts burning fat. If you are physically or mentally very active (and not diabetic), these ketone bodies made by fat cells are not related to the high blood sugars you'll see in diabetic ketoacidosis.

On the other hand, if you have diabetes and are taking insulin or any medication that increases insulin production, these can cause hypoglycemia/low blood sugar if your meds were not taken correctly, if there is an increase in physical activity, or if meals were missed. The most common culprits in this case are the sulfonylurea drugs like glipizide, glyburide, and glimepiride.

Alcohol is another reason for the development of hypoglycemia/low blood sugar. If you drink alcohol (especially without food), you risk having a significant drop in blood sugar about 8-10 hours later. This is why alcohol will make you feel very hungry the next morning.

Alcohol stresses the liver, keeping it from making glucose in the fasting state. As a result, you will not be able to get a boost in blood sugars from the liver during fasting when you drink alcohol. Your hunger stems from having such low blood sugars the following morning.

Excessive alcohol intake (> 3 drinks over a few hours), especially from hard liquors without cocktails, will stress the liver, keeping it from making glucose in the fasting state. As a result, you will not be able to get a boost in blood sugars from the liver during fasting when you drink alcohol.

The hunger you get when drinking too much alcohol stems from having such low blood sugars the next morning. Having food and some carbs with alcohol will help prevent low blood sugar later; however, avoiding excessive alcohol is a better idea. The best alcoholic beverage for a diabetic would be to have 1 to 2 glasses of wine with dinner.

Also, if you have severe chronic kidney disease or liver disease, you may be more prone to having low blood sugar. That is because both the liver and kidney contribute to making glucose when you fast.

Others who have chronic pancreatitis disease may not be able to absorb glucose, which can also cause low blood sugars.

Factors That Contribute To Low Blood Sugar

Several factors contribute to low blood sugar/hypoglycemia. Some of these are unavoidable and can't be changed. Others are due to frequent errors many diabetics make that can be changed to avoid repeated episodes. Here are the main contributing factors:

- *Longer duration of diabetes:* The longer you have diabetes, the less able you are to make glucagon to counteract low blood sugars. This is more prominent in type I diabetics. Glucagon is the main hormone that protects against low blood sugar.

- *Older age:* Symptoms of low blood sugar may not be as prominent in older individuals. As a result, the risk of low blood sugar is much higher in older individuals who have type 1 or type 2 diabetes.

- *The blood sugar is in tight control with medications:* Of course, the goal is to have the blood sugars as close to the normal range as possible. But some individuals and their doctors use medications that are too strong or are in doses too high. This mistake will increase the risk of hypoglycemia/low blood sugars. Common drugs that do this are the sulfonylurea drugs and certain types of insulin.

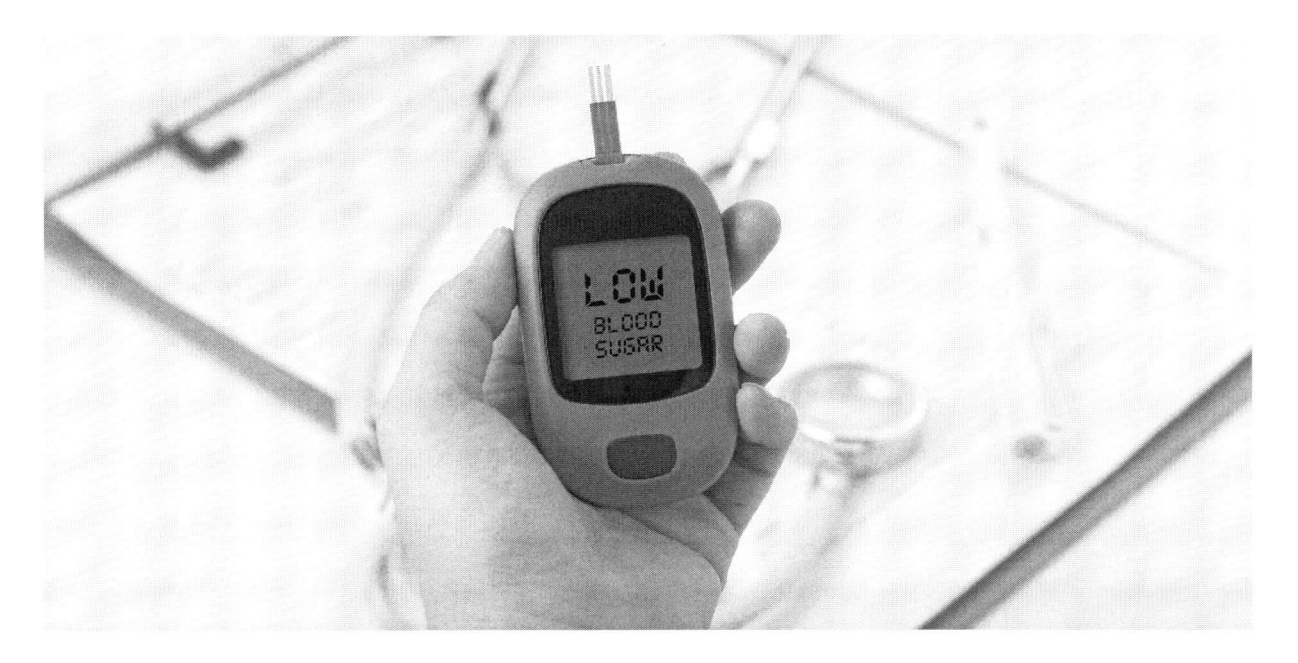

- ***Erratic timing of meals, including missed meals and low carbohydrate content of meals:*** This is very important in individuals taking insulin at mealtimes. It is also true for individuals taking sulfonylureas, repaglinide, or nateglinide. When people take insulin or any of these oral medications, the risk of low blood sugar increases dramatically if they do not eat but still take the medication.

- *History of recent severe hypoglycemia:* If the individual recently had an episode of low blood sugar in the recent past and did not change the cause of the problem, it's more than likely that another episode will occur soon.

- *Exercise:* Exercise can increase the risk of low blood sugar, especially in the setting of insulin and sulfonylureas. Even so, this isn't a good reason to stop getting out there and using your muscles. It just means that you need expert help, perhaps to figure out how to exercise safely to avoid this complication.

- ***Alcohol ingestion:*** Remember that drinking alcohol will stress the liver and prevent adequate liver production when glucagon tries to bring the glucose level up again. The liver is the ultimate glucose-storing organ in the body and is what is most activated when you need a burst of glucose. A poorly functioning liver will not respond to signals telling it to send more glucose out of storage and into the bloodstream. Excessive alcohol intake suppresses the liver, keeping it from releasing glucose.

- ***Chronic kidney disease:*** People with chronic kidney disease also are susceptible to low blood sugar. This is because kidneys also contribute to gluconeogenesis (making glucose similar to the liver). It isn't the major organ for gluconeogenesis, so it isn't as noticeable if it fails in the diabetic individual.

  In addition to being unable to generate glucose in damaged kidneys, individuals with chronic kidney disease tend to accumulate insulin and some other diabetic medications such as sulfonylureas drugs. This leads to an increased risk for hypoglycemia among type I and type 2 diabetics with chronic kidney disease.

- ***Malnutrition with glycogen depletion:*** If the individual with diabetes is not eating well, the glucose stores in the liver and kidneys will be depleted very quickly. Also, if you are on medications with a known increased risk of causing low blood sugar, being malnourished will definitely increase the risk of low blood sugars.

- ***Autonomic failure with hypoglycemia unawareness:*** This happens mostly in people who have type 1 diabetes. It happens because the individual has had frequent hypoglycemia/low blood sugar episodes. In some cases, the person stops responding to their low blood sugar episodes over time.

  This is undoubtedly a dangerous situation because the individual doesn't realize they have very low blood sugar. It happens because the autonomic nervous system has become impaired by diabetes. It's this system that allows an individual to have symptoms that would tell them their blood sugar is low (like shaking, sweating, and heart palpitations).

What Can You Do To Manage Low Blood Sugars?

These are tips you'll want to remember:

1. *Check your blood sugar:*
   Anytime you feel like your blood sugar is too low, you should check it immediately with a glucose meter if you can. Even if you are wearing a continuous glucose monitoring system, it is still a good idea to confirm the low blood sugar with a fingerstick reading.

2. *Eat carbs:*
   If you find that it is low and you are sure you can keep food down, you should eat a simple carbohydrate that can quickly raise your blood sugar. This is the opposite of what we normally recommend a diabetic take as part of their regular diet. However, in this emergency situation, you really need something that will increase blood sugar rapidly. This could be crackers, juice, candies, white bread, or regular soda.

3. *Keep your glucose meter handy:*
   Keep in mind that this type of complication can happen at any time—even when you are away from home. Keeping a glucose meter handy for when you are at work or away from home for any reason is a good idea. You should also carry some source of simple carbs with you. You can purchase glucose tablets or gel for this purpose or carry a package of some quickly-absorbing candy.

4. *Follow the 15-20 protocol:*
   I advise patients to use a 15-20 protocol. This means you eat 15 to 20 g of carbohydrates as soon as you know your blood sugars are low. Then recheck your blood sugar in 15 to 20 minutes. If blood sugars are up by 15 to 20 mg/dL (0.8-1.1 mmol/l) above your baseline, the protocol is complete, and you can resume your normal routine.

5. *Do not overcorrect:*
   Don't overdo it by eating too many carbohydrates, which is a common mistake. If you do this, you might find that your blood sugar is as high

as 300-400 mg/dL (16.7-22.2 mmol/l) after eating too many carbs. Depending on the carbohydrate you chose, this often happens about 1-2 hours later. Avoid the urge to do this, even if you feel hungry. Instead, use your blood sugar numbers to guide your management of low blood sugar.

6. ***Do not eat foods that contain fat to correct a low sugar:***
You won't be able to manage low blood sugars by eating high-fat foods like chocolate or peanut butter. The fat in these foods delays the absorption of carbs that need to absorb faster than that.

   If you can correct your hypoglycemia/low blood sugar with the 15-20 protocol, you should recover at home. If there is a family member around and you are too confused to think about what you need to do, they can be taught to administer glucagon to raise your blood sugars.

   Glucagon is available nowadays in a vial, pen, and nasal application. If they follow the protocol and your blood sugars continue to stay low, then someone needs to call 911. Of course, if there is no glucagon nearby and the person has passed out, calling 911 should be the first step.

7. ***Go to the ER if low blood sugar persists.***
If you do have low blood sugar or have had low blood sugar, and you still have low glucose after correcting, it is not a good idea to drive to the hospital yourself. Someone can take you to the hospital if needed, or an ambulance should be called.

   For those who are prone to have low blood sugar after fasting, it is not a bad idea to eat frequently. The diet should consist of protein, fat, and carbohydrates instead of just simple carbohydrates.

Low Blood Sugars Without Symptoms

I generally suggest some type of defensive actions when you monitor your sugars yourself and find that your glucose level is less than 70 mg/dL (3.9 mmol/L). Defensive options I recommend include repeating the measurement within

15 to 60 minutes, avoiding critical tasks such as driving. You can't predict, for example, that your blood sugar isn't headed in the wrong direction, so treatment with some carbohydrate-containing food is essential.

This is why I love using continuous glucose monitoring systems (CGM) such as Freestyle Libre, Dexcom, or the Guardian/Medtronic systems. The systems not only detect low blood sugar when it happens, but they can also predict a low blood sugar up to 30 to 60 minutes before it develops. This gives you time to take action.

Every person who is on insulin or a sulfonylurea drug should have glucagon available. Diabetics should always make sure that their glucagon is not expired. They should also make sure their family members and friends know how to use glucagon correctly.

How Can You Avoid Low Blood Sugars In The First Place?

There are many ways you can avoid getting low blood sugars. If you follow these tips, you'll do better and avoid the complication of low blood sugar altogether:

1. *Avoid alcohol:*
   If alcohol is the reason you have hypoglycemia/low blood sugar, you should make sure that you don't drink it alone. Instead, mix alcohol with some type of carbohydrates at the same time. My personal recommendation to my diabetic patients, however, is to avoid alcohol altogether.

2. *Avoid sulfonylurea and insulin when possible:*
   If you have diabetes, you may need to avoid using insulin or sulfonylurea such as glipizide, glimepiride, and glyburide to treat your diabetes. These medications are most likely to contribute to low blood sugars. You can ask your physician to possibly change your medications if this is a problem for you. If changing the medication is not an option, you will need to understand how insulin works and how the medications work so you can avoid a reaction from them.

3. *Adjust sulfonylurea and insulin medications when physically more active:*
   For example, if you take long-acting insulin such as Lantus, Levemir, Toujeo, or Tresiba, you should know how and when to reduce your insulin dose. If your blood sugar is normally in the 100-120 range in the morning, you should consider reducing the long-acting insulin dose by 20% to 30% on the days you have been physically more active.

4. *Try to adhere to the diet schedule:*
   If you are taking sulfonylurea agents, you should stay on a strict and regular diet schedule. Missing a meal when you take sulfonylurea agents is definitely an invitation for hypoglycemia/ow blood sugars.

5. *Watch blood sugar more often after starting a new medication:*
   If you are on insulin or sulfonylurea agents and your doctor starts you on a new diabetic medication, you should be careful as well. Even if the new medication would not cause hypoglycemia/low blood sugar, adding the new medication on top of insulin or sulfonylurea definitely can. Your endocrinologist should be able to adjust your other medications to avoid a hypoglycemic reaction.

6. *Be consistent with carbohydrate intake:*
   If you are on mealtime insulin, you should be very careful about being consistent in your carbohydrate intake if you are on a fixed-dose regimen. If you are counting carbs, being right on in terms of your carbohydrate counting will reduce the chances of hypoglycemia/low blood sugar.

Why Do The Symptoms Of Low Blood Sugar Differ Between Individuals?

A lot of the symptoms depend on the degree of insulin resistance the person has. For example, if your blood sugars range from 90-120 mg/dL (5-6.7 mmol/l) (a typical range for most normal people), then a blood sugar less than 70 mg/dL (3.9 mmol/l) may make you feel irritable or hungry. Most of the time, people do not even know that their blood sugars are less than 70 mg/dL (3.9 mmol/l), but they know that they are extremely hungry. Some people will report shaking in the hands or even a foggy mind.

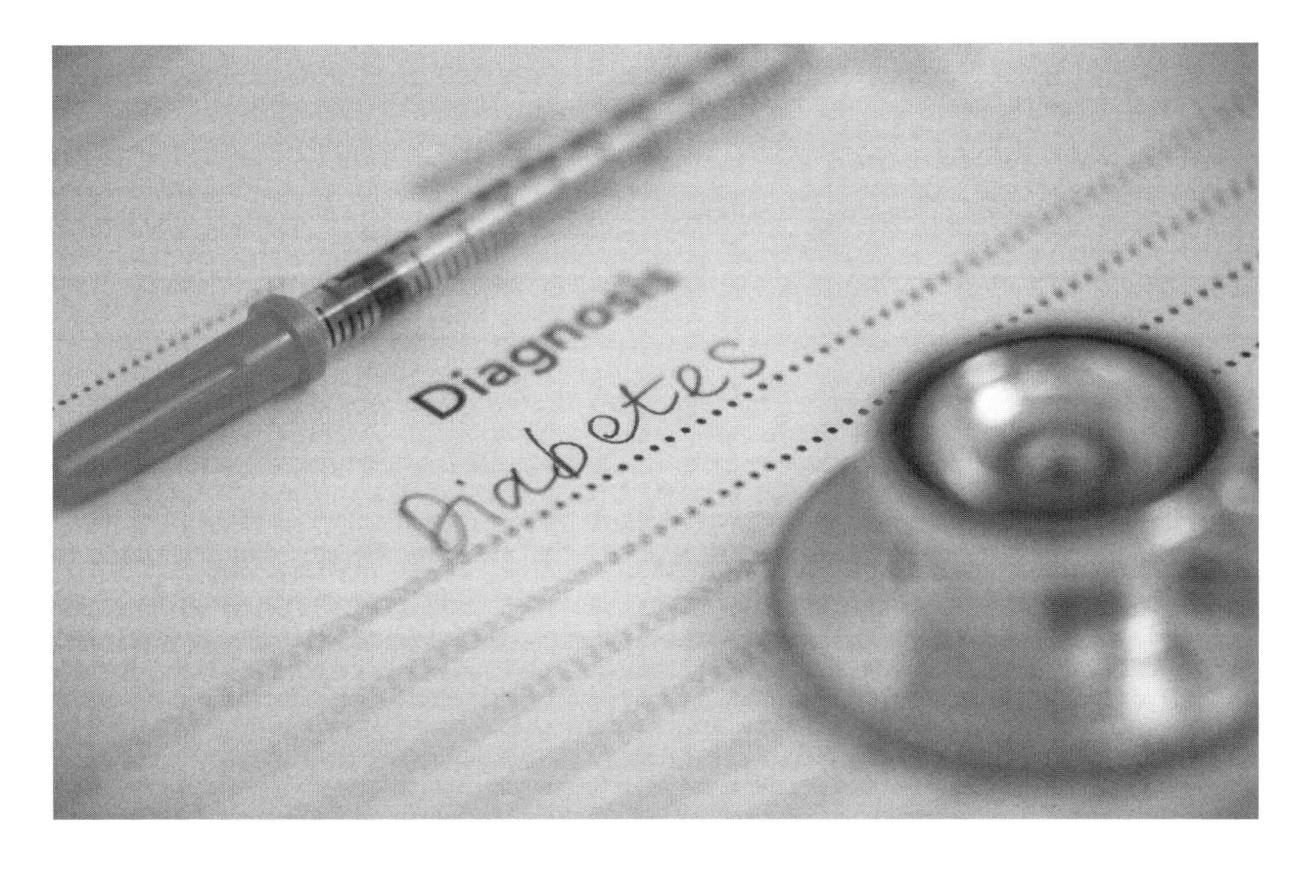

For very skinny people that are quite sensitive to insulin, the definition of low blood sugar is somewhat different. Some of these people can actually drop down to 60 mg/dL (3.3 mmol/l) blood sugar without any symptoms.

On the other hand, insulin-resistant people will experience blood sugar differences even when their blood sugar is in the normal range. For example, the person with diabetes may feel hypoglycemia/low blood sugar symptoms when the blood sugar drops from 300 mg/dl (16.6 mmol/l) down to 150 mg/dL (8.3 mmol/dL0. This is because the body differentiates the changes in the glucose environment rather than the absolute blood sugar value.
If a diabetic person's blood sugar is running between 200-300 mg/dL (11.1-

16.6 mmol/l) on average but then quickly drops to sugars in the range of 120-150 mg/dL (6.7-8.3 mmol/l), this blood sugar level would feel low for that person. The good news is that our body is very adaptable, and a "new normal" will be reestablished when the person loses weight or changes their lifestyle in ways that keep their blood sugars in the near-normal range. When this happens and is maintained, the symptoms of hypoglycemia will disappear.

The bottom line is that hypoglycemia/low blood sugar is a very complex phenomenon that can happen to anyone. It happens mostly in people with diabetes due to the effects of real-life situations who also have complex medication regimens. The most common hypoglycemia/low blood sugar events happen in individuals taking multiple daily injections of insulin.

Insulin And Sulfonylurea Drugs Increase The Risk Of Low Blood Sugar!

If you are on insulin or a sulfonylurea drug, it is very important to regularly monitor your blood sugars. This could be done via fingerstick or continuous glucose monitoring systems. Regardless of the monitoring system you are using, the blood sugars you obtain must be interpreted by someone who understands what they mean. This means establishing contact with an endocrinologist to help you.

Continuous Glucose Monitoring Systems Help A Lot

I believe remote glucose monitoring is the best way to manage patients on a day-to-day basis. Keeping blood sugar logs is helpful; however, waiting months to see the doctor to show him or her all of the hypoglycemic episodes you have can be costly. Having to be hospitalized for low blood sugars is also costly.

Hypoglycemia is a serious event that can cause hospitalization, coma, and death. Understand what causes hypoglycemia in your case. Know what you need to do to treat hypoglycemia. Make sure you have the latest technology to keep you safe.

Diabetic Drugs That Don'T Cause Low Blood Sugar

You can take some diabetic drugs that don't have hypoglycemia/low blood sugar as a side effect. If you have a problem with low blood sugar or are worried about it, talk to your endocrinologist about switching to one of these medications:

- » Metformin
- » Alpha-glucosidase inhibitors such as acarbose
- » Thiazolidinediones such as pioglitazone (Actos)
- » Glucagon-like peptide-1 (GLP-1) receptor agonists such as Rybelsus, Ozempic, Bydureon, and Trulicity
- » Dipeptidyl peptidase-4 (DPP-4) inhibitors such as Januvia and Tradjenta
- » Sodium-glucose co-transporter 2 (SGLT2) inhibitors such as Jardiance, Invokana, Farxiga, and Steglatro

What Other Measures You Can You Take To Prevent And Control Low Blood Sugar?

In addition to the general measures we discussed preventing low blood sugars, I believe the prevention of hypoglycemia involves first assessing your risk factors and tailoring a personalized treatment program for those at the greatest risk for episodes of hypoglycemia. As I mentioned, every individual is different and will have various risk factors, medications, and lifestyle issues that need to be taken into consideration.

In my practice, I look holistically at every patient to ensure that the medications I prescribe will not worsen the frequency of these types of episodes. I monitor patients either through continuous glucose monitoring systems such as Dexcom G6, Freestyle Libre, or Freestyle Libre 2.

I still use traditional finger prick glucose monitoring for patients who may not be able to obtain these devices. We offer cellular technology that allows data to be transferred to our diabetes center directly and immediately so we can monitor patients continuously and intervene as soon as possible.

Most individuals, however, are on their own to monitor their blood sugars at home but have the option to use our SugarMD app for free. It helps them to keep a nice record that they can share with their doctors or loved ones. Even if they do not have a service like ours, patients should monitor their sugars as frequently as possible, especially if they are on a sulfonylurea agent or insulin. An endocrinologist should determine the frequency of monitoring.

If one of my patients has frequent low blood sugars, I generally change their diabetes medication regimen. The patient also should attend classes that focus on lifestyle changes designed to help the individual improve their dietary and exercise regimen. I also believe our YouTube channel called SugarMD has filled a huge education gap for many people. It's very important to incorporate the individual's diet, medication schedule, and level of exercise into any decision about hypoglycemia management.

The management of hypoglycemia is highly individualized. For example, the elderly person with chronic kidney disease and other health problems should have a more relaxed glucose goal to avoid low blood sugars that can be severe enough to cause more harm than benefit.

Fear Of Hypoglycemia (Low Blood Sugar)

Hypoglycemia can be a scary, unpleasant, and potentially lethal complication of diabetes. I understand this common fear of having a low blood sugar reading. As a result, I always encourage diabetics to be aware of early symptoms and to ingest carbohydrates before symptoms progress.

In some cases, however, having a fear of hypoglycemia can become a major barrier to lowering blood glucose concentrations substantially. In those individuals, I try to change the medications they are taking, especially if they are on medications that can drastically increase the risk of low blood sugars.

A good endocrinologist will definitely pay attention to low blood sugars while treating diabetes. One study found that patients who had a frightening episode of severe hypoglycemia in the previous year often became so fearful that they kept their blood glucose excessively high for several months afterward.

I really want you to overcome this fear if you have it; it is not a good idea to have such high blood sugars just because you fear having an episode of low blood sugar.

What Causes Blood Sugar Fluctuations?

These are the main reasons why your blood sugars might fluctuate a lot. Keep them in mind when you find your numbers aren't what you expect them to be:

- ***Taking excessive or inadequate amount of diabetes medication:*** Say, for example, that you take 10 units of insulin before every meal and you eat a bagel every morning, but this morning you decided to eat something different. You instead decide to eat two eggs, cucumbers, and yogurt because you are in the mood for a healthy breakfast. What you may not have realized is that a bagel has 50 g of carbs while yogurt and cucumbers probably have less than 20 g of carbs.

  As you can imagine, if you didn't make any changes in your insulin dose and still took 10 units of insulin, your body will respond differently with fewer carbs in your breakfast. Your blood sugar will likely be too low after the second breakfast. This is a great example of taking too much of a medication based on your lifestyle change.

  The opposite would happen if you decided to eat two glazed donuts for breakfast on the second day. Your insulin then will be inadequate to cover the carb load you've eaten. You have to be very careful when it comes to taking short-acting insulins or similar short-acting medications, including NovoLog, Humalog, Fiasp, Starlix, repaglinide, and sometimes glipizide and glyburide.

If you make a mistake one day and take short-acting insulin inadvertently instead of long-acting insulin, you will more than likely have a very low blood sugar shortly after that. This seems to be a no-brainer; however, it is a common mistake. For example, consider what would happen if you were taking Lantus and Humalog and took 50 units of Humalog instead of 50 units of Lantus. You will almost certainly have severely low blood sugars within an hour or two of making that mistake.

- ***Changes in dietary patterns or food content such as eating fried food or a lot of carbohydrates:*** Most people know that eating a lot of carbs in your diet will spike their blood sugars. However, not everyone knows about the glycemic index. The Glycemic Index (GI) is an indicator of how fast your blood sugar will spike compared to other carbohydrates.

For example, if you eat 30 grams of carbohydrates in an apple versus a similar 30 grams of carbohydrates in your breakfast cereal, your blood sugar will be different after each of these meals. In fact, the blood sugar may spike 2-3 times faster with the breakfast cereal compared to the apple—even though they have the same amount of carbohydrates. This is because the glycemic index of an apple is much lower than the cereal.

Another thing you have to think about is the fat content in the food. Anytime you eat carbohydrates along with a high amount of animal fat, your blood sugars will spike much higher. Still, it will be delayed by many hours because fat slows the digestive system, and food will stay in the stomach longer (where it isn't absorbed yet).

On the other hand, if you decide to eat very healthy and eat very little carbs one day, the medications you have been taking regularly may suddenly be too much, especially if you are on sulfonylureas or short-acting insulins.

So to prevent blood sugar fluctuations caused by your diet, you should pay attention to the glycemic index and fat content in your diet in addition to paying attention to carbohydrate load. I will talk more about this in the next chapter.

- ***Change in your activity level, such as starting a new activity or exercise:*** When you exercise, your body uses more glucose, and you become almost immediately more sensitive to insulin. As a result, any medication that increases your insulin levels will be more effective in reducing your blood sugars. This is true for those who take injectable insulin or sulfonylureas.

  For example, if you normally take 40 units of Tresiba (which is a long-acting insulin) every day and you decide to go to the gym today, you are likely to have a low blood sugar reading after midnight. This complication is more likely to happen if you normally wake up with blood sugars less than 100-120 mg/dL (5.5-6.7 mmol/l). This is because you already have less of a buffer or safety zone to prevent low blood sugars. In this case, you may want to reduce the amount of Tresiba by 20% to 30% or more, depending on the amount of exercise you have had.

  Monitoring your blood sugar closely when you exercise will help you better understand your blood sugar patterns after exercise. Remember, exercise can influence your sugars in the short-term and for up to 24 hours following exercise. I don't want to say you shouldn't exercise because you need to if you can. The goal is to determine how much medication you should take on the days you are more strenuous about exercising.

- ***Stress and anxiety:*** Unfortunately, when you are under stress and have anxiety, your body produces stress hormones. The most common stress hormones are cortisol and adrenaline. These are the same hormones that cause the increase in blood sugars you'll see in the dawn phenomenon. However, when these hormones are chronically elevated, this can lead to a reduction in the action of insulin in your body. Pain is another reason your blood sugar levels might increase due to the activation of your stress hormones. Thinking positively and finding ways to reduce stress and anxiety can definitely improve your blood sugar levels.

- ***Variability in diabetes medication absorption:*** Many people with diabetes do not know or understand that the bioavailability of medications we take again and again is not necessarily the same. In other words, the same dose of the same medication may be absorbed differently every time we take the medication. Most insulin injections have a possible variability in absorption of up to 20% after an injection. This variability can change from 5% to 20%.

  At higher levels of insulin, the absolute number of insulin units you receive will change significantly. For example, if you take 10 units of insulin, the maximum variability may result in the absorption of 8-12 units of insulin. On the other hand, if you are taking 100 units of insulin, you may be getting a "real" dose of 80-120 units. Obviously, this can create significant changes in your blood sugar levels. The injection site, type of needle, and injection technique can also make a difference in the variability of insulin absorption.

  Besides insulin, other medications can have variability in the absorption through the GI tract. This can potentially cause severe blood sugar fluctuations. Taking metformin with food can improve the absorption significantly, compared to taking metformin on an empty stomach.

- ***Variability in carbohydrate consumption and incorrect nutritional labels:*** Unfortunately, regulatory agencies do not always disclose certain facts. One of these is that nutrition facts can be less than 100% accurate. This is completely legal. This uncertainty can also be as much as 20%. If you are counting carbs, this significant inaccuracy in food labels will make it extremely difficult for you to stay on track and prevent blood sugar fluctuations. It means that 100 grams of carbs reported on a nutrition label can actually be 80-120 g of carbohydrates. Of course, given the variability in the insulin absorption and the variability in the nutrition facts, you can see how you might have a significant risk of developing blood sugars that are too high or low—even if you've otherwise done everything correctly. This lack of accuracy is even more of a problem for type 1 diabetics.

- ***Brittle diabetes:*** Patients with type 1 diabetes are particularly high risk of having extreme blood sugar fluctuations. That is because they are typically only on insulin and are subject to variability in the absorption I just discussed. They also miss another significant hormone (glucagon). Remember that glucagon opposes the action of insulin and raises the blood sugar level. In type 2 diabetics, glucagon is still present, so there is some regulation happening, even when the insulin levels are low.

  Without glucagon, individuals with type 1 diabetes are more prone to developing low blood sugars they can't regulate themselves. Also, if they are not counting carbohydrates correctly, extreme blood sugar fluctuations are inevitable. For these people, called "brittle type 1 diabetics", I strongly recommend using a continuous glucose monitoring system such as Dexcom G6 or Freestyle Libre 2. These devices help prevent huge fluctuations in blood sugars by alerting the patient regarding extremes and by predicting future highs or lows in blood sugar readings.

The Bottom Line On Blood Sugar Fluctuations

If your blood sugars are all over the place, then maybe you need to pay closer attention to your diet so you can improve its consistency each day. Carbohydrate counting will also help. If you're taking 10 units of insulin for breakfast each morning, for example, and your blood sugar ranges from 90-190 mg/dL (5-10.5 mmol/l) after this meal on two consecutive days, it often means you aren't consistent with your diet. While it would be nice to eat whatever you want, your diabetes will be better managed if you stay consistent in the number of carbs you eat each meal.

Lowering the total carbohydrate amount you eat in your meals will also prevent errors or miscalculations in your insulin estimations. Also, when you need to take higher doses of insulin, the effect of the injected insulin may vary up to 20% each time, leading to variable results in your blood sugar control. If you need fewer units of insulin, the variability in your blood sugars will be naturally less noticeable. Of course, having a better handle on your stress and anxiety will help prevent these fluctuations in your blood sugars.

What Is HbA1C?

As I mentioned, the hemoglobin A1c, A1c, or HbA1c test measures the amount of sugar on red blood cells. It is a good measure of a person's average blood sugar over the past three months. It is measured in percentages or the percent of your red blood cells with sugar attached to them. A1c is purely a reflection of average blood sugars.

For example, 7% A1c corresponds to an average blood sugar of 150mg/dL (8.3 mmol/l). 6% A1c corresponds to average blood sugars of 120 mg/dL (6.7 mmol/l). An A1c of 8% corresponds to 180 g/dL (10 mmol/l) in average blood sugars. As you may have noticed, every 1% change in A1c reflects a 30 mg/dL (2.1 mmol/l) change in average blood sugars.

The A1c is a widely used clinical test because it is a good measure of blood sugar over time rather than at a specific moment in time. There is no need for special preparation such as fasting, which is an added plus. The A1c is used to diagnose diabetes and monitor treatment for type 1 diabetes and type 2 diabetes. It is a handy clinical test with many advantages. Even so, you should know there are some disadvantages that make it impractical to use as the only test in the management of diabetes.

The reason the test is called "hemoglobin A1c" is easy to remember. Hemoglobin is the protein that carries oxygen in the bloodstream. It is formed in new red blood cells that freely allow glucose to enter them. As a result, glucose irreversibly attaches to the hemoglobin. The more glucose you have, the more glucose binds to the hemoglobin. Since the average lifespan of hemoglobin is 120 days, A1c reflects average glucose levels within the last three months.

Keep in mind that A1c only reflects the average blood sugars. When you talk about the average, you automatically disregard very high and very low blood sugars. For example, if your blood sugars were between 50 mg/dL (2.8 mmol/l) and 250 mg/dL (13.9 mmol/l), your average would be 150 g/dL (8.3 mmol/l). That would give you an A1c of 7%. Although it seems to be a success, it does not tell you about very high and very low blood sugar as it only reports the average blood sugars. This why home monitoring is still important.

Even with its disadvantages, the A1c test is a handy clinical tool. You can still say that 7% A1c is much better than 9% because 9% suggests at least 60 mg/dL higher average blood sugars in any given individual.

Please take a look at the table below to better understand the average blood sugars corresponding to each A1c level:

Hemoglobin A1c:	Corresponding average blood sugars (mg/dL):
5%	90
6%	120
7%	150
8%	180
9%	210
10%	240
11%	270
12%	300
13%	330
14%	360

What Is A Good A1c Goal?

Typically, if your A1c is above 5.7% but less than 6.5%, it means you have prediabetes. If the A1c is more than 6.5%, then you have diabetes. The goal of diabetic control depends on your situation. For some people, a good goal is anything less than 6.5%. For others, a good goal is a number that is less than 8%. Your endocrinologist will determine your A1c target.

Why have a goal for A1c so high for some people but not for others? Part of this is that your goal is determined based on multiple clinical factors that make a higher A1c reasonable for some individuals. Multiple clinical factors such as life expectancy, duration of diabetes, risk of hypoglycemia (low blood sugar), and the presence of advanced diabetes complications including heart attacks, strokes, chronic kidney disease, neuropathy (diabetic nerve damage), and retinopathy (diabetic eye disease) determine one's A1c goals.

The older and the sicker an individual is, the higher I tend to set the A1c goal. On the other hand, the younger and healthier individual will have a much lower A1c goal. Because small vessel diseases such as kidney or eye disease take decades to appear, and because most large vessel diseases, such as heart disease, happen early in the course, I want young people to have the lowest A1c goals as possible.

Therefore, it does not make sense to try to implement tough sugar control measures on an 80-year-old frail patient who already has heart disease and has recently been diagnosed with diabetes. We generally do not expect this person to live long enough to develop small vessel disease. Moreover, the older individual in this example can suffer more harm than benefit from excessive treatment, which often leads to severely low blood sugars. This complication may cause severe damage to her body that runs the risk of being lethal.

On the other hand, it is also absurd to have a target A1c target of more than 7% in a 50-year-old type 2 diabetic male who is healthy overall. In some of my type 1 diabetic patients, low blood sugar is so difficult to manage that I allow the blood sugar to run a little higher for the individual's safety.

Another example is the individual with type 1 diabetes who has frequent episodes of low blood sugar. I generally set a target A1c goal of 7.5% instead of 6 to 6.5%. The bottom line here is that we try to bring the target A1c as low as is both reasonable and as safe as possible. For this reason, you need to make sure that you discuss your A1c target with your endocrinologist. You need to clearly understand what goals make sense for you.

Using The A1c Level To Help Manage Your Diabetes

Some people wonder if it makes any sense to check the A1c level more often than every three months. In my practice, I sometimes do this. If used correctly, performing this test more frequently than every three months can still be helpful. This is because 50% of the change in A1c happens within the first 30 days, even though the lifespan of the red blood cells is triple that number.

For example, if your A1c has improved 1% within one month, that can imply that it will improve another 1 to 1.5% in the next three months. On the other hand, Medicare only allows A1c testing every three months, so it may not be possible to do this cheaply for some of my patients. Although monthly A1c testing can help make intensive changes in a person's diabetic treatment plan, limitations like insurance coverage may be a problem in doing more frequent A1c testing.

You may have noticed that an A1c checked in your primary care doctor's office may be a little different than the reading you get at another lab or another clinic. The difference happens due to variability in the testing method each laboratory uses. Every test has a slight margin of error. For example, when repeated, the A1C test result may be higher or lower than the first test. Let us assume that the first test was an A1c of 6.9%. Repeat tests could be reported in a range from 6.5% to 7.3% in the same blood sample.

Another caveat to keep in mind about the precision of these test results is that every test reported has a confidence interval. The confidence interval is a statistical term used to say how confident you are that the value is accurate. To make it easier to understand, let's let look at an example. When the lab reports your A1c as 7%, the assumption is that the average blood sugar is 150 mg/dL (8.3 mmol/l). If you know the confidence interval of any test value, you can determine the range of numbers the lab can say they are 95 percent sure the real value is.

What you'd get with an A1c of 7% might actually be "7% +/- 0.2%". It means the real value would be between 6.8% and 7.2%. No test is perfect, so there will always be this range where you can be 95 percent confident of the "real" answer. The lab won't report this confidence interval, but you should know that there is one for every lab. It means you shouldn't be concerned if you get two separate values from two different labs that are slightly different from one another.

Advantages And Disadvantages Of The A1c Test

There are advantages and disadvantages to using the A1c in monitoring your diabetes. You should know that the concept of A1c wasn't even understood until 1969, and most doctors didn't start using the test in clinical practice until the mid-1980s. It took a long time before the medical community to trust that the test would help manage their diabetic patients and for the test to be recommended by major medical organizations. We now know it can be an extremely helpful test.

The main advantages of the A1c are these:

- *It is a nationally and internationally standardized test.* It allows clinicians across the globe to communicate and understand blood sugar control in patients with diabetes.

- *Multiple large clinical studies have used this test to determine the outcomes of blood sugar control.* For example, one large study found that every 1% improvement in the A1c prevented complications of diabetes by 30%. So, if your A1c comes down from 10% to 7%, your diabetes complication risk goes down by 90%.

- ***Most diabetes care centers do the test in the outpatient setting with a single finger prick.*** Results are typically provided within 5 minutes. This rapid result allows clinicians to understand longstanding average glucose numbers in any diabetic patient immediately.

<u>There are some disadvantages of trusting the A1c completely in managing diabetes.</u> Like any other testing in medicine, there can be technical errors in interpreting the A1c levels. These errors can lead to misleading results or assumptions.

Also, the lifespan of hemoglobin can influence the test results. The test result will be falsely high when the red blood cell turnover is lower. A1c levels will be falsely low when the red blood cell turnover is higher.

So if your blood cells' average life in the bloodstream on average is longer, it gives you a falsely high A1c result. On the other hand, if the average lifespan of your red blood cells is shorter (such as with hemolytic anemia, where blood cells are destroyed before their natural lifespan ends), this will lead to falsely low A1c levels. These things will affect the A1c level.

Let's review what I mean by all the possible hemoglobin lifespan problems with the test:

- » Falsely high A1c test results tend to occur more in patients with untreated iron deficiency anemia, vitamin B12 deficiency, and folate deficiency anemia.

- » Patients who have severe kidney disease taking erythropoietin will have a falsely low A1c result. Erythropoietin stimulates the production of younger red blood cells.

- » Depending upon the testing methodology, the values may be falsely high in patients with abnormal hemoglobin types, such as is seen in sickle cell anemia or thalassemia.

- » Racial differences can also affect the ability of the test to be complexly accurate. A1c levels are typically higher in African-

American, Hispanic, and Asian populations, even with the same corresponding blood sugar levels as Caucasians.

What Are Some Alternatives To A1c Measurements?

We can do some other tests to get an idea of what the average blood sugars look like. Some provide the same glucose averages as you'll get with an A1c measurement. Others will allow you to better understand when your blood sugars trend high and low during the day and with different activities like exercise and dietary changes. These are the tests I sometimes use:

- *Fructosamine:* Just like hemoglobin, many other proteins also can attach to glucose. Your serum albumin is one of these. This glucose interaction and attachment can lead to a similar interpretation you will see with the A1c level. It means these can also be used to estimate your glucose control.

  Generally, there is a good correlation between A1c values and fructosamine levels. However, there are some problems with the use of fructosamine as well. For example, because the turnover of serum albumin is more rapid than hemoglobin, fructosamine values reflect your average glucose values over a much shorter time. Fructosamine survives about 1-2 weeks, so its measurement will say how the blood sugars have averaged during this time.

- *Glycomark (1,5-anhydroglucitol):* 1,5-anhydroglucitol is a polyol (a type of alcohol) present in your diet. The kidneys completely reabsorb this in normal individuals after it is first filtered into the urine. As a result, its concentration in the blood is usually stable in normal individuals. When glucose levels go up, the kidney can't reabsorb this molecule as well. As a result, 1,5-anhydroglucitol levels will go down as glucose levels go up (because more of it is in the urine instead).

  The test that measures the 1,5-anhydroglucitol level in the blood is called Glycomark. Glycomark reflects blood sugar spikes after meals better than A1c.

Sometimes endocrinologists will use this test as a complementary test to A1c to help improve blood sugar spikes that happen after meals. That is because blood sugar spikes after meals are more challenging to control than fasting blood sugars.

- ***Continuous glucose monitoring systems:*** Continuous glucose monitoring (CGM) systems such as Dexcom, Freestyle Libre, or Medtronic Guardian systems can also give you continuous blood glucose readings that correspond well to the A1c level. Since these systems will also give you an average blood sugar reading, if your average blood sugars on CGM are 150 mg/dL (8.3 mmol/l), you can safely assume that your A1c is about 7%.

Why Is My A1c Not Coming Down Below 7%?

Some people are concerned that their A1c isn't coming down below 7%--even when they have made many changes in their lifestyle and medications. This problem can be easily explained. Unfortunately, it is a lot easier to bring the A1c from 10% down to 8% than it is to get lower than 8% to levels around 7% instead. Normally, the goal for a person with mild to moderate diabetes is to have an A1c level of around 6.5%. This isn't very easy to do, however.

The main barrier to achieving this goal of 6.5% or less is the presence of blood sugar spikes after meals. You will not notice this unless you check your blood sugars 2 hours after meals. If you want to get your A1c below 7%, you need to make sure that your fasting blood sugars are less than 130 mg/dL (7.2 mmol/l) and that your blood sugar two hours after a meal is less than 180 mg/dL (10 mmol/l) at all times.

This goal can be achieved with certain non-insulin or insulin-containing medications when your dietary changes are not enough. Your endocrinologist should discuss your options with you. Once your fasting blood sugars are less than 130 mg/dL (7.2 mmol/l), you need to shift your focus on the blood sugars you obtain after meals.

A1c Testing During Pregnancy

Lastly, the A1c test can be useful in early pregnancy to diagnose preexisting diabetes in pregnant women. Some women don't know they have diabetes, but the A1c test will show this early in the pregnancy. If the woman has already developed diabetes before pregnancy, A1c testing is typically not very helpful to follow during the pregnancy because the amount of hemoglobin and blood volume changes during the pregnancy. Typically, your endocrinologist will use a glucose tolerance test and follow you with glucose testing using fingerstick checking of the blood sugar or using continuous glucose monitoring systems.

Final Thoughts On The A1c Level

Endocrinologists and primary care doctors commonly use the A1c test to diagnose, treat, and monitor diabetes. It reflects your average blood sugars within the last three months. This is because the test relies on hemoglobin turnover that is typically three months. If there are problems with your red blood cells or hemoglobin due to various reasons, the test may not be reliable. There are also many caveats related to A1c testing that endocrinologists and diabetic patients should keep in mind when interpreting these test results.

In general, the lower the A1c, the fewer are the diabetic complications. Your personal A1c goal depends on your individual characteristics, such as the duration of the disease, the number of diabetic complications, and your risk of hypoglycemia (low blood sugar).

Regardless of how you decide to monitor yourself and your blood sugars, it has been proven multiple times that people who monitor their sugars frequently and who communicate with their endocrinologists regularly do much better in getting their A1c to their goal. No matter what glucose monitoring plan you use, intervening and correcting high blood sugars immediately will prevent unwanted increases in the A1c and reduce your risk of diabetic complications in the long term.

Individualized Blood Sugar Goals

Remember that normal blood sugar levels for patients without diabetes and normal blood sugars for individuals with diabetes are different. The same thing applies to normal or target/goal A1c levels. Even within the diabetic population, A1c goals will have to be individualized.

The blood sugars you want to aim for are entirely individualized. At this point, you will need to discuss your individualized goals with your endocrinologist. I cannot tell you one number that can fit every reader. For example, I may tell an 85-year-old frail type 1 diabetic that having a 150 mg/dL (8.3 mmol/l) blood sugar in the morning and 200 mg/dL (11.1 mmol/l) after eating are perfectly okay.

On the other hand, a blood sugar goal for a 22-year-old pregnant woman would be less than 90 mg/dL in the morning and less than 120 mg/dL (6.7 mmol/l) 2 hours after meals. Do you see the contrast here? Because of these differences, you should not make your own decisions about what your goal blood sugars should be. Instead, trust your endocrinologist.

What Is A Normal Goal For The HbA1c?

Like many major guidelines put out by different national agencies, there is not 100% agreement among them. The general agreement, however, for a normal HbA1c in diabetic adults who are not pregnant is 7%. A lower goal, such as less than 6.5% or even 6%, may be appropriate for some people.

Lower A1c goals are expected for those who have a shorter duration of time with diabetes, younger people, and among those without heart disease, and/or who have type 2 diabetes treated with lifestyle or metformin only. A higher HbA1C goal, even above 8%, may be better for people with a history of frequent or severe hypoglycemia or a limited life expectancy.

Other reasons for higher A1c goals include having advanced diabetes complications, multiple other illnesses, or among those who can't achieve a lower HbA1C safely. People with diabetes need to discuss their target blood sugar goals with their endocrinologist. This is a very important conversation to have.

Final Thoughts

This chapter was all about your "toolbox"—those things you need to do to manage your diabetes using lifestyle measures and the right medications. You can do many things without medications, including watching your carb intake, exercising regularly, and managing stress. Many people do well with lifestyle changes alone; they may eventually need medications at some point, but can put that off for an extended period of time.

There is no reason you can't do everything nondiabetics do as long as you know your body and its limitations, track your sugars, and make adjustments when necessary to account for high or low blood sugars. It isn't easy in the beginning; you should always look for trends and patterns in your blood sugars as you navigate any changes in your life.

Certainly, many factors can influence your blood sugar, such as the dawn phenomenon, the Somogyi effect, heavy exercise, your fat and carbohydrate intake, illness, and others. This is why I recommend you look carefully at my recommendations on how often you should check your blood sugars, depending on your own situation.

The goal is to make sure you have an individualized diabetes management plan that works for you. Your personalized diabetes care plan depends on what type of diabetes you have, your age and other risk factors, the medications you take, and your ability to do things like exercise daily. What works for someone else with diabetes will often not be one I would recommend for you. This is exactly why self-managing your diabetes without the help of your doctor is not recommended.

CHAPTER 4
DIABETES MANAGEMENT

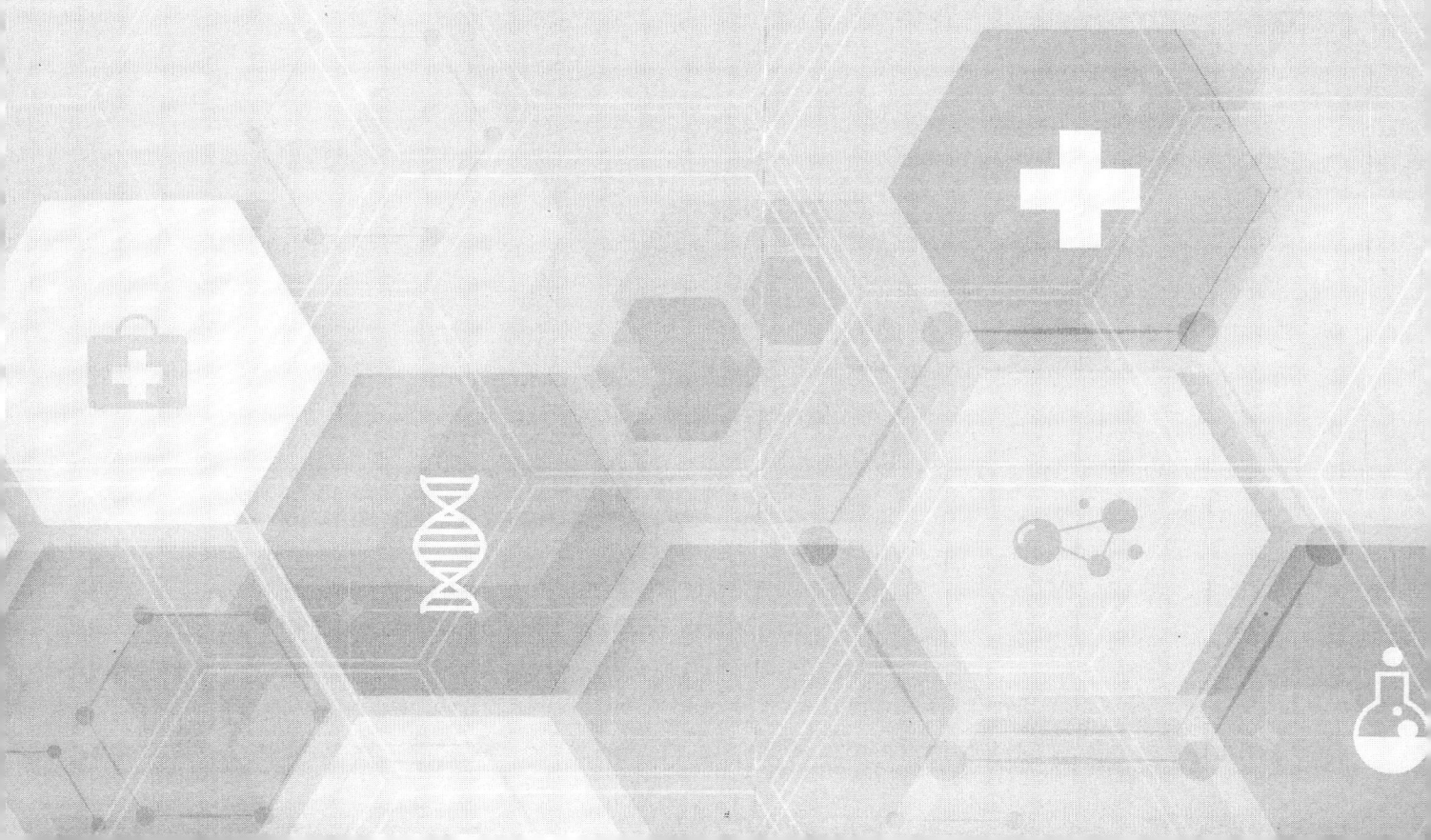

CHAPTER 4
DIABETES MANAGEMENT

Now that you are armed with the knowledge of important facts—like when to check your sugars, things that affect these sugars, and what to do if a value you get is too high or too low, there is much more you can do with this information. It's one thing to monitor your blood sugars but an altogether different thing to feel empowered in managing these numbers.

Ultimately, if it was all about "managing numbers," doing what it takes to help yourself and control your diabetes would be boring and unsatisfying. You need to think beyond the numbers and realize what you are really doing in changing your lifestyle so dramatically: you are deciding you want to live a long and healthy life. When you think of it that way, it all becomes much more important and far more interesting.

In this chapter, we will look mostly at lifestyle measures and diabetes management techniques you can add to your daily life. You can do these things to turn around a great deal of your diabetes. These things are far more important for type 1 and type 2 diabetics and for those who have insulin resistance or prediabetes. You already have an idea that it's important to do these things, but it will soon be clear to you how you can go about it.

You will see that diabetes management involves a multi-faceted approach that includes diet, exercise, medications, and managing the varying circumstances in your life. Even managing stress will affect your diabetes. I will also talk about the different diabetes complications you could develop if the diabetes isn't well controlled.

Remember this as you read this chapter: *Every tiny change you make will help you.* Make one small change every few days, especially if it all seems too overwhelming to do at once. Then adjust to the change and add something else. Before you know it, you will see the kinds of effects on your diabetes you need to see. You'll see in the numbers, yes, but you'll also see you have more energy, better sleep, and an improved ability to enjoy your life to the fullest.

6 Pillars Of Diabetes Control: What You Need To Know To Be Fully Prepared To Manage Your Diabetes Easily

Now I'll talk about what you most likely want to know, which are solutions and strategies to overcome diabetes. I'll start by summarizing everything you need to know about the different lifestyle changes you can make; these things are necessary to turn your diabetes around. I think both type 1 and type 2 require a holistic approach, so I'll talk about these things first.

We will go over topics like healthy eating, being active, glucose monitoring, taking medications, problem-solving, healthy coping, and reducing risks. Let's get started…

1. Eat Healthy

Let's talk about healthy eating tips to help control your diabetes. Having diabetes doesn't mean you have to give up all of your favorite foods suddenly. But you need to know how the foods you eat affect your blood sugar.

But what is healthy eating in reality? You need to know that it is entirely possible to create a healthy eating plan for yourself that still satisfies and keeps your taste buds alive. You just have to keep an eye on foods with added sugars, saturated and trans fats, sodium, and alcohol in your everyday diet. In this chapter, I will talk in great detail about the different dietary strategies that we know work effectively.

There are three main types of nutrients in food: carbohydrates, proteins, and fats. You need to include some of each of these three nutrients in each meal. When you do this, your body gets all the nutrients it needs, and you improve your blood sugar numbers at the same time. There is no one single diet that fits everyone. I will also talk about which one I think is most effective for diabetes, but you need to work with your dietitian to develop a diet that will fit your specific needs.

I am going to talk about different types of diets more in detail later on. I will only talk about scientifically proven diets that are known to help manage diabetes. There are some dietary principles, however, that apply to all of us.

<u>Here are some basic diet plans for any diabetic:</u>

1. ***Set realistic, achievable healthy eating goals.*** Eliminating carbohydrates totally from your diet, for example, may not be achievable or maintainable in the long-term. Rather you should focus on eliminating carbohydrates that are processed, avoiding simple sugars (like table sugar and high fructose corn syrup), and sticking with natural sources. Pay attention to the glycemic index and understand the differences between simple and complex carbohydrates.

2. ***Consider a variety of healthy eating options.*** There are so many recipes and so many different food types that you may not be aware of. Always look for alternatives to carbohydrates that raise your blood sugar if you do not or cannot eliminate that food from your diet. For example, you can adapt to a slice of whole-grain bread instead of white bread (as white bread has a higher glycemic index compared to whole-grain bread).

3. *Develop a meal plan that fits your lifestyle.* If you try to adapt to a completely different diet that you have never tried before, the chances of failing are very high. Rather, try to stick with food groups that you like and try to find healthier options. For example, use olive oil instead of butter or hydrogenated oils.

4. *Learn about appropriate portion sizes.* Try to reduce the size of your plate. Avoid overfilling your plate. Never go over one-third of your plate for your carbohydrates. Use this picture as a simple guide for all the different foods you eat:

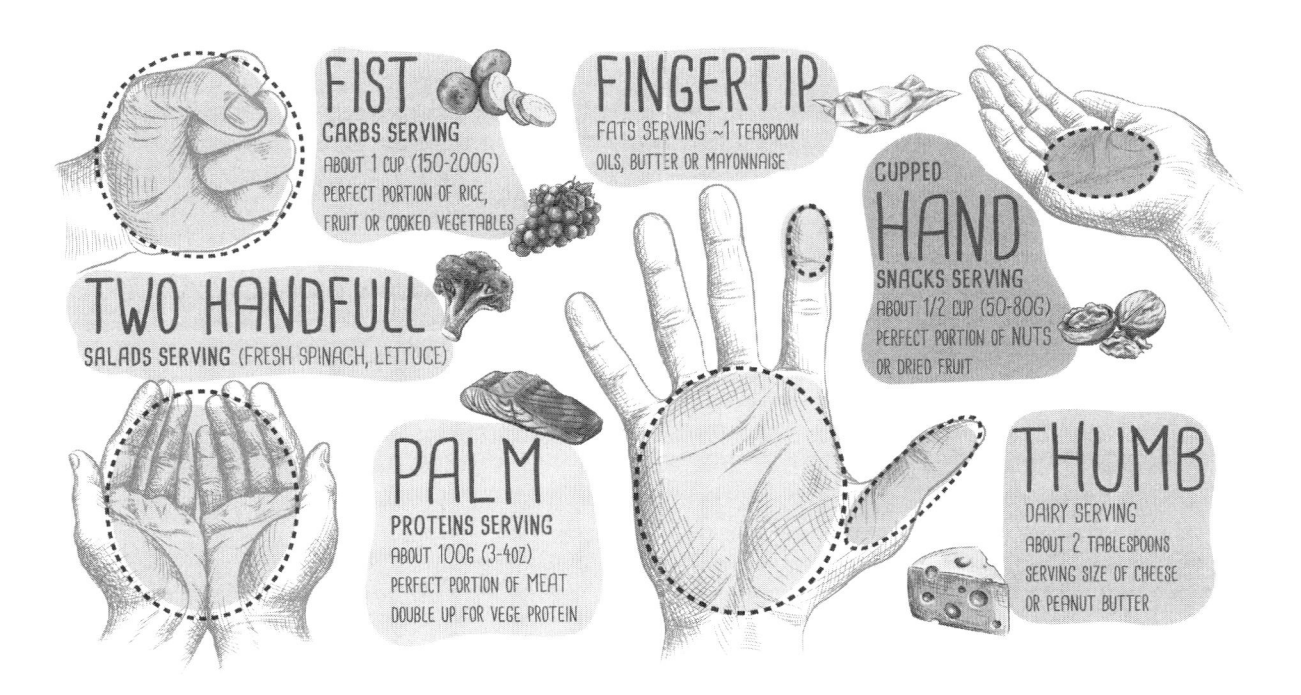

FIST — CARBS SERVING. ABOUT 1 CUP (150-200G) PERFECT PORTION OF RICE, FRUIT OR COOKED VEGETABLES.

FINGERTIP — FATS SERVING ~1 TEASPOON OILS, BUTTER OR MAYONNAISE

CUPPED HAND — SNACKS SERVING. ABOUT 1/2 CUP (50-80G) PERFECT PORTION OF NUTS OR DRIED FRUIT

TWO HANDFULL — SALADS SERVING (FRESH SPINACH, LETTUCE)

PALM — PROTEINS SERVING. ABOUT 100G (3-4OZ) PERFECT PORTION OF MEAT. DOUBLE UP FOR VEGE PROTEIN

THUMB — DAIRY SERVING. ABOUT 2 TABLESPOONS SERVING SIZE OF CHEESE OR PEANUT BUTTER

5. *Try to eliminate carbohydrate snacking.* The problem with carbohydrate snacking is twofold. First, most carbohydrate snacks are not very nutritious. Things like chips, cookies, and crackers have almost no nutritional value and a lot of calories. Second, a lot of carbohydrate snacks are somewhat addicting. When, for example, did you take only 18 potato chips (one serving) out of the bag and put the bag away?

These foods are "munchies" that are emotionally satisfying but very bad for your waistline.

6. ***Understand the Nutrition Facts Label to make healthy choices.*** Most people are still confused about the difference between total carbohydrates and the sugar contents listed on the food label. Remember to look at the total carbohydrates on the label. Try to eat foods high in fiber, which will help reduce the effects of carbohydrates on your blood sugar. Also, remember that nutrition facts are not solid facts. <u>Typically there is a 10 to 20% chance of an error in nutritional labels, which can significantly affect your blood sugars, especially for individuals with type 1 diabetes.</u>

7. ***Be aware of sodium and saturated/trans-fat content of foods/beverages.*** As diabetes is a cardiovascular risk factor, you will need to avoid any food groups that can increase your risk of heart disease or worsen your insulin resistance. Healthy fats are okay to eat; however, saturated and trans-fats are definitely very toxic for your heart.

8. ***Adjust meal plans for physical activity, holidays, and travel.*** Remember that physical activity will reduce your blood sugar. It will also reduce the need for medications. So you may need to adjust your medications if you exercise a great deal. If you tend to have low blood sugars after physical activity, you will need to eat a healthy carbohydrate snack before or during physical activity, so you can avoid low blood sugars.

   You need to know that taking a short walk after a meal can significantly help your blood sugars more than you think. Being sedentary after a carbohydrate-heavy meal is an open invitation for very high blood sugars.

9. ***When you go on vacation or travel, you need to be mindful of your diabetes.*** This includes remembering to pack your medicines, keeping them at an appropriate temperature, and remembering to take them. Remember, you are going out on vacation and not a "drug holiday." Staying healthy and keeping your blood sugars regulated while traveling will keep your energy level high as well.

Should I Lose Weight, And If So, How Much?

I recommend losing just 5 to 10% of your body weight, at least in the beginning. Although it seems like a small amount, it can make a big difference in your blood sugar levels, cholesterol levels, and blood pressure. To achieve weight loss, I recommend decreasing your caloric intake by 10 to 12 calories per pound per day. Although your caloric needs may change, most everybody will be able to lose weight with this guidance.

Fast Fact

While 5-10% of your body weight is great for improving your diabetes, if you feel like you could continue, you might want to reach for a weight closer to what's considered normal. If you can achieve this weight (having a BMI of less than 25-27), your chances of needing diabetic medications and having diabetic complications go way down.

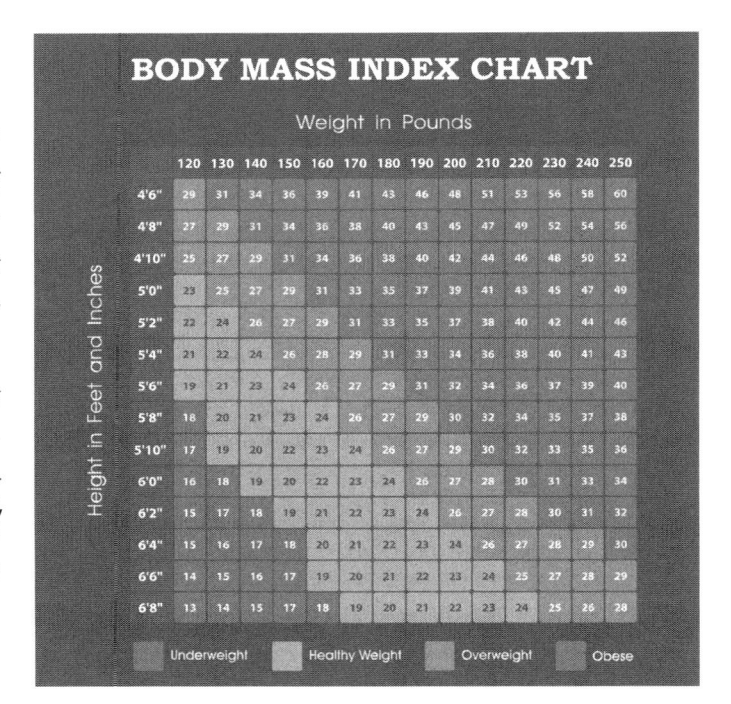

What Is The Best Diabetic Diet?

I want to talk more about type 2 diabetes and your diet. My patients constantly ask, "What should I eat for my diabetes?" or "How much carbohydrates/carbs should I eat in my diet for type 2 diabetes?". They want to know if they can still eat their favorite foods and wonder which foods will spike their blood sugar the least.

There are special diets I want to talk about for diabetes. There are many more I won't talk about because they have not been proven to help improve diabetic outcomes. Still, diets like the DASH diet are also helpful for the person who needs to watch the salt intake in their diet if they have high blood pressure, too.

Specific Diabetic Diets

I certainly have my favorite diets I recommend to most of my patients. Even so, there are other diets out there that some people use to manage their diabetes. Some of these are specific to certain disorders, such as the ADA diet put out by the American Diabetes Association.

There is nothing wrong with using the DASH diet If you have high blood pressure, but you might want to be creative and combine the best of the DASH diet, for example, with the best of the Mediterranean diet. Talk to a registered dietician if you have special needs to consider concerning your diet.

Keto Diet

The ketogenic or "keto" diet is a diet that is high in fat and low in carbs, which can be beneficial for diabetics. The biggest downside of the keto diet, however, is that it is difficult to maintain. Any diet that is difficult to maintain will not be a permanent solution to put your diabetes into remission or at least keep it under control. When my patients ask about a ketogenic diet, I tell them that they can use this diet to lose weight fairly quickly, and then they can gradually start introducing healthy carbs in smaller portions into their diet.

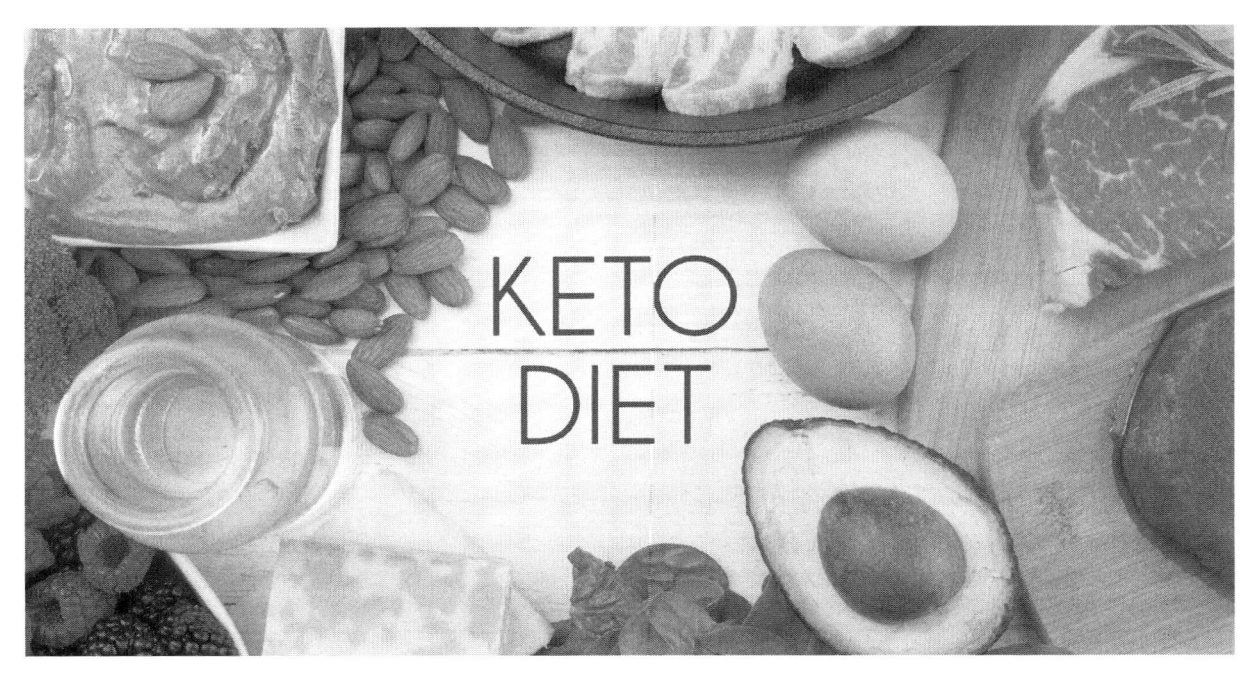

Low carbohydrate or ketogenic diets are thought to lower insulin levels, which you know is *a critical hormone that produces an anabolic state, inducing weight gain.* Keto diets may questionably and indirectly improve cardiometabolic function and induce weight loss.

Ketogenic diets restrict carbohydrates to cause your body to make ketones. It generally limits your carb intake to 20-50 grams daily. Restricting carbs also induces the depletion of glycogen (the storage form of glucose in the liver) and enhances ketone production due to the mobilization of fat stored in fat tissue.

Following a ketogenic diet may improve blood sugar levels while also reducing the need for insulin. However, as with most diets, the keto diet carries its own risks. This is particularly true for diabetics on insulin who have to be extremely careful. These folks really need to consult with an endocrinologist before starting this diet.

The ultimate goal for any weight loss diet is to reduce total daily calories. The whole purpose of the ketogenic diet is to make the body use fat for energy versus carbohydrates or glucose. This is what leads to ketosis. During the transition from glucose metabolism to fat metabolism, you will feel hunger, but the hunger will dissipate once you are in ketosis. This will help you consume fewer calories.

The idea behind the ketogenic diet is that simple carbs with minimal fiber content are rapidly absorbed and turned into fat unless these immediate energy sources are used by the body. Since the body does not want to go into this state of ketosis, you will feel hunger and continue to eat carbs, which could turn into a vicious cycle, causing a lot of weight gain.

However, with the keto diet, fats are absorbed much more slowly and allow the body to go into ketosis. Again, when energy is needed in a situation where no carbohydrates are available, your body will mainly burn fat. A byproduct of this metabolism is ketone production.

On the other hand, healthy carbs should not induce insulin spikes and subsequent fat storage, especially if you eat small portions of healthy carbs with high fiber content such as chia seeds, steel-cut oats, apples, green leafy vegetables, etc.

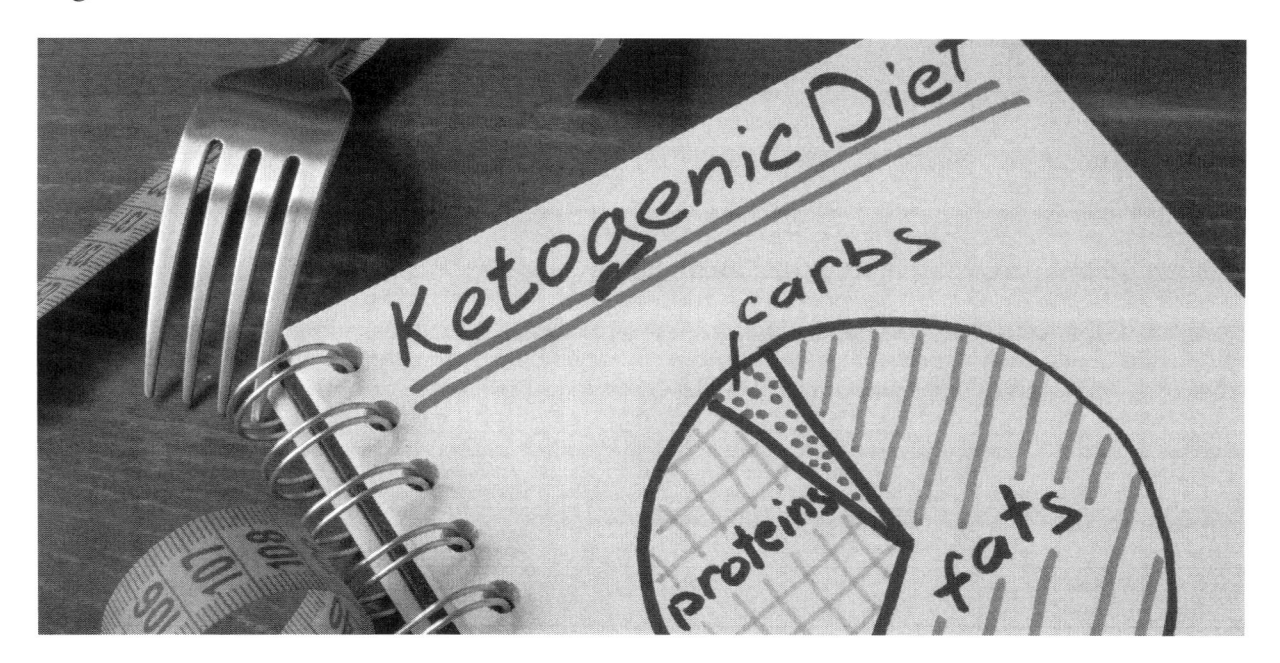

What Types Of Fats Are In The Keto Diet?

The best fats in this diet are those that are the most heart-healthy. Some healthy fats that are commonly included in the ketogenic diet are:

- » Fish such as salmon
- » Avocado
- » Olives and olive oil
- » Nuts and nut butter
- » Seeds

You need to stay away from animal fats, especially red meat and butter.

What Are The Effects Of A Ketogenic Diet On Blood Sugar?

The ketogenic diet has the potential to decrease blood sugar levels. But managing the carbohydrate intake is recommended more often for people with type 2 diabetes because carbohydrates are almost inevitably present in a normal human diet, and healthy carbs have many vitamins and minerals you do not want to miss out on.

If you already have high blood sugars, eating too many carbs can be risky. By switching your focus to healthy fats and fewer carbs, you can actually reduce your blood sugar this way.

Is There A Downside To The Keto Diet?

When you have too many ketones in the bloodstream, you could be at risk for developing diabetic ketoacidosis (DKA). DKA is most prevalent in type 1 diabetes when the blood glucose is too high in the absence of enough insulin. Although rare, DKA is possible in type 2 diabetes if the ketones are too high. Being ill while on a low-carb diet may also increase your risk for DKA.

If you're on the ketogenic diet, be sure to test blood sugar levels throughout the day to ensure they are within their target range.

DKA is a medical emergency. If you're experiencing the symptoms of DKA, see your doctor immediately. Complications can cause a diabetic coma. Signs and symptoms to look out for include these:

- » Consistently high blood sugar
- » Dry mouth
- » Frequent urination
- » Nausea
- » Breath that has a fruit-like odor
- » Breathing difficulties

What Not To Eat On A Ketogenic Diet

To eat a healthy diet, you should avoid or limit some things on a keto diet. These include

- *Certain types of fats*—there are different types of fats. Some types of fats are better for your body than others. Saturated fats, for example, should be avoided at all times. Most saturated fats come from animal fat.
- *Trans fats*—these are especially unhealthy for you. They are found in margarine, many fast foods, and some store-bought baked goods. Trans fats can raise your cholesterol level and your chance of getting heart disease. Try to avoid eating foods with these types of fats.

"Polyunsaturated" fats found in fish are healthy and can reduce your chance of getting heart disease. Other polyunsaturated fats might also be good for your health. When you cook, it's best to use oils with some healthier fats in them, such as olive oil and canola oil.

Studies indicate that 85% of patients with diabetes eat more than the recommended amount of fat in their diet. Increased saturated fat causes insulin resistance and a reduced effect of the insulin you take. High saturated and trans-fats found in red meat, margarine, butter, bakery products, etc., in the diet also increase blood sugar, increase your weight, and raise your cholesterol levels.

The type of fat you eat is also extremely important if you want to prevent heart attacks and strokes. Trans fats (hydrogenated fats) are never recommended because they cause blockage of the arteries. Mono and polyunsaturated fats (particularly omega-3 fatty acids), on the other hand, protect the arteries from blood clots and cholesterol plaques. If you instead replace saturated fats with polyunsaturated fats, you will reduce both your blood sugars and insulin resistance. Also, replacing carbohydrates, saturated fat, or monounsaturated fat with mono and polyunsaturated fat improves your ability to secrete insulin.

So, a low carb diet is not just a low-carb or low-fat diet. It is about eating good fats and good carbs. Also, it is very important to keep the total calories consumed daily on the low side, no matter what the content of the diet is. I recommend less than 1200 calories for women above the age of 40 and less than 1800 calories a day for men age above 50.

Monitoring Your Diabetes On A Keto Diet

The ketogenic diet seems like any other "specialty" diet; eat specific types of food and avoid certain foods…simple enough, right? Well, unlike a typical low-calorie diet, a high-fat diet requires careful monitoring for reasons I just mentioned.

Your doctor needs to monitor both your blood glucose and ketone levels to make sure that the diet isn't causing any harmful effects. Once your body adjusts to the diet, you still need to see your doctor for testing and to see if you need any potential medication adjustments.

Even if you think you are stable, it's still important to keep up with regular blood glucose monitoring. For type 2 diabetes, the testing frequency varies. Be sure to check with your doctor to determine what testing schedule is best for you.

Is There Any Evidence To Back Up The Benefits Of A Keto Diet?

"In 2008, researchers conducted a 24-week study to determine the effects of a low-carbohydrate diet on people with type 2 diabetes and obesity. At the end of the study, participants who followed the ketogenic diet saw greater improvements in glycemic control and medication reduction compared to those who followed a low-glycemic diet."

"A 2013 review reported that a ketogenic diet can lead to more significant improvements in blood sugar control, A1c, weight loss, and discontinued insulin requirements than other diets."

"A 2017 study also found the ketogenic diet outperformed a conventional, low-fat diabetes diet over 32 weeks regarding weight loss and A1c."

The Final Word On The Keto Diet...

Reducing your carbohydrate intake with a ketogenic diet can be effective in reducing body weight and improving glycemic control in people with type 2 diabetes. Type 2 diabetics tend to have a stronger effect on blood sugars than type 1 with a very low carb diet.

On the other hand, a keto diet may not be appropriate for all individuals. In people with type 2 diabetes, there is a necessary balance between the potential increase in cardiovascular risk because of the unfavorable lipid profile from eating unhealthy fats. The benefits from weight loss and improvement of glycemic control in this diet may be short-lived. It is hard to have any long-term compliance with such a low carb diet.

For those with type 1 diabetes, there is no evidence that a keto diet delays or prevents the onset of the disease. These diets can improve metabolic control, but individuals with diabetes should be careful because of the increased risk of DKA or worsening the lipid profile.

In many studies among the general population, a higher carb intake in diabetes was associated with worse outcomes; however, consuming healthier carbs such as oats, chia seeds, fruits, and vegetables in your diet is associated with a decreased risk of death from cardiovascular disease and other diseases. When a healthy low-fat diet was compared to a healthy low carb diet, good results in terms of weight loss were observed with both diets.

Therefore, the source of the carbs, proteins, and fats and their quality are important. Choosing high-fiber and nutrient-rich foods is a good option for everyone. For this reason, it is important to evaluate not only the number of carbs eaten but also their type.

To summarize, the ketogenic diet may offer some help for people with type 2 diabetes who have difficulty controlling their symptoms or losing weight. Not only do many people feel better with fewer diabetic symptoms, but they may also be less dependent on medications.

Still, not everyone has success on this diet. Many may find the restrictions too difficult to follow over the long term.

Please keep in mind that "high-fat" dieting can be dangerous for your glucose control, especially because of the potential for severely low blood sugars if you are on certain medications such as insulin or sulfonylureas.

My advice to my own patients is that they should only start the ketogenic diet if they're sure they can commit to it. Your dietician or doctor can help you determine the best diet choice for managing your diabetes.

Intermittent Fasting

For people who are not a big fan of the keto diet or those who cannot maintain this kind of diet but still want to have similar benefits, intermittent fasting may be a great alternative. Intermittent fasting is fasting for a long period of time in a given day; typically, it is 16 to 20 hours a day. Some people prefer fasting for a shorter time, such as 8 to 12 hours, but that's not necessarily the same as 16 hours of fasting when it comes to the health benefits you'll see with longer fasts. Intermittent fasting 16 to 20 hours a day can help reverse insulin resistance and put diabetes into remission.

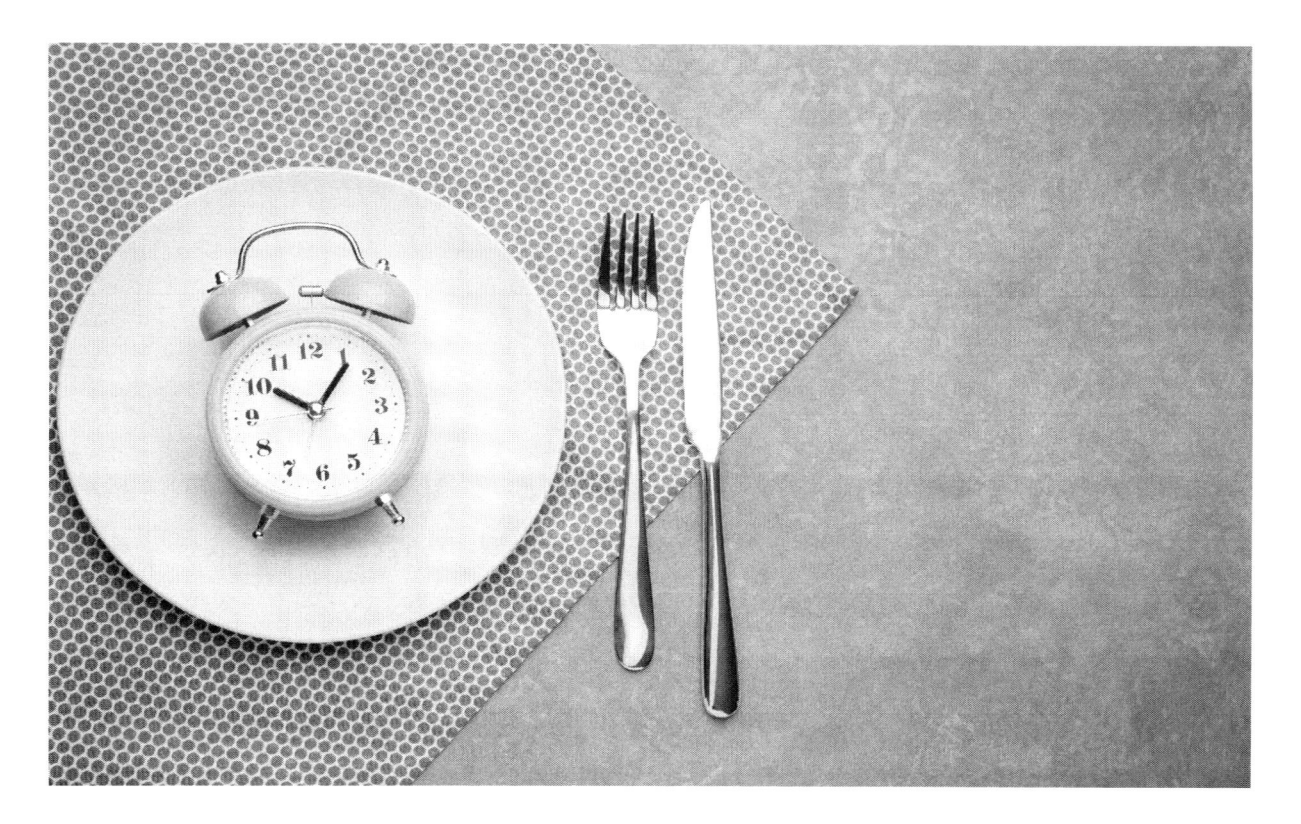

This type of intermittent fasting isn't the same as fasting for two to three days. After 2 to 3 days of fasting, you will feel very weak, and it isn't any more beneficial than fasting for 16 to 20 hours in one day. It also isn't the same as dry fasting because you get to drink water.

You can do your 16 hours of fasting at any time during a 24-hour day, depending on your schedule and your eating habits. You are giving yourself 4-8 hours of eating; it depends on the length of time you fast.

An important caveat is that you should not binge-eat after 16 hours of fasting. This means you will still need to control your calorie intake. The idea is that you need to make sure you are restricting your calories significantly during the days of intermittent fasting, so you're typically eating between 800-1200 cal/day. Some people do the 5: 2 rule, which is two days of fasting out of seven days a week. Others do three days of fasting and four days of regular eating.

What Is The Difference Between Reducing Calorie Diet Versus Intermittent Fasting?

Cutting your calories or counting calories down to 1200 to 1500 calories per day versus intermittent fasting can result in similar weight loss, but there are major differences between these two eating strategies.

Studies show that if you are fasting 16 to 20 hours two to three times a week, your insulin resistance will dramatically improve, and you may actually go into diabetes remission. Studies show that people who reduce their total intake on a more consistent basis can still lose weight, but improvement in insulin resistance and diabetes remission does not necessarily happen in all cases.

The bottom line is that it has been proven that by eating pretty much nothing and just drinking non-caloric beverages during that 16-20 hour period, you are going to have a major benefit, especially if you can do that twice or three times a week.

Remember, this isn't the same as fasting for the entire week. You just need to do intermittent fasting 2-3 days out of seven days. You can pick your days. Choose days you're not super-busy or super-active to do this. You need to make sure that on those days, your goal is not to eat anything solid or even liquid calories for 16 to 20 hours. Believe me, you're going to see a dramatic improvement in your insulin resistance.

Studies also show that even if you don't lose weight at all while doing intermittent fasting for 2 to 3 days a week, your insulin resistance will still improve. You might be eating too many calories during the times you are eating. Even so, you're going to lose abdominal/visceral fat.

Will I Lose Muscle While Intermittent Fasting?

Muscle loss will be very minimal compared to the fat you'll lose by reducing your calories this way. If you are actually doing intermittent fasting twice a week, you will keep your muscle mass and lose more abdominal/visceral fat in the process.

Intermittent fasting is very doable for diabetics. It means that you will not have to take as many medications or that you will not have to take insulin anymore. This kind of fasting is a good bargain for diabetics because it's not the same as cutting everything out, fasting every day, or going on a keto diet. You will see the difference without having to suffer.

What Changes Happen In Your Body When You Fast?

Your body is burning glucose during the first 8 to 12 hours of fasting. Then you start burning fatty acids from your fat cells. Your muscles are full of these fatty acids, along with the storage form of glucose (glycogen). If, for example, you eat on a regular basis, glucose is always going to your muscles. If your muscles do not use this glucose during periods of physical inactivity, those excessive glucose calories become triglycerides or stored fat.

Your body starts using triglycerides in a fasting state by turning them into fatty acids that your body burns. Your body can only do this after you deplete the glucose you eat and your glycogen stores first. Then, once the fatty acids get burned, ketone bodies are made as waste products. Finally, you burn the ketones too.

Intermittent Fasting Results

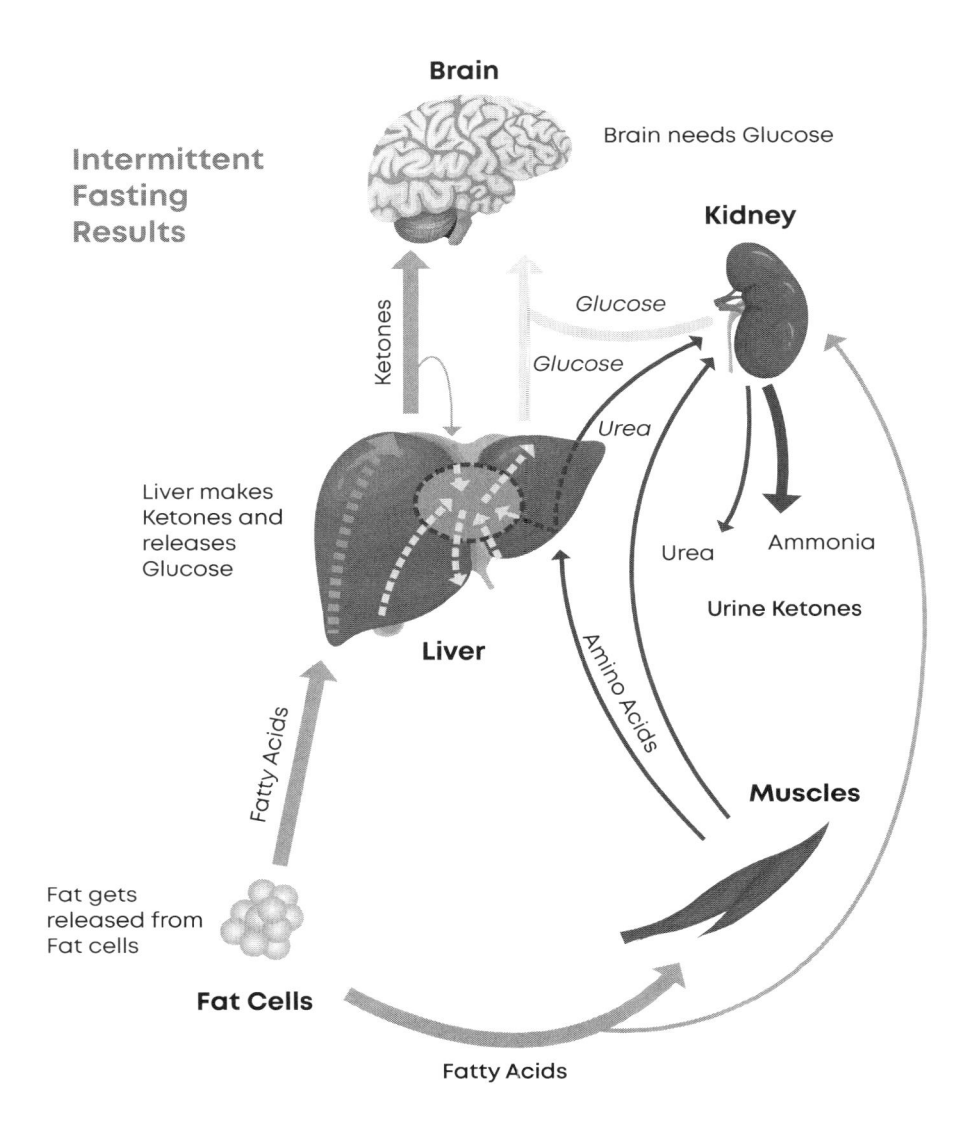

What Are The Benefits Of Using Ketones As A Source Of Energy?

Ketones are not necessarily just a breakdown product of fatty acids. Ketones have many major functions in the body. Ketones or "ketone bodies" are like housekeepers or police officers in your body. They stimulate certain proteins and molecules in the body to repair the damage from oxidative stress. During fasting, cells activate pathways that enhance defenses against oxidative and metabolic stress. They help remove or repair damaged molecules.

Think about it: Have you thought about the fact that you work 8 hours and rest 16 hours a day? What would happen if you work 16 hours a day every day instead of 8 hours? You would burn out, become too stressed, and end up getting sick. So you are working eight hours a day, and the rest of the time you're resting; this is because your body needs to recover from the stress of the work so you can regenerate muscle and brain activity.

In a very real sense, your body needs a break from eating because every time you eat, you're introducing potentially toxic chemicals into your body. Sometimes those toxic chemicals come from the metabolism of the food you eat. These toxic chemicals create what we call "oxidative stress." Oxidative stress can damage healthy tissues. Ketones help eliminate oxidative stress so your tissues can be healthier.

The cells in your body also need to regenerate. We call that process autophagy. Autophagy means that your cells must destroy old cells so that the new ones can come in and replace the old ones. Ketone bodies also induce that process. Ketones also help create hormones and chemical messengers called cytokines (such as adiponectin). Adiponectin has been shown to reduce insulin resistance. Ketone bodies also help eliminate inflammatory cytokines you don't want to have, such as TNF alpha.

As a result of this reduction in inflammation, ketones can help patients with epilepsy or other inflammatory disorders such as rheumatoid arthritis, inflammatory bowel disorders, arthritis, and others.

Remember, diabetes and insulin resistance are also inflammatory states. When you are overweight, your protective adiponectin levels go down, and inflammation goes up. Fat cells are very inflammatory when they are too full of fat and stressed from this.

Ketone bodies are the only way for fat cells to unload. In the absence of fasting and when you engage in constant calorie intake, fat cells fill up and go into a state of metabolic and oxidative stress. Lack of protection from ketone bodies makes the situation worse.

The moment you go into a fasting state, suddenly the ketone bodies start repairing the inflammation. When the inflammation goes down, your insulin resistance improves. Another benefit of ketogenesis during intermittent fasting is the protection of the endothelial cells, which are the cells inside your arteries. This translates into a reduction in cardiovascular disease because your arteries don't get inflamed and blocked by lipid-containing plaques.

How Do I Deal With The Side Effects Of Intermittent Fasting?

When you fast for 16 hours, you are going to be irritable. You are going to feel weak. You are also going to have a little bit of mental fog. The good news is that the symptoms will go away within the first 2 to 4 weeks of intermittent fasting practice.

You will see similar symptoms when you start exercising after a sedentary lifestyle. In the beginning, when you start working out in the gym, you can often feel like all of your muscles are failing. However, if you keep going to the gym, your body will learn to recover from the stress response, and you will have stronger muscles and feel much fitter and recover more easily.

The process is not any different than going through alcohol withdrawal or stopping smoking. At first, you are not going to feel good because your body is not used to fasting for a long time.

Once you go through the initial uncomfortable symptoms of intermittent fasting, you're going to be a new person in a few weeks. You need to be patient for the side effects to go away. In the meantime, you're going to be irritable. You also have to control yourself; it's your body that is going through this, so your spouse and family won't understand. You don't have to put other people through the same stress you're going through.

It is not a bad idea for you to explain to people around you what you are going through is a temporary symptomatic process.

Can I Exercise During Intermittent Fasting?

Yes, you can, but I have a very important suggestion. You have to stay hydrated and listen to your body. Also, do not force yourself if you feel too fatigued. You can do a milder cardio workout that you normally do if you can. It will help you a lot with weight loss because you're already burning fat during fasting. This only gets more prominent if you exercise, so it will be useful to you if you can do it.

When it comes to weightlifting, the fasting state may not be the best time to lift because your muscles will be totally depleted of glycogen. Typically with resistance exercises, your muscles use glycogen or glucose preferably so, without these molecules, your performance will be very limited. Therefore, I would suggest doing your lifting in the fed state, maybe two hours after eating.

Important Points For Diabetics Trying Intermittent Fasting...

If you are contemplating doing intermittent fasting, you should talk to your endocrinologist. Those who are on short-acting or fast-acting insulin need to be very careful; this is because if you take a short-acting or fast-acting insulin when you're not eating, you run the risk of severe hypoglycemia (low blood sugar).

On the other hand, if you're taking long-acting insulin, you still have to be also very careful, even though the results you get will not be as disastrous as using fast-acting insulin. You will require less basal insulin during intermittent fasting and in the days that follow because your insulin resistance will go down dramatically. As a result, you really need to monitor your blood sugars very closely. <u>On those days that you're not going to eat anything for 16 to 20 hours, you must remember to reduce the basal insulin amount.</u>

The most common basal insulins are Tresiba, Toujeo, Lantus, Levemir, Novolin N, and Humulin N. Whatever you're on, you should reduce your basal insulin by 20%, especially if your blood sugars are not above 200 in the morning to begin with. I also do not recommend stopping the basal insulin prematurely. Remember, be sure to discuss any medication changes with your endocrinologist first.

Unfortunately, a lot of people don't understand the role of basal insulin. Because of insulin resistance, type 2 diabetics still need some insulin as a baseline to maintain their blood sugar stable without an increase in these numbers. People with type 1 diabetes also need basal insulin at all times because they do not produce any, no matter what the circumstances. Basal insulin helps keep the liver from making too much sugar. On the other hand, excessive basal insulin can totally stop glucose production from the liver, leading to severely low blood sugar.

People who are on sulfonylureas such as glipizide, glimepiride, or glyburide need to be extremely careful. Since these oral pills have unpredictable effects on insulin production, patients may develop severely low blood sugars when they do not eat. Make sure to talk to your doctor to see if there is an alternative medication to sulfonylurea agents you can take.

GLP-1 class medications such as Ozempic, Trulicity, Rybelsus, Victoza, and Bydureon do not lower your blood sugars to dangerous levels, so you can still take those medications to regulate your blood sugars, especially if you find that your blood sugars are going up without taking them.

Other mediation types that can be relatively safe are the SGLT-2 inhibitors, such as Jardiance, Farxiga, Invokana, and Steglatro. Although there is a small risk of diabetic ketoacidosis with these agents, there is no evidence that fasting will increase that risk. Pioglitazone is another safe agent you can use during intermittent fasting.

The bottom line is that intermittent fasting 2-3 times a week, around 16 to 20 hours a day, is a great way of reducing insulin resistance and putting diabetes into remission. If diabetes remission is not possible, intermittent fasting will reduce at least the amount of medications taken and potentially eliminate the need for insulin for type 2 diabetics. Intermittent fasting also has other benefits, such as reducing inflammation and reducing cancer risk.

Mediterranean Diet

<u>In my opinion, and with the evidence we know about the effects of diet on diabetes, I can safely say that the low carb Mediterranean diet is the best diabetic diet! It is one of the few diets proven in studies to improve glycemic control in those with diabetes. It also reduces mortality from heart attacks and strokes, which are the main reasons for death among people with diabetes.</u>

In the research that has been done on diets and diabetes, the Mediterranean diet was compared with other diets such as low-fat, nonrestricted calorie, low carbohydrate, high carbohydrate, and usual diets. In one of those studies, participants with diabetes who were on the Mediterranean diet were much less likely to use diabetic or non-diabetic medications compared to patients on other diets.

In this study, 44% of patients on the Mediterranean diet for diabetes took medications for their diabetes compared to 77% of patients on other diets. At the end of the study, there was no difference in terms of weight changes after 3 to 4 years among the different diets.

The main features of the diet are the frequent use of olive oil, eating several vegetables every day (such as onions, garlic, onions, peppers, and tomatoes), whole fresh fruit, whole grains, legumes, and nuts. Moderate amounts of red wine, seafood, chicken, eggs, cheese, and yogurt are also allowed. They do not recommend much red meat, and they don't recommend any refined carbohydrates, sweets, or processed meats.

Diabetic Diet Basics

Let's talk about diet in general and how it affects your diabetes.

What Are The Different Food Groups, And How Do They Affect Your Blood Sugar?

I will talk about carbohydrates more in detail later as this group has the most effect on blood sugar. On the other hand, proteins and fats can also affect blood sugar, although in a less predictable way.

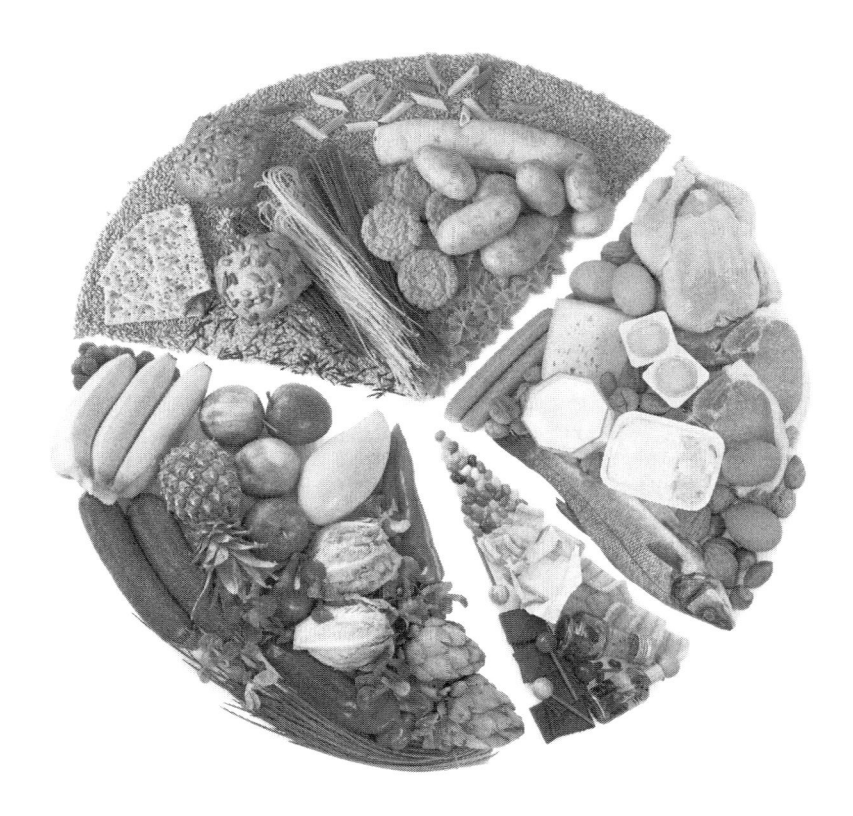

How Does Protein Affect Blood Sugar?

What we do know about the effect of protein is that in individuals who do NOT have diabetes, protein consumption can stimulate insulin release, which decreases glucose while also causing glucagon release. This increases blood glucose by causing the release of stored glucose from the liver.

Unfortunately, type 1 diabetic individuals do not produce insulin; however, they continue to produce glucagon. As a result, protein consumption can trigger glucagon release, which increases blood sugar. This can happen 3 to 5 hours after a meal and can frustrate glucose management. It is not uncommon for my patients to ask why their blood sugars are still spiking, although they are not eating carbs.

On the other hand, the effect of protein on your blood sugar is not easily predictable. That is why I do not recommend a very high protein diet, especially for type 1 diabetics. Instead, I recommend that they have a balanced diet that includes a healthy amount of proteins, carbs, and healthy fats. For insulin-resistant type 2 diabetics, the same rules apply. Protein intake can cause a modest glucose increase, and the exact amount of this increase can be unpredictable. Most type 2 diabetics tend to secrete more glucagon after a high protein meal, which can still raise blood sugar.

What Are Carbohydrates?

Carbohydrates are one of the three macronutrients in our diet, along with protein and fat. When we talk about carbohydrates, we usually mean things like sugar, fruits, vegetables, tubers (potatoes, carrots, and beets), and legumes (peanuts and beans). They are the main source of energy for your body.

While there are many types of carbohydrates, your diet benefits most when you take a specific subset of carbohydrates. There really are good carbs and bad carbs. As a diabetic, you should know the difference in order to make the right dietary choices for yourself.

You may have heard that "Not All Carbs Are Made Equal." This is actually true. The more you know about which carbs are better for you as a diabetic, the better able you will be to make in-the-moment choices about which ones to incorporate into your diet. I will teach you what you need to know about this important macronutrient in this part of the chapter.

Are All Carbohydrates The Same?

While many fitness blogs compel us to resent carbohydrates, you need to rethink whether or not you want to go by those kinds of biased recommendations. Ask yourself, do you really know all you need to know about that mouth-watering morsel we call a carbohydrate?

If a diet plan (and there are many of these) requires you to sacrifice it for a good three months, would you blindly conform to it? Or would you dig deeper into why it's out of the diet regimen in the first place? And if possible, would you figure out if there are any healthy carbs that you can safely squeeze into your diet?

Anyone who loves carbs – that makes most of us – will do the latter. Yes, it's a lot of work, but it's worth it. As you'll soon see, not all carbs are created the same, and it is possible to find carbs you can comfortably eat. Many are not only very tasty, but they're good for you as well. Doesn't that make you feel better?

How Do Carbohydrates Metabolize In The Body?

A lot of carbohydrate metabolism boils down to the molecular structure of these molecules. At their very foundation, they metabolize into weight-gaining sugars in the body. Most starchy foods like potatoes, some fruits, and processed grains have a very high glycemic index (GI). I will talk more about the glycemic index soon but, with regard to this number, a high GI-food is not optimal for diabetes. This is because they can spike blood sugar levels and insulin in the body after you eat them.

Refined carbs, such as the ones in the bakery products, have consequential and often adverse effects on your metabolism, blood sugar, and overall health. Besides being mostly carbs and fats, these kinds of foods offer you essentially no important nutrients. If you doubt this, take a look at this comparison:

Nutrient/Feature	Donut	Apple
Calories	450 calories	95 calories
Carbs	51 grams	25 grams
Fat	25 grams	0.3 grams
Protein	5 grams	0.2 grams
Fiber	1.3 grams	4 grams
Vitamin C % RDI	1%	14%
Vitamin K % RDI	5%	5%
Potassium % RDA	5%	6%
High in other vitamin and minerals	Calcium, Phosphorus, Manganese	Manganese, Copper, Vitamins A, B1, B2, B6, and E, Antioxidants

Even though there are great differences among the different types, carbohydrates are your body's primary energy source and a vital part of any diet across the world. These are not only one of the three "macronutrients" that your body relies on for proper functioning – they are the major building blocks of energy.

What Do Carbohydrates Do?

Carbohydrates provide the only fuel for your central nervous system and are the major energy your muscles need to function. The body cannot produce these macronutrients from scratch like plants can; you can only access them through certain foods in your diet.

A healthy intake of carbs can do these important things for you:

- » Provide energy
- » Protect against diseases
- » Help in weight control

The foods you eat primarily contain three different types of carbohydrates consisting of starches, fiber, and sugars. Let's start by exploring what they are and how they affect your body.

What Are Complex And Simple Carbohydrates?

To make it easy, we will divide them into simple and complex carbohydrates.

Complex Carbohydrates

"Complex carbohydrates" – also known as polysaccharides – are a bunch of sugar molecules strung together in a long, complex chain. Just imagine a bunch of sugar cubes all holding hands.

Due to the complexity of these types of carbohydrates, they take longer to break down in the body. Since complex carbs are digested more slowly than simple carbohydrates, they tend not to cause spikes in your blood sugar levels after you eat them. Yet, not all complex carbs are the same. You will need to choose complex carbs low in the glycemic index, which we will discuss shortly.

Whole grains (non-refined) like, barley, quinoa, bulgur, steel-cut oatmeal, and chickpeas, non-starchy vegetables, and beans are the best food choices. These all contain complex carbohydrates that are low in glycemic index.

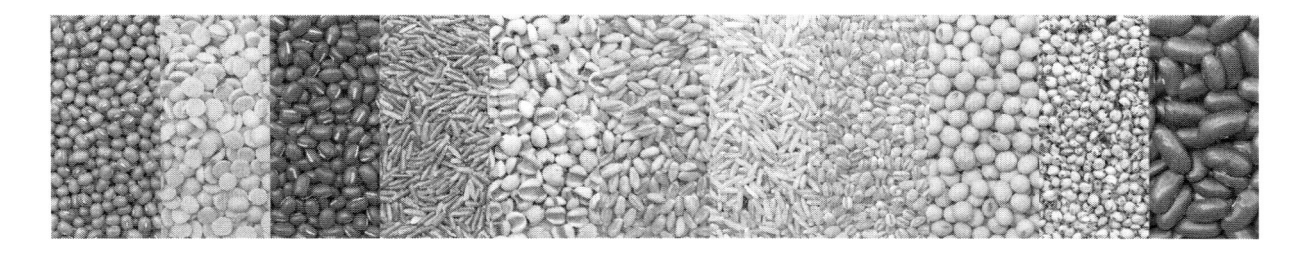

CHAPTER 4 - DIABETES MANAGEMENT

Examples Of Complex Carbohydrates

Examples of starchy vegetables are potatoes, including sweet potatoes, corn, and peas. So when nutritionists tell you to eat complex carbohydrates, they are referring to whole grain foods and non-starchy vegetables.

An individual with diabetes should stick to non-starchy vegetables and carbohydrates that have a low glycemic index and low glycemic load. My favorite vegetables for diabetic individuals are leafy greens such as spinach, romaine, swiss chard, kale, cauliflower, cabbage, eggplant, celery, onion, green bean, bell pepper, and Brussels sprouts.

My least favorite starchy vegetables are potatoes and corn. Whole grains and legumes are always good choices. For example, I love farro, kidney beans, lentils, cauliflower rice, hummus, or falafel (made from chickpeas and tahini).

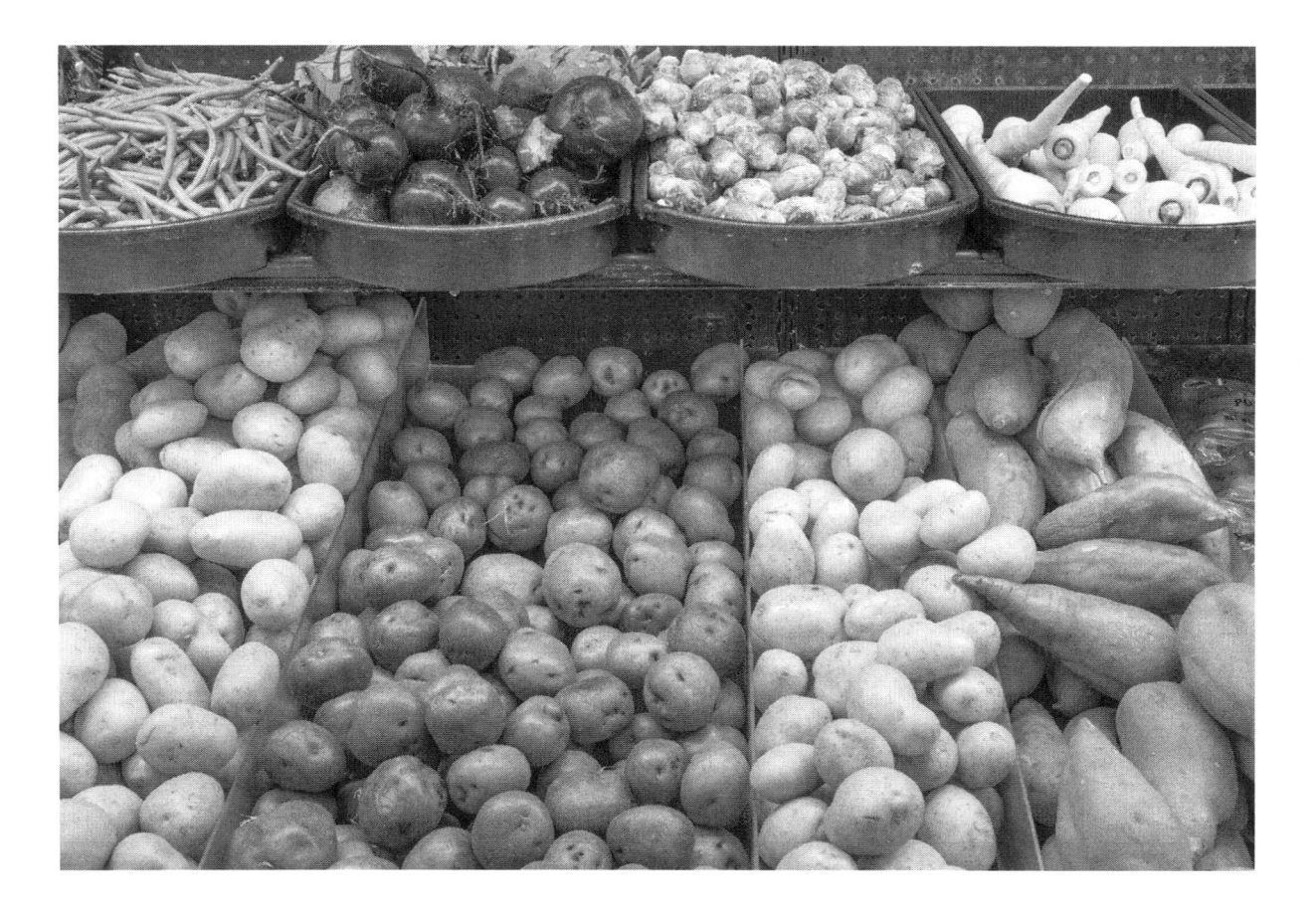

Simple Carbohydrates

On the other hand, simple carbohydrates are already broken down and quickly digested by the body as the name suggests. They are naturally found in most foods like milk, dairy products, fruits, and refined sugars. Table sugars, corn syrups, sodas, bakery products, and store-bought candies are processed carbs that come under this category.

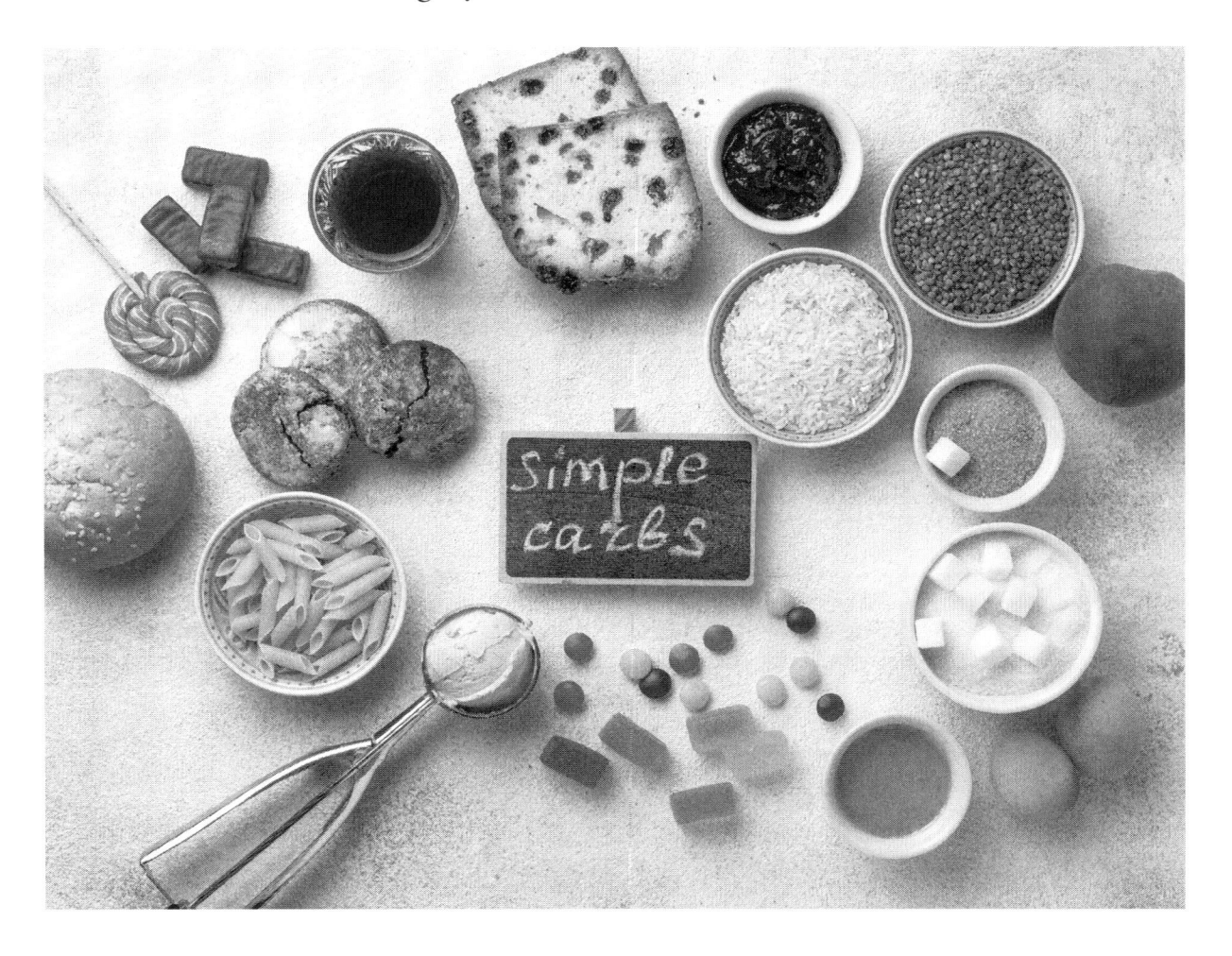

Although simples carbs are typically more rapidly absorbed and their glycemic index matters, the glycemic load of these carbs can make a big difference. Glycemic load is somewhat different than the glycemic index. Let's learn more about the glycemic index and glycemic load.

What Are The Glycemic Index And Glycemic Load? And How To Use The Glycemic Index To Your Advantage?

When it comes to carbohydrates, it's important to know that the rate of breakdown and absorption is key to managing blood glucose levels. But how can you tell what foods will have the greatest impact on your next blood sugar reading? The glycemic index is here to help.

The glycemic index is a system of assigning a number to carbohydrate-containing foods according to how fast each food increases blood sugar. The Glycemic Index is scored from 0 to 100; carbs with a low glycemic index value (55 or less) are slowly absorbed by our bodies as compared to carbs with a high GI. They cause blood glucose levels to rise slowly, and therefore, insulin levels rise slowly as well. Carbohydrates with middle to high values get absorbed much faster, which is why they cause a spike in blood sugar.

On the other hand, glycemic load measures the rise in blood sugar based on the number of carbohydrates the food contains in an average serving while accounting for glycemic index. The glycemic load can actually be more reliable than the glycemic index. For example, watermelon has a glycemic index of watermelon is 72, which is very high. This means it can spike blood sugar rapidly; however, watermelon is mostly water, so the total carbohydrates in one cup of watermelon are low. The glycemic load in a serving of watermelon is only 4, which is extremely low, as the carbohydrate content of watermelon is very small. Foods with a glycemic load between 4-10 have a very low glycemic load, which is the safest range. A glycemic load between 10 and 20 is moderate. They can spike your blood sugar to some degree but will not keep your blood glucose levels elevated for long periods of time. Foods with a glycemic load higher than 20, however, should be eaten sporadically, as they will spike blood sugar levels and keep them elevated for longer.

My patients are often so surprised to see their blood sugars spiking from 110 mg/dL (6.1 mmol/l) in the morning to 230 mg/dL (12.6mmol/l) one hour after eating cereal or a piece of toast. Yes, if you are insulin resistant, 30 grams of carbs in an apple versus in 2 pieces of toast can make a difference of up to 100 mg/dL (5.5 mmol/l) in the blood glucose levels after each of these meals.

If you want foods that have a low GI, go for whole-grain foods. On the opposite end of the spectrum, avoid refined carbs at all costs, which have a high GI. When calculating the GI of carbohydrates, you might want to use an app that does it for you. There are many applications found on both iPhone and Android phones; these provide a search function that allows you to search for specific foods to automatically calculate the GI. I personally prefer to use the glycemic load of a given food as it gives you a better picture of the carb load you are getting from the food. Take a look at the table below.

	Food	Glycemic Load
Low	1 oz peanuts	1
	1 cup diced carrots	2
	1 medium pear	4
	1 large slice pumpernickel bread	5
	2 tsp white sugar	6
	1 cup boiled kidney beans	8
	1 cup All-Bran cereal	10
Medium	1 slice white bread	10
	4 soda crackers	12
	1 cup banana	13
	Sara Lee blueberry muffin	15
	3 puffed rice cakes	17
	Campbell's minestrone soup	18
High	1 cup cornflakes	20
	1 oz jelly beans	22
	Clif Bar (Chocolate Brownie)	22
	1 cup boiled white spaghetti	24
	1 white bagel	24
	2 oz dried dates	25
	Milky Way candy bar	26
	1 medium russet baked potato	33
	1 cup boiled white rice	35

Low GI Food	Medium GI Food	High GI Food
45 or less	Between 45 and 70	More than 70

The Glycemic Load of food is based both on the glycemic index and the quantity of food you eat. It is a good measure of how many of the carbs you are eating will get rapidly absorbed into the bloodstream. The definition of a low GL, moderate GL, and high GL food is different from the glycemic index. It looks like this:

Low GL Food	Medium GL Food	High GL Food
10 or less	Between 11 and 19	20 or greater

How many carbs you eat depends on you, your doctor, and your dietitian. You should all be on the same page as to what's appropriate for you. There is no cookie-cutter approach to diabetes care. This is why a diabetes coach is an essential component of your long-term success.

Unfortunately, insurance companies prefer not to pay for diabetes coaching services. They will, though, pay for expensive medications costing thousands of dollars, which doesn't make much sense. Even so, it is something you might consider when you get stuck on what kind of diet you should be on.

The Essential Role Of Fiber In Carbohydrates

As I just mentioned, complex carbs are far healthier and safer for the body than simple ones. Here's why. The rich fiber content, vitamins, and minerals are what make these carbs a diet-friendly food. Whole grains, non-starchy vegetables, and beans all provide a substantial amount of fiber and essential minerals.

Fiber is a critical component of any diet, but it is especially important for people with diabetes. Fiber helps keep your blood sugar levels from spiking too high. It can help regulate your cholesterol levels and is extremely important for intestinal health. It improves the internal gut environment, which is fundamental for healthy digestion.

Recommendations On Fiber Intake

Even when the Academy of Nutrition and Dietetics advise a much higher RDI (Recommended Dietary Intake) for fiber, the majority of adults only consume 15 grams a day on average. So, if you're looking for a short-cut to a high-fiber diet, then complex carbs are the way to go, of course in moderation while watching your glucose levels.

Refined starches or carbohydrates, such as white bread and white pasta, are starches that have undergone processing. Processing removes the bran and germ of the grain, stripping them of fiber, vitamins, and minerals. What you want to eat instead are whole-grain foods that have not been so heavily processed.

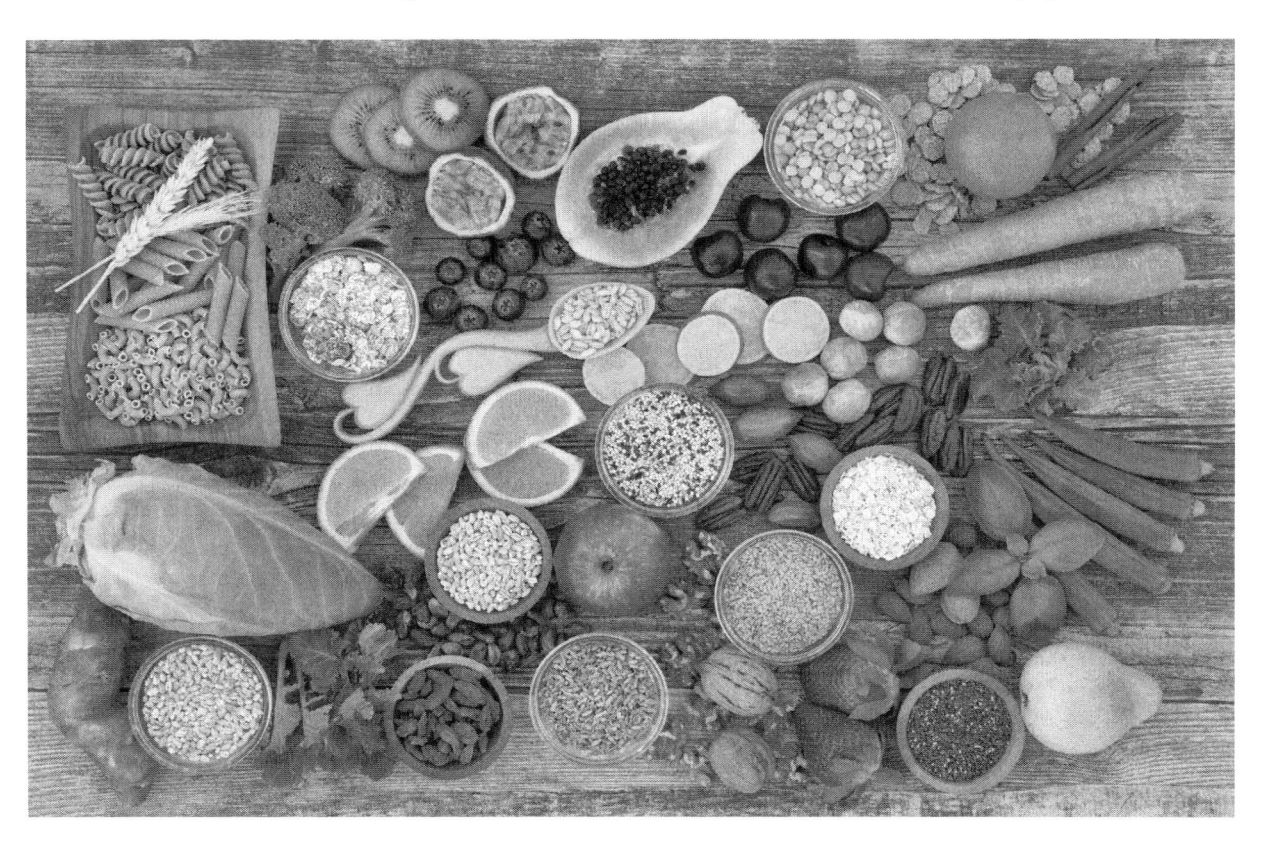

Quick Tip

When in doubt, choose unprocessed grains and those you can "see" in your bread. The more refined the grain, the less brain/fiber in the grain. Fiber does many things for the diet but, for diabetes, it means it "holds onto" glucose in the GI tract, meaning it can't be rapidly absorbed into your bloodstream.

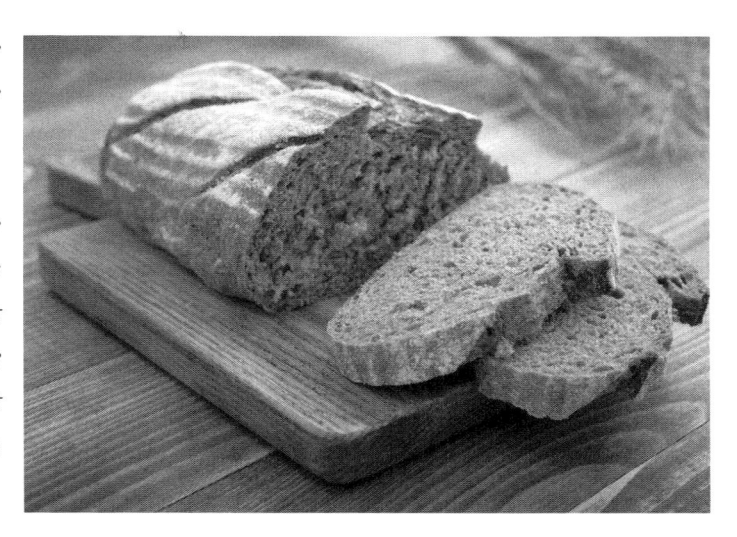

Why Does The Body Absorb Refined Carbohydrates Very Quickly And Raise Blood Sugars?

The reason why refined carbohydrates are rapidly digested and absorbed into the bloodstream is that there is no protein, fiber, or fat content present in them. You need fat and fiber to slow the digestive process down. They're basically "empty calories." This can contribute to blood sugar and insulin spikes after you eat them. Remember that complex carbohydrates include all starches, regardless of whether they are whole, refined, or have a high fiber content.

In summary, complex carbohydrates such as whole grains are considered "good" carbs because they take much longer to break down in your gut before they are absorbed into the bloodstream. This means you will get lower amounts of sugars released at a more consistent rate instead of a rapid influx of sugar all at once. They typically have a low glycemic index and low glycemic load as well. If in doubt, quickly check it online or in your carb book.

These complex carbs also keep you feeling full and going throughout the day. They can still increase your blood sugars; however, I do not recommend totally avoiding all of these nutritious carbohydrates. Rather, I would pay more attention to portion control, increasing activity level, and taking medications when necessary to overcome sugar spikes.

Quick tip

According to the American Diabetes Association, nutritional labels do not differentiate between the different types of carbohydrates. The term "total carbohydrates" includes all three types of carbohydrates we discussed. This is the number you should pay attention to if you are carb counting. You might also want to pay attention to the "total sugars" and "added sugars." These represent simple sugars. While you count carbs with the total carbohydrates listed, you want to stay away from those with a lot of sugar or added sugars.

Nutrition Facts

4 servings per container

Serving size	1 cup (180g)

Amount per serving

Calories 245

% Daily Value*

Total Fat 12g	14%
Saturated Fat 2g	10%
Trans Fat 0g	
Cholesterol 8mg	3%
Sodium 210mg	9%
Total Carbohydrate 34g	12%
Dietary Fiber 7g	25%
Total Sugars 5g	
Includes 4g Added Sugars	8%
Protein 11g	

Vit. D 4mcg 20%	·	Calcium 210mg 16%
Iron 3mg 15%	·	Potas. 380mg 8%
Vit. A 84mcg 9%	·	Vit. C 10mg 11%
Zinc 7mg 17%	·	Iodine 15mcg 10%

*The % Daily Value (DV) tells you how much a nutrient in a serving of food contributes to a daily diet. 2,000 calories a day is used for general nutrition advice.

The Role Of Your Diabetes Coach And Endocrinologist

Whatever guidance you can get from the endocrinologist you see will help you learn more about carbohydrates. So, you can apply this information to your own diabetes management. This information will also make a great difference in your A1c values.

I strongly recommend that you work with both a diabetes coach and an endocrinologist who can advise you on your diet and monitor your exercise very closely. Think of these individuals as a good friend keeping an eye on you. That way, you can often avoid taking costly diabetic medications that can also have serious side effects.

Even when you are on medications for your diabetes, you should know how to be consistent with your diet regarding the carbohydrates you consume with every meal. It will be a challenge initially, but once you get the hang of it, you will feel more self-control over your diet.

Soon enough, the practice of mindful eating will become second nature.

It's funny how people think about what type of gas they're putting in their cars and have no understanding of what type of food is going in their tummies. Well, it's time to make that decision.

In Summary

Successful self-management of diabetes is the simple difference between choosing a healthy, complex carb and a refined sugary treat. It will challenge your self-control, but once you get on with healthy eating, there's no going back.

Here are some ways to improve your intake of healthy carbs and self-regulate your blood sugars:

- Increase your water intake
- Eat more beans, legumes, and peas to increase the variety of minerals, fiber, and proteins in your diet
- Have a decent portion of fiber-rich veggies and fruits with every meal
- Reduce your dairy intake or stick to low-fat versions (although you can consume whole-milk dairy products made from goat milk safely)
- Cut down or limit added sugars like candies, soft drinks, white pasta, French fries, etc.
- Have a limited amount of dried fruits like figs, dates, and raisins
- Make a conscious effort to choose whole grains like brown rice, brown pasta, and wholegrain bread for breakfast and lunch. You will be surprised at how this little change will go a long way in regulating blood

sugar levels. Instead of having a bowl of cereal, switch it up with quinoa or healthy granola.

With these simple changes, prepare to be amazed at how well your body begins to manage your diabetes.

How Many Carbs Should A Diabetic Have?

A type 2 diabetic should eat anywhere between 15-60 grams of carbs per meal to control and manage blood sugars effectively. *It depends a lot on your age, caloric needs, activity level, and the duration of your diabetes. Individual goals can vary. You need to understand what your individual needs are.*

How many carbs you should eat per day is a personal decision you need to make. It's all between you, your endocrinologist, and your diabetes coach., We will go over the basics of the carbohydrate needs of the average diabetic.

What Does "Counting Carbs" Mean?

Counting carbs (also called "carb counting") is a type of meal planning. Some patients with diabetes use this with precision, especially when they are on insulin. Counting carbs means knowing the number of carbs you plan to eat or have just eaten. When patients with diabetes count carbs, they keep track of how many carbs they eat for each meal and snack.

People with diabetes need to know how many carbs they eat because eating carbs raises the blood sugar levels. There are reasons why "carb counting" is particularly important for diabetics taking insulin for every meal. This is because diabetic patients will need to adjust their insulin doses according to the carbohydrate content of the food they plan on eating. However, even for those who do not take insulin, carb counting can help keep blood sugar levels from getting too low or too high. It increases your awareness of the carbs in your diet, which helps control the caloric intake as well.

How Do I Count Carbs?

If your food has a nutrition label, please make sure to check out the information on the label. You need to look at certain things. A common misconception is that patients look at the amount of "sugar" or glucose on the label and disregard total carbohydrates. As I mentioned earlier, you should note that all the carbohydrates you read on the label turn into sugar (except the fiber content). There are other tricks you need to understand about carb counting, including these:

- *Total carbohydrates:* Let's say you are on a diet for diabetes and want to count carbs to help manage it. You look at nutrition labels and find the total carbohydrates on the label. Total carbohydrate on the label will tell you how many carbs are in 1 serving of the food. For example, if you see a number of 27 grams, it means one serving of that food has 27 grams of total carbohydrates. If one serving is one piece of that food, having two pieces will give you 54 grams of carbohydrates.

- *Serving size:* This tells you how much food is in 1 serving. If you have two servings, the number of carbs will be two times the number of carbohydrates listed.

- *Dietary fiber:* Fiber is a carbohydrate that is not digested. As a result, it does not raise your blood sugars. Foods with a lot of fiber can help control the blood sugar of patients with diabetes. If a food has more than 5 grams (g) of fiber, less insulin is needed for that food. You can subtract the fiber grams from the total carbohydrates to count your carb intake. If there is 5 g of fiber in 1 serving and 30 g of total carbohydrates are listed, you can safely use 25 g of carbs in your calculation of how much insulin you need.

- *Foods without labels:* Unfortunately, many foods, such as fresh fruits and vegetables, don't have a nutrition label. For these foods, you will need to learn about the usual serving sizes of different foods. You can easily do so by searching the item in Google or using phone applications that provide the same data or old school carb counting books.

You will also need to learn how many carbs are in one serving in those fruits and vegetables. For example, it is straightforward to learn that one small apple and one small orange are each only 15 g. After you get to know how many carbs are in these fruits and vegetables, you will be able to memorize very easily how many carbs are in the foods you commonly eat.

Do I Have To Count Carbs For Diabetes Or Are There Any Other Alternative Ways To Manage My Diet?

Yes, there are. One way I sometimes recommend is called exchange planning in a diabetic diet. With exchange planning, you can categorize all the foods you eat as carbohydrate, meat or meat substitute, or fat. In this system, one serving of sugar (like one small orange, which is 15 g) can be exchanged for any other sugar (like 1/3 cup of rice). You can do that because both portions contain about 15 grams of carbohydrate. As a result, you can also easily find out the total carbohydrate content of your meals and snacks using the exchange method.

Do I Have To Eat At The Same Time Every Day?

Meal timing can be very important. For some patients with diabetes, eating at the same time every day is crucial. This is because certain medications cause low blood sugar if you skip a meal. For patients who are on mealtime insulin, however, meal timing is not as important. If you are on sulfonylurea agents such as glipizide, glyburide, glimepiride, which are not taken in direct relation to your meals, sticking to consistent mealtimes can be very important.

Diabetics who take medications that do not cause low blood sugar, such as metformin, Ozempic, Trulicity, Rybelsus, Jardiance, Farxiga, and Invokana, have more flexibility with their diet and timing after meals. For those individuals, skipping or delaying a meal will not usually increase their risk of developing low blood sugar.

How Do I Determine The Number Of Carbs I Need?

How many carbs you can eat is largely based on your gender, age, activity status, and the duration and severity of your diabetes.

I'm going to give you an example. Let's say you have been a diabetic for 20 years, and you are a 65-year-old woman. You are on three oral medications along with basal insulin injections. You are inactive, and you have problems such as joint pain. Mostly, you just sit at home, not doing much. As a result, you weigh 230 pounds (which is in the obese range).

In this case, how many carbs should you eat? My answer to that would be to eat very few carbs(15-20 gr per meal). I recommend this because I can imagine you are very insulin resistant. Anytime you eat even a few carbs, your blood sugar may skyrocket. I definitely do not let this happen to my patients and help them with medications to improve their blood sugar control.

On the other hand, my advice in the office with my own patients is not intended to underestimate the power of knowledge and coaching in your diabetes management. That is one of the main reasons I have decided to write this book. You should know more about diet and diabetes so you can have more meaningful discussions with your coach or doctor.

On the other hand, physically active men with diabetes can have 30 to 75 grams of carbohydrates per meal in their diet. Like everyone with diabetes, it depends on the usual things: age, level of exercise, type of diabetes, and the severity and length of diabetes.

For example, consider the man with diabetes who has a very active, physical job. He is 35 and has type 1.5 diabetes (LADA). He is on one long-acting insulin and two oral agents. (Some type 1.5 diabetics do not end up on insulin right away) This individual is doing well with his lifestyle and also goes to the gym five times a week and works out one hour on those five days.

I would tell this individual that my conservative goal for him could be as low as 30 grams of carbs per meal if he wants to go on a really low-carb diet. This approach also helps reduce the number of diabetic medications he might need. On the other hand, if he works out a lot, he will eat carbs for his endurance and to prevent low blood sugar. Glucose is what your muscles are burning. If you do not eat any carbs, you're going to have significant fatigue with exercise. So for this very active man, I can allow up to 75 g of carbs per meal even if he is a diabetic.

Do Men And Women Have Different Carbohydrate Goals?

For a woman, my maximum carbohydrate recommendation is 45 grams of carbohydrates per meal in a diabetic diet compared to men who can eat up to 75 grams of carbs, provided that they are physically active, as discussed earlier. Again, the exact amount depends on you and your lifestyle. Most of the time, women need fewer calories and fewer carbs than men.

In most cases, if you're looking from a carbohydrate standpoint, you're looking mostly at carbs as a percentage of total calorie intake. So, if you want to be on the low carb side of things, you may drop down to 30 percent of your total calories. If you want to be more generous about carbs, especially if you're physically very active (working out more than 3 hours a week), you may be able to increase your carb intake to 35 to 45 percent of your total calories as carbohydrates. That is true for both men and women.

The basic thing you need to understand is that if you want to keep your blood sugar under control while eating healthy carbs, you also need to be physically active. If you're not physically active, then your goal if you are a woman is to eat 15 to 20 grams of carbs per meal. If you are a man who isn't physically active, you should stick to less than 30-45 grams of carbs per meal. On the other hand, this goal can be as high as 60 to 75 gr of carbs per meal for men and women who are extremely physically active.

How Many Carbs Should A Diabetic Person Eat Later In Life?

On the other end of the spectrum, people who are extremely frail and elderly, who are already losing weight unintentionally, and who are at an advanced age are a different class of diabetics. I will not be very strict with their blood sugars or carb intake. I often allow blood sugars after meals to be as much as 180 mg/dL (180 mmol/l). Part of the problem is that these are people who don't have a good appetite anyway, so it doesn't make much sense to further restrict their diet. Others have diseases like cancer, so they need all the nutrition they can get. Their blood sugar can still reasonably controlled with medications.

On the other hand, cancer cells are driven by sugar, so if they reduce their carbohydrate intake, they can improve their survival from this medical problem. If this is a person who isn't expected to survive their cancer, there is no reason to have them suffer further by limiting carb intake. In such situations, I am most guided by the cancer doctor who can tell me the patient's chances of survival.

Can I Go With No Carbs To Cure My Diabetes?

A no-carb or very low carb diet can help put diabetes in remission or mask it but will not cure diabetes in the long term. There are other things you should do to help put your diabetes into remission besides cutting carbs completely. Exercise, for example, also has many benefits. If you are going to have regular exercise, you have to have some healthy carbs in your diet to ensure that you have enough fuel for your muscles during exercise.

Are Artificial Sweeteners Safe For Diabetics To Take?

A lot of people use artificial sweeteners to avoid calories that can come from table sugar. People with type 1 and type 2 diabetes are especially likely to use artificial sweeteners frequently. Are they really helpful? Are there any serious side effects of these sweeteners diabetics should worry about? How much of an artificial sweetener is safe to consume? Let's take a look at these questions and answer them.

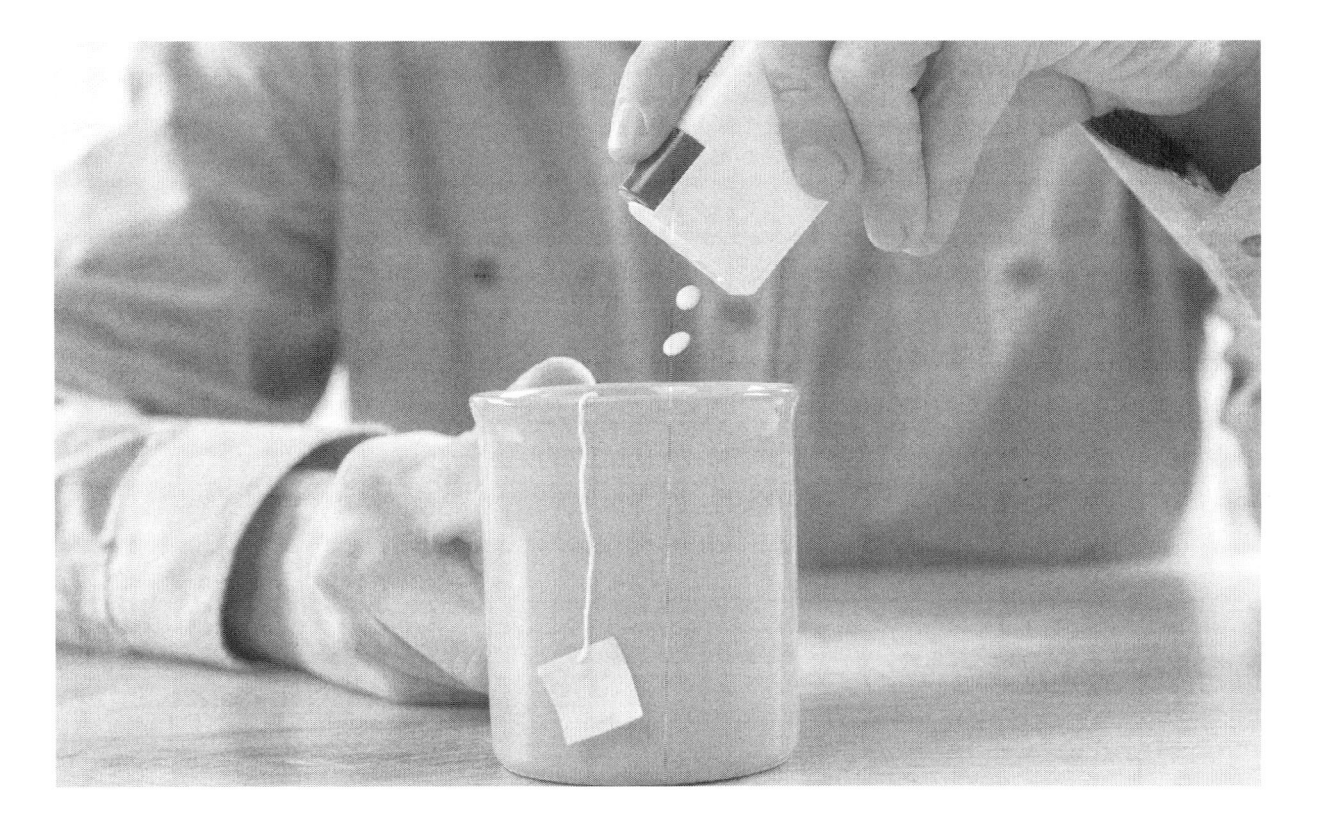

Because of the increased incidence of obesity, diabetes, and metabolic syndrome, and enhanced public awareness of the effects of regular sugar on these disorders, more artificial sweeteners were made and used by the public in recent years. They can generate very intense sweetness with few or no calories. The food industry uses them in foods, beverages, drugs, and even mouthwashes.

Most of these artificial sweeteners are not broken down by the body, and as a result, they often do not provide any calories for the consumer. For some people, these products are great alternatives to sugar. The potential decrease in calories and carbohydrates could help bring about long-term blood sugar control, weight management, and a reduction in cardiovascular disease risks.

Remember, artificial sweeteners such as Splenda, Stevia, and Sweet' N Low themselves may not add calories. Still, many foods that use these sweeteners may have other sources of calories and carbs. Label claims you'll see, such as "sugar-free," "reduced sugar," or "no sugar added," do not necessarily indicate that these are going to be carb-free foods. You must look at the entire nutrition facts label to understand how many carbs you are eating.

Do Artificial Sweeteners Help With Weight Loss?

Studies show that low-calorie sweeteners can actually help with weight loss unless people make up the calories they save with low-calorie sweeteners by eating other carbohydrate-containing foods. This has been researched, with most studies showing no weight loss among those using artificial sweeteners. Many people compensate for the calories made up by using artificial sweeteners by eating other carbohydrates and sugars.

The good news is that the current evidence also does not support the idea that artificial sweeteners can lead to weight gain, diabetes, or changes in appetite. If you use artificial sweeteners carefully without adding further calories from other carbohydrate-containing foods or beverages, it can significantly help your diabetes and weight management.

Do Artificial Sweeteners Cause Cancer?

No major studies show any evidence that the most common artificial sweeteners cause cancer. Saccharin, aspartame, stevia, and sucralose have been studied and proven to be safe.

Questions about artificial sweeteners and cancer arose when early studies showed saccharin caused bladder cancer in rats. However, results from the human studies that followed regarding this sweetener have not shown evidence of an association with cancer in humans.

What Are The Disadvantages Of Artificial Sweeteners?

Overstimulation of sugar receptors from frequent use of artificial sweeteners may cause desensitization of the taste buds, and so people may start to find less intensely sweet foods not as appealing; foods like vegetables (that aren't sweet at all) are almost unpalatable. As a result, this can, in turn, cause people to turn to high sugar foods.

Artificial sweeteners may prevent you from associating sweetness with caloric intake. Therefore, people may crave the taste of sweet foods. This can cause you to choose sweet stuff over nutritious food. This eventually leads to weight gain because more calories are eaten.

Like everything else, I would recommend using artificial sweeteners in moderation. They are not free food, and I would not use artificial sweeteners to make any beverage or food taste super-sweet.

What About Sugar Alcohols?

Sugar alcohols are naturally found in certain fruits and vegetables. Some of them can also be manufactured. Sugar alcohols do not contain any real alcohol (which is ethanol). You can easily identify sugar alcohols in nutrition labels because they all and with "ol", such as sorbitol.

Sugar alcohols aren't considered intense sweeteners because they aren't sweeter than sugar. In fact, some are less sweet than sugar. This can be an advantage because, as I said, having too much of a sweet taste can desensitize you from tasting the sweetness in natural foods.

Sugar alcohols also contain calories. However, they have fewer calories than regular table sugar. On the other hand, these benefits come at an expense as most sugar alcohols create gastrointestinal distress such as bloating and diarrhea. In summary, everyone uses artificial sweeteners these days—fat, thin, diabetic, and nondiabetic adults and children alike. Health awareness in the US and extensive marketing by food companies have increased the use of artificial sweeteners. They allow more food choices for the health-conscious population and increase the palatability of the many foods these are added to.

However, many of their proposed beneficial effects are still uncertain, based on the clinical studies we have so far. If carefully used by diabetic and insulin-resistant individuals, it may help reduce the total caloric intake. If total caloric intake does not go down with artificial sweeteners, using them may cause the exact opposite effect and can actually worsen insulin resistance and obesity in some cases.

How Much Pasta Can A Diabetic Have? Are There Any Pasta Alternatives Diabetics Can Eat?

Diabetics should stay away from pasta; however, there are many other alternatives such as Shirataki Noodles, spaghetti squash, and zucchini noodles.

You love pasta, right? But some of our favorite comfort foods like those containing pasta are detrimental to a diabetic-approved diet. My favorite alternative to standard pasta is "Shirataki Noodles." These noodles have many different names, including Miracle Noodle and Pasta Zero. The Shirataki noodle is made from a type of fiber called Glucomannan that comes from Japanese konjac yam. The noodle will take on the flavor of whatever sauce or seasoning you use along with it, making them extremely versatile.

The benefits of incorporating this type of noodle into a diabetic diet include the fact that glucomannan has been shown to help lower blood sugar levels in people with diabetes and insulin resistance. Because viscous fiber delays stomach emptying, blood sugar and insulin levels rise more gradually. The nutrients are much more gradually absorbed into your bloodstream. In summary, Shirataki noodles can delay stomach emptying, which may help prevent blood sugar spikes after meals.

One serving of Shirataki Noodles contains 15 calories and 4g of total carbs with 3g of fiber! That is only 1g of net carbs! Compared to 220 calories and 43g of carbs per serving of your standard box pasta.

*****Note:** These amazing noodles come in a variety of shapes like fettuccine, spaghetti, and rice! Yes! They also have this available in a rice shape!

Another great alternative to pasta for diabetics is spaghetti squash. This starchy vegetable has a yellow-orange color. Once cooked, it can be separated with a fork into strings that look like spaghetti noodles. At 6.5 grams of carbs per 3.5 ounces (100 grams), spaghetti squash only has about 20% of the carbs in the same amount of pasta. Also, squash is richer in vitamins A, C, E, K, and B vitamins.

Zucchini noodles (called Zoodles), Eggplant lasagna, and cabbage noodles are other alternatives to your regular pasta.

How Much Rice Can A Diabetic Eat And Is There A Rice Alternative For Diabetics?

Shirataki rice is a great alternative to white rice. Cauliflower can also be "riced" and is very versatile due to its mild flavor. These alternatives can help replace the infamous carb we all love to indulge in…rice. As mentioned, you can even find cauliflower in a riced form in the frozen section at the grocery store.

A little-known ancient grain called Farro can also substitute for rice in your dishes. Farro has a "nutty" flavor and is soft and chewy in texture. It's packed with fiber, protein, vitamins, minerals, and antioxidants. That's what makes Farro a "good" carb versus a "bad" carb, such as white rice. Since Farro has such high fiber content, it helps to prevent blood sugar spikes. A 1/4 cup serving of Farro contains about 140 calories and 27g net carbs versus 160 calories and 35g of net carbs found in white rice.

Quinoa is also a popular rice substitute with much more protein in it than rice and is high in fiber. A 1/2-cup (92-gram) serving of cooked quinoa provides 4 grams of protein — double the amount found in the same serving of white rice. Most grains don't contain all the amino acids to build a protein. However, quinoa has all the essential amino acids. The Glycemic Index of quinoa is much lower than rice, making it a great choice for diabetics to prevent blood sugar spikes.

Barley is a grain that's similar to wheat or rye. Barley resembles oats and has a chewy texture and an earthy taste. With about 100 calories, a 1/2-cup (81-gram) serving of cooked barley is equal to a full cup of rice, so you can enjoy more. Also, it contains a little more protein and fiber than regular rice.

Can Diabetics Eat A Potato? Is Sweet Potato Better Than A Regular Potato?

No! Absolutely, no! And sweet potatoes are not much better than regular potatoes either.

I get it. Who doesn't love anything with potatoes in it? Potatoes go great with many meat dishes like pot roast, but potatoes can put you over your recommended carb intake in just one serving.

So the next time you are looking to make mashed potatoes, try using cauliflower instead. You can boil, steam, or roast it. It's very low in carbs, making it a great option for diabetics and anyone following a low carb diet. Root vegetables like

Taro and parsnip are another great alternative to the traditional potato. Try steaming these alternatives and mashing them with garlic and other seasonings for a healthy side dish.

As I said, a great alternative to the potato for diabetics is parsnips. They have a sweet taste similar to a carrot. They are also very high in fiber content. Mashed butternut squash is also a very tasty alternative to potato. The last good alternative to the potato for diabetics would be mashed carrots.

Beware, sweet potatoes are not a good alternative to regular potatoes. Both will spike your blood sugar to the sky.

Can Diabetics Eat Oatmeal Or Cereal?

Cereals such as corn flakes, puffed rice, bran flakes, and pre-packaged instant oatmeal have a high glycemic index with a value of 70 or more. Alternatives with a low glycemic index of 55 or less could be steel-cut oatmeal, rolled oatmeal, and oat bran.

On hectic, busy mornings, many people rely on quick breakfast foods like cereal or pre-packaged oatmeal. Unfortunately, cereal can lead to blood sugar spikes after you eat them. Boxed cereals contain added sugars and are high in carbohydrates. Pre-packaged instant oatmeal is also loaded with added sugars that can throw your blood sugars into a frenzy!

Something to remember with any cereals or oats is the glycemic index. I'll talk about oatmeal and why steel-cut oats are better than regular oatmeal in a little bit. Many people don't look at oatmeal as a savory option, but it can be! Try savory oatmeal in the morning to switch it up. Top your oats with and an over-easy egg and incorporate some healthy veggies—season to taste.

Oatmeal is reasonably good if you want to have carbs in your breakfast. It's better than having white bread, and it's better than having pastries for breakfast. Oatmeal is an extremely heart-healthy food. There are substances in oatmeal that help your heart. All you need to understand is how many carbs you're getting when you eat oatmeal.

For example, one cup of cooked oatmeal is around 30 grams of carbs. So if you're only allowed to have 30 grams of carbs per meal, that's all you can have with that meal. You cannot have anything else, and if you start adding stuff on top of oatmeal, such as other fruits and bananas, then you have to consider those things as well since you're adding those carbs together.

Are Oatmeals A Low Glycemic Index Food?

Yes and no. Steel-cut oatmeal is a low glycemic index food because it is absorbed more slowly. This means that this kind of oatmeal does not necessarily spike your blood sugar as quickly. Yet, it will still spike your blood sugar if you have a high enough glycemic load; it's just doesn't do this as quickly as other oatmeals. That's a good thing because if you're taking medications, they sometimes take time to get into your bloodstream. If your blood sugar spikes before your medications kick in, that will be a problem, and you'll see some spiking of blood sugar.

The glycemic index of steel-cut oatmeal is good; it's below 55. On the other hand, not every oatmeal is the same. Regular instant oatmeal, for example, has a score of 79. This means that, among oatmeals, steel-cut oatmeal is the best choice, even though it takes almost 30 minutes to cook unless you have a pressure cooker, which only takes 5 minutes to cook.

I strongly suggest using an Instant Pot or pressure cooker that can cook oatmeal in less than five minutes. It's still not going to be a one-minute cooking time like you'll see with instant oatmeal. Although instant oatmeal still keeps the nutritional value of regular oatmeal, it loses all its fiber during manufacturing.

I know this might not sound too exciting, but you can learn to prepare them in a fast, flavorful way. If time is an issue in the morning, try to prepare a larger batch of steel-cut oatmeal and store it for the week ahead. Your Instant Pot will prepare steel-cut oats much faster with a lot less effort. Try adding cinnamon, nuts, and a sweetener such as Splenda. For some seasonal flare, season your steel-cut oats using spice blends like a pumpkin pie spice mix. Experiment and see what works for you.

I consider all instant oatmeal to be too heavily processed. For this reason, I would not recommend eating any oatmeal that is not steel-cut oatmeal. That includes rolled oats, instant oats, and any other oats out there.
Chia seeds are a wonderful food for people with diabetes. They're extremely high in fiber yet low in digestible carbs. I love a nice cold chia seed pudding topped with berries in the mornings.

Can Diabetics Eat Bread? What Types Of Bread Are Good For Diabetics?

A great choice for sliced bread is a "Sprouted Grain Bread," which is high in protein and fiber and easier to digest. Don't be fooled by whole-wheat pieces of bread. Whole wheat bread is different from whole grain bread and differs in its nutritional benefits. What you want to choose is a whole grain bread.

Bread and bakery items are also quite hard for my patients to part with. You don't have to completely break up with them! You just need to be smart about what options are available as alternatives.

Another option that's a great substitute for a bun or English muffin is almond flour bread. Did you know you can make one of these with just 90 seconds in the microwave?! The recipe is so simple anyone can make it, and again, it's quick.

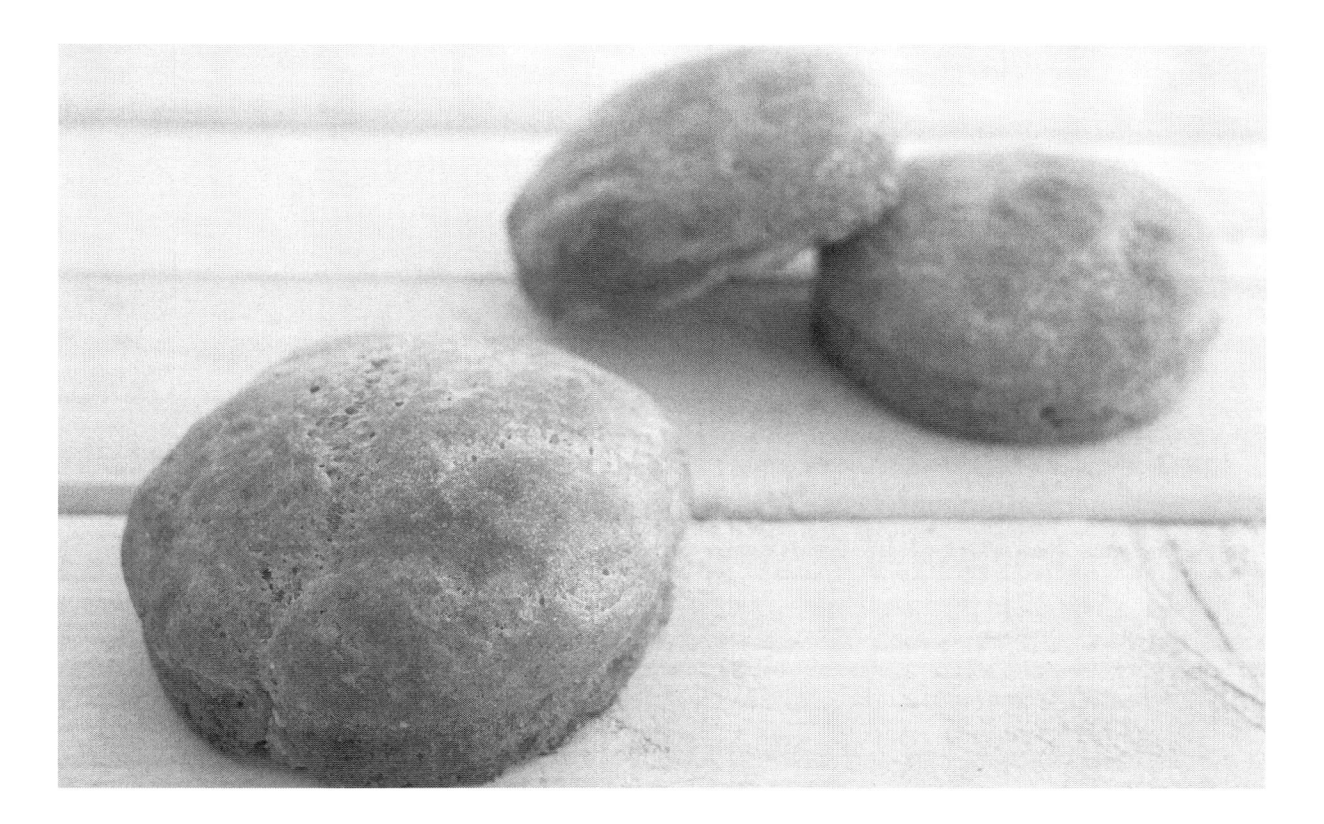

Mini-Almond Flour Bread

» 1 Egg

» 1 Tablespoon butter or oil

» 2 Tablespoons Almond Flour

» 1/2 teaspoon baking powder

To make these pieces of bread, which look like English muffins, just mix all of the ingredients in a small bowl and pour into a greased microwave-safe bowl or ramekin. Microwave for 90 seconds.

Flip out of the ramekin and slice in half. Toast them and butter as needed.

Other bread alternatives to white bread:

- ***Ezekiel bread.*** Ezekiel bread is one of the healthiest types of bread available. Ezekiel bread contains sprouted grains and legumes, including wheat, soybeans, millet, barley, spelt, and lentils.

- ***Rye bread*** is made from rye, a type of grain that is related to wheat. Rye bread is denser than regular bread, as well as much higher in fiber. Rye bread causes a slower rise in blood sugar than wheat bread. However, it also has a stronger, more unique flavor. You may need to acquire its taste.

- ***Pumpernickel bread:*** Pumpernickel is a type of bread made using a sourdough starter, rye flour, and whole rye grains. At least one recent study has shown that consuming pumpernickel results in significantly lower peak glucose levels than other bread, including white, whole wheat, buttermilk, and wholegrain bread. It also produced a lower peak insulin response than white or wholegrain bread.

Calories And Calorie Distribution On A Diabetic Diet

We've talked about carbohydrate recommendations but not about calories or the distribution of these calories in the optimal diabetic diet. There are some basic recommendations you should follow:

> » Men and active women: 15 calories/lb. minus 500 calories
>
> » Most women, sedentary men, and adults over 55 years: 13 calories/lb. minus 500 calories
>
> » Sedentary women and obese adults: 10 calories/lb. minus 500 calories
>
> » Pregnant or Breastfeeding women: 15 to 17 calories/lb. minus 500 calories

Patients should carry a log, which can easily be done via phone applications today. This helps keep track of total daily calories. The distribution of calories is also very important. A reasonable distribution of calories would be 40% of calories taken with breakfast, 30% with lunch, and another 30% with dinner. Although difficult yet not impossible, some individuals can skip dinner. Skipping dinner creates an intermittent fasting period. If possible, Skipping dinner can also allow you to be more successful at staying within your glucose control range.

You should always know your portion sizes and the number of calories you consume per meal. Consistency is another key factor in a good diabetic diet, especially for those taking mealtime insulin. If the calories and carbohydrates taken do not match the insulin injected, glucose control will be almost impossible.

For example, if you eat 60g of carbohydrates with breakfast and take 10 units of mealtime insulin today and then eat just 30g of carbohydrates tomorrow for breakfast, still taking the same 10 units of mealtime insulin, you will have a good chance of having low blood sugar the second time, especially if your sugars were stable the first day.

Let us move on to the fat content of your diet. You should understand that fat consumption can drastically increase insulin resistance.

For example, compare the person who eats a slice of bread with another person who eats a slice of bread with butter. These people will see a totally different blood sugar number when they check it. In reality, the carbohydrate amount is the same in both foods. *Remember, your body will need to make 30% more insulin for the same carbohydrate that is mixed with fat.* This is because the fat causes insulin resistance in the person's body.

But I Only Had A Salad...

Occasionally, my patients will complain that they only had a salad with chicken that day and that their blood sugar still went up. When asked, however, they will admit that they had chicken wings instead of chicken breast. Chicken wings contain a significant amount of animal fat, leading to insulin resistance.

As a result, even the small amount of carbs in the salad will cause blood sugar elevation due to the fat content of the chicken wings.

Dressing on the salads can also contain a significant amount of sugar and fat. Most patients ignore this fact and get frustrated over not being able to lose weight or control their blood sugars.

It is not uncommon for patients to be unhappy over not being able to lose weight or control their diabetes. They think that they are eating a lot of vegetables and fruits. A fact not commonly known by many is that eating too much food even with low carb content can trigger a glucose spike due to glucagon release. Glucagon is disproportionately released more than insulin after a large meal causing high blood sugars even after eating just lettuce. Also, many "high-fluid" fruits such as watermelon, honeydew, and grapes are high in carbohydrates when you eat a lot of them. This is called the glycemic load, as mentioned previously.

In summary, an ideal diet or the best diet for diabetes is composed of 30-40% of healthy low glycemic index carbohydrates, 30% of healthy proteins, and 20-40% of healthy fat, which is what we see in Mediterranean diets. _**The best diet for diabetes is also a diet low in calories. The only scientifically proven diet that reduces the risk of heart attack and stroke, along with lowering blood sugars and cholesterol, is the Mediterranean diet. Portion and calorie control, awareness of glycemic index/load, and consistency are the major components of diabetes control.**_

What Are The Other Important Things Besides Carbs In Anyone'S Diet Living With Diabetes?

- It's a good idea to get protein from lean meats, fish eggs, beans, soy, and nuts, and to limit the amount of red meat you eat. The recommended total protein for a sedentary man is around 55 to 56 grams per day. With advanced kidney disease, the protein intake may also need to be limited.

- Having a diet low in sodium and high in fruits, vegetables, and low-fat dairy products will help maintain good blood pressure control.

- Although artificial sweeteners do not affect blood glucose levels, I recommend consuming these in moderation in a diabetic diet. Beverages such as diet soda can be a short-term solution. However, the best approach is to avoid both sugar-sweetened and artificially sweetened beverages. Try instead to drink more water or electrolyte waters.

In the past, I have recommended to my patients that they not eat carbohydrates at all in their diabetic diet and that they limit their sugar intake to almost none. This is not true anymore. With the medications now available, lifestyle adjustments, and diet education, healthy carbohydrates can be a great source of energy in anyone's diet.

Do not fall for products that are labeled "sugar-free" or "fat-free." They do not necessarily have a reduced number of calories or carbohydrates. Read all nutrition labels carefully to see the correct amount of carbs in your diabetic diet.

Always compare your food choices with other similar products on the shelf to find out which product has the best balance of carbohydrates, fat, and fiber as well as total calories.

There are also some sugar-free foods, such as sugar-free gelatin and sugar-free gum. They have a limited number of calories, so they are considered "free foods." Also, any food with less than 20 calories and 5 grams of carbohydrate per serving is regarded as a free meal or snack, meaning that it does not affect body weight, nor does it require an adjustment to your medication.

2. Being Active

Exercise is crucial in managing diabetes. In type 2 diabetes, it promotes the necessary weight loss to maintain a normal body weight. In all diabetes, blood sugar can be maintained more effectively—mostly because carbs are burned instead of allowing excess sugar to be stored as fat. Blood glucose management with exercise in type 1 diabetes can be more challenging because of the necessary insulin adjustments you need to make. Still, nearly all of the same benefits are possible for type 1 diabetics as well. The benefits of exercise for diabetics and even those at risk for diabetes due to insulin resistance can be summed up in this list:

- » Can prevent or delay type 2 diabetes onset
- » Can reduce complications of diabetes
- » Better control of diabetes than medicine
- » Improves the activity of insulin
- » Reduced blood sugar levels
- » Promotes weight loss
- » Reduced blood pressure
- » Improves HDL (good cholesterol)
- » Prevents diabetes progression
- » Reduces medications needed for diabetes

All of these things are related to one another and add up to a pronounced reduction in long-term complications. _While having good blood sugars and reduced symptoms of diabetes is important, the main goal of treating your diabetes is to prevent complications._

How To Exercise For Diabetes

There are many aspects of exercise that one should consider before starting an exercise program.

Many Americans do not meet the recommended guidelines for physical activity. Just 39% of adults with diabetes are physically active. We define exercise as a moderate or vigorous activity that raises your pulse and breathing rate. This activity should last for at least 30 minutes, 3-5 times per week. The most common recommendation is 150 minutes of weekly exercise time. For athletes or those who intensely exercise during their workouts, the total duration can be shorter. For example, if you intensely exercise for 20 minutes a day, 3-4 times a week, you will have the same benefit you would see with moderate exercise of 30 minutes a day, five times a week.

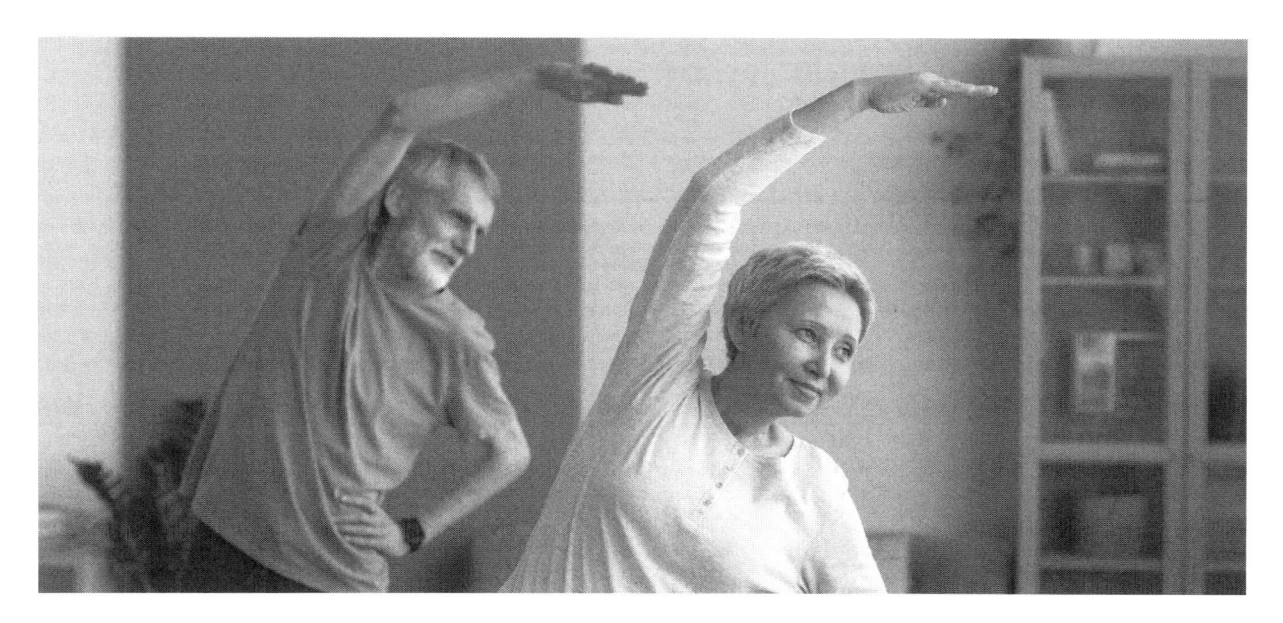

For most people with any type of diabetes, exercise can be undertaken safely; most also find it helps manage blood glucose levels effectively.

Consider being under the supervision of a doctor who understands exercise for those with diabetes, especially if you already have evidence of heart disease or poor circulation in your legs.

Activity Tips To Help Control Your Diabetes:

1. *Choose your favorite activities:* You can choose anything you enjoy doing. Things like walking, swimming, running, or gardening are perfectly acceptable. Think of activities you are more likely going to stick with over the long-term. For patients who are disabled or not able to easily move, I highly recommend learning sitting exercises on the chair.

2. *Take it slow.* No need to rush things. You are not trying to run a marathon next month. Start with five or 10 minutes of exercise and slowly improve your workout time to 30 minutes at a time, five days a week (or more, if you can).

3. *Don't overdo it!* During exercise, you should be able to speak short sentences during the activity, but you may not be able to have a conversation. That is the intensity you want to stick with unless your fitness allows for more intense exercise. Check your blood glucose before and after exercise. If the activity is more than 30 minutes, check it during the exercise to make sure your blood sugar remains in a safe range.

4. *Keep track of your activity.* This will help you keep motivated and encourage you to achieve your goals. Find a buddy if you can who you can exercise with. You can push each other to stick with the activity. Taking a class at the gym can also keep you motivated. Always be on the lookout for what the community has to offer. There may be a variety of activities in your local health club, etc.

How Do I Transition From Being Sedentary To Active?

I recommend moderate-to vigorous-intensity physical activity. This type of exercise for diabetes helps achieve aerobic and metabolic improvements. Yet, safe exercise participation can be complicated by the presence of diabetes-related health issues. There are many of these issues, such as cardiovascular disease, hypertension, neuropathy, and others not necessarily relate to being diabetic.

For those who wish to participate in low-intensity activities like walking first, your doctor may be able to help. He or she will use their clinical judgment in deciding whether to recommend pre-exercise testing. Commonly recommended tests before embarking on an exercise program include an ECG or cardiac stress testing. These should be completed in high-risk individuals before starting an exercise program.

Before undertaking higher intensity physical activity, almost all diabetics should undergo a detailed medical evaluation. It is important to account for blood glucose levels, physical limitations, and medications. Your doctor will search your medical history for signs of vascular problems. Vascular problems include problems with the heart, blood vessels, eyes, kidneys, feet, and nervous system.

On the other hand, asymptomatic individuals who are receiving good diabetes care are lucky. If they only wish to begin low-or moderate-intensity physical activity, they can, although it should not exceed the demands of brisk walking or activities of everyday living. If this is all the exercise they are doing, there is no need for medical clearance. So, it is very important to be evaluated by a diabetes expert before deciding to exercise if you are currently sedentary.

Developing A Structured Diabetes Exercise Program

Structured exercise sessions generally have three parts:

1. *Warm-up*—this phase includes doing 5 to 10 minutes of activity at a slower speed or lower intensity than your exercise will be. Warming up before moderate- or vigorous-intensity aerobic activity allows you to have a gradual increase in heart rate. It also helps you catch your breath more easily at the start of the exercise.

2. *Conditioning*—this phase includes activities you do to enhance cardiac and respiratory fitness, muscle strength, endurance, or flexibility. This is when you work at the maximal rate you have planned to do.

3. *Cool-down*—this phase lasts at least 3 to 5 minutes. It involves doing a lower intensity activity to help the body gradually recover from the

exercise. It also helps to transition your body safely back to a resting state. Doing so helps prevent blood from pooling in the arms and legs and removes metabolic waste immediately after exercise. It will also help to reduce fatigue and muscle soreness after exercise. If you are walking, for example, you simply slow your pace gradually until you are not short of breath, and when you feel your heart is slowing down.

Types Of Exercises That Are Helpful For People With Diabetes

There are two main types of exercise you might decide to engage in. Most endocrinologists will recommend doing mostly aerobic exercise and a little bit of strength or resistance training.

- *Aerobic exercise:* Aerobic exercise is defined as a continuous, dynamic exercise you do over an extended time period. With aerobic exercise, you mainly use your large muscle groups, such as your arms and legs. Examples include walking, jogging, biking, swimming. If you are interested in something different, you can do water aerobics, cycling, rollerblading, and skiing. Aerobic exercise is the most common prescription for diabetes management and prevention. The goal is to get your heart rate up, keep it elevated during the exercise, and do exercises that get oxygen to your active muscles.

- *Resistance/strength training:* Resistance exercise or strength training also improves musculoskeletal health and insulin resistance. It helps you maintain independence in performing daily activities. It also reduces the possibility of injury. Properly designed resistance programs may improve heart function, glucose levels, and strength. The goal is to strengthen your muscles through lifting weights or using resistance bands. Most people don't "bulk up" with these exercises but have stronger and more resilient muscles.

<u>Individuals with unstable diabetic eye disease should avoid activities that dramatically elevate blood pressure. These activities include intense resistance training, such as heavy lifting. You should also avoid jumping, jarring, head-</u>

down, or breath-holding activities. These can worsen the visual outcomes in those with unstable eye disease.

Before starting resistance training, individuals with diabetes and heart disease need to have an ejection fraction testing of >45% and a fitness level of 7 METs. These are determined through special testing with a cardiologist. Do not do resistance training if you have abnormalities in your ECG testing, serious arrhythmias, or symptoms of serious heart disease.

Safety Precautions For Diabetics Deciding To Undertake Exercise:

1. Warm-up and cool-down.
2. Careful selection and progression of exercise program.
3. Monitor blood glucose pre-and post-exercise.
4. During prolonged activities, adjust medications and food intake to prevent hypoglycemia.
5. Consult with your doctor about any changes you wish to make regarding exercise

Determining The Intensity Of Exercise For Diabetes

It is often a challenge for me to recommend a standard starting intensity range for sedentary people. This is because sedentary/deconditioned individuals often can improve their cardiorespiratory fitness at lower intensities. On the other hand, individuals with greater fitness levels to begin with typically require a higher minimum threshold.

I prescribe the optimal intensity range for my diabetic patients based on certain criteria. These include one's fitness level, duration of diabetes, degree of complications, and individual goals. Because of the high prevalence of cardiovascular disease in diabetes, I err on the side of caution when applying standard heart rate formulas to my diabetic patients.

The Rating Of Perceived Exertion (RPE)

The rating of perceived exertion (RPE) is another useful guide for estimating exercise intensity. When we use RPE, we recommend patients to focus on full-body feelings of exertion and general fatigue. While performing the activity within your target exercise intensity, I ask you to identify feelings of exertion and fatigue.

Rating of Perceived Exertion (RPE) Scale

Number		
2	I'm relaxed, chilling out, and watching TV. I might just take a nap.	
4	My body is moving, but it's all cool. I think I could do this kind of activity indefinitely.	
6	I'm definitely active, and I'm not sweating yet. I feel like I'm breathing a bit harder. I don't think I could do this all day	
8	I'm definitely sweating and breathing hard but I can still carry on a decent conversation while doing my activity.	
10	I'm a little uncomfortable, sweating, and breathing hard, but I can carry on a conversation for a brief period of time.	
12	I can talk a little, but I am breathing very hard and sweating a lot. I feel my heart rate is up there. I can still continue for a while though.	
14	Don't talk to me even though I can probably answer you. I am sweating profusely and am really working hard right now.	
16	There is no way I can keep this up for long. I can only grunt and am working at what feels like my maximal activity level.	
18	I am overexerting for sure, can't go on, and feel like this exercise might kill me.	
20	I feel completely dead and think I am going to die if I don't stop this immediately.	

Generally, a moderate-to-vigorous exercise intensity RPE ranges from 12 to 16 on a scale of 1-20. A high correlation exists between a person's perceived exertion rating (6-20 scale) multiplied by 10 and the actual heart rate during physical activity. For example, an RPE rating of 13 × 10 = a heart rate of approximately 130. This works best for younger individuals whose maximal heart rate (HR) is near 200 bpm.

This means that the RPE or perceived exertion may provide a fairly good estimate of your actual heart rate during activity. This practice does not apply to people taking medication that affects heart rate. The most common drugs in this area are beta-blockers, which artificially slow your heart rate at all times. Even so, your perceived exercise exertion is still valid to use with caution in these cases and among people with altered HR due to autonomic neuropathy.

How Long Should I Exercise To Benefit My Diabetes?

Do you want to burn the most calories and reduce your blood sugar more effectively? If so, you should perform lower intensity exercise for longer periods of time rather than shorter and higher intensity exercise over a shorter time period.

The recommended guidelines from the American Heart Association and the CDC are as follows:

- For older adults, they recommend 150 minutes of moderate activity (30 minutes, five days per week).

- For all other adults, they recommend 60 minutes of vigorous physical activity (20 minutes on three days).

- Most diabetic individuals will not be able to engage in vigorous physical activity due to physical or medical limitations. For these people, it is recommended that most individuals with type 2 diabetes perform at least 150 minutes of moderate aerobic exercise per week. This helps achieve optimal cardiovascular risk reduction.

- Add moderate- to high-intensity muscle-strengthening activity (such as resistance or weights) on at least two days per week.
- When adults with disabilities cannot meet the guidelines, they should engage in regular physical activity according to their abilities and avoid inactivity.

Individuals with diabetes should undertake physical activity for at least three nonconsecutive days per week. Up to 7 sessions of moderate activity per week will likely be even more beneficial. More exercise will improve glucose control and fitness. It will help in achieving target caloric expenditure. An exercise that is limited to 2 days per week generally does not result in significant improvements.

For individuals taking insulin, being active daily may help balance caloric needs with insulin dosing. Exercise also helps maintain higher levels of insulin sensitivity to allow for less insulin dosing.

In Summary

1. *Physical activity is a vital part of better diabetes control.* It has a positive effect on blood pressure and blood cholesterol. It aids in the prevention of type 2 diabetes as well. Choose an activity you enjoy! Involve family or friends in a swim class, biking, or hiking trip, even some Zumba.

2. *Contact your healthcare provider for approval of an exercise plan.* Let them know if you have high blood pressure or any other complications (such as neuropathy or arthritis).

3. *Wear diabetes identification.* Test blood glucose before and after activity. Create a network of friends and family who will support you. Ask them to keep you accountable, partner with you, and motivate you to get going. Make sure to talk to your healthcare team about your physical activity routine. Report any pain associated with it, any challenges, and the impact on your health.

CHAPTER 4 - DIABETES MANAGEMENT

4. ***Exercise with a frequency of a minimum of 3 days per week. Remember, the additional benefits are better if you exercise 7 days a week.*** Do not go without exercise for more than two consecutive days. Keep your total exercise duration to a minimum of 150 minutes weekly. Spread the exercise throughout the week. You can shorten the total time to as little as 60-90 min if you exercise more intensely each time. Move from moderate to vigorous activity as fitness levels allow.

5. ***Strength training 2-3 times a week also helps improve diabetes control.*** For resistance/strength training, you can use machines, free weights, resistance bands, and/or your own body weight as resistance exercises. Perform 8 to 10 exercises that cover all the major muscle groups. Try to do 3 sets of 8 to 15 repetitions is ideal.

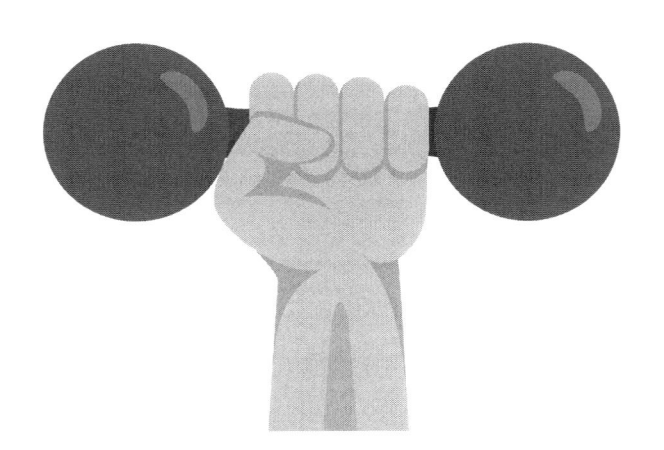

If you lift this weight 12 times:
This equals **12 reps.**
This will also equal **1 set.**

If you do this 10 times over again:
This equals **10 sets.**
It also equals **120 reps** total.
10 sets x 12 reps = 120 reps

Quick tip

If you are always wondering if you are getting your heart rate up, try purchasing a fitness watch or other device for monitoring your heart rate. These are great devices that don't need to be expensive. Some are waterproof, so you can track your fitness levels if you are into water activities.

Avoid Exercise-Induced Low Blood Sugar

Exercise-induced hypoglycemia can occur during, shortly after, or many hours after exercise. This means that diabetic exercisers should remain vigilant for its occurrence, including frequent self-checks or using a CGM device like Dexcom and Freestyle Libre.

Your endocrinologist can help you take measures to reduce early post-exercise hypoglycemia. These measures may include interchanging brief episodes of intense exercise (which tends to raise glucose concentrations), adding carbohydrate snacks such as 0.5 g/pound of body weight per hour, and reducing insulin doses.

Exercise increases glucose utilization by your muscles. Therefore, exercise can cause hypoglycemia in patients with near-normal or moderately elevated blood glucose levels at the start of the exercise.

3. Checking Blood Sugars (Monitoring)

Checking sugars are an important part of diabetes management. There is a lot to learn in a short period of time. One main source of confusion is how to check the blood sugar accurately, why you need to do it, and how often you need to check your sugars. Checking your blood sugars regularly is an essential component of proper diabetes management. Here are some facts you may want to understand about how and when you should check your sugars to improve your diabetes control.

These are the reasons why self-monitoring of blood sugars are so important:

- » Self-monitoring of blood glucose plays a key role in supporting self-care behaviors and decision-making in all diabetics.
- » Self-monitoring of blood glucose provides people with diabetes the information they need to assess how food, physical activity, and medications affect their blood glucose levels in the short term.

» Structured blood glucose monitoring schedules are necessary to help you interpret the effects of food, physical activity, and medications on glycemic control over the long term.

» In addition to blood glucose monitoring as a way to manage blood sugars, continuous glucose monitoring (CGM) has become a useful tool for filling in glucose data gaps.

In my opinion, the best way to monitor blood sugar nowadays is through continuous glucose monitoring systems that are available in the market. The systems mostly allow users to see glucose data through a device or even a smartphone app continuously without having to do a fingerstick blood sugar measurement. I will talk more about the CGM systems later; however, if your insurance covers these devices or if you can afford to buy them out-of-pocket, I would highly recommend using these devices to help understand your blood sugar patterns and how a variety of factors affect your blood sugars such as diet, exercise, stress, etc.

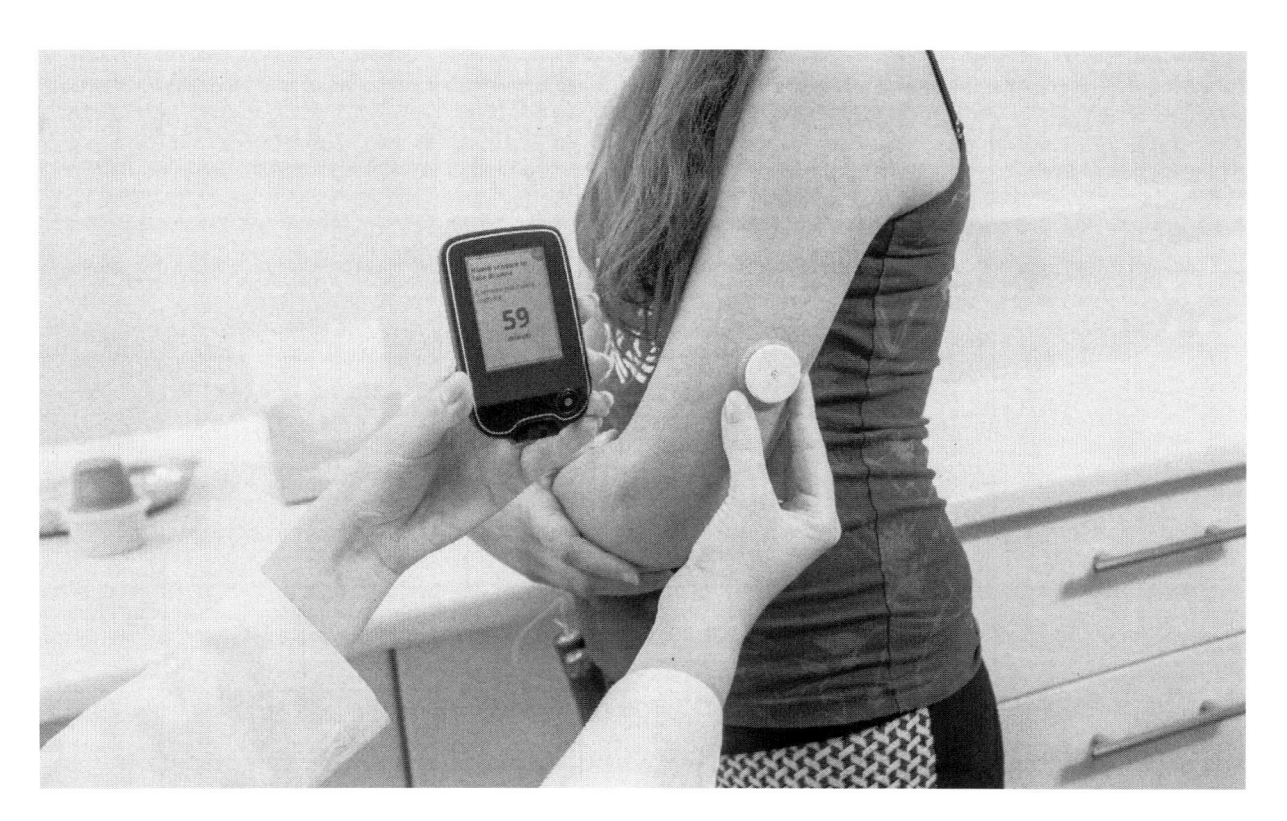

What Can Frequent Monitoring Glucose Do For You?

There are many benefits of this simple process that can make checking your sugars something you will want to incorporate as part of your daily program, just as you take time to brush your teeth, bathe, and take your medications. Some benefits you should know about self-monitoring are these:

- » Achieving and maintaining target goals for blood glucose levels. You may focus on the A1c as a general guide of how you are doing with your diabetes, but it's only through daily monitoring that you can get an idea of which things impact your blood sugar the most.

- » Preventing and detecting hypoglycemia (low blood glucose). Not everyone knows they are having an episode and the symptoms of both high and low blood sugars have some overlapping features. Any time you just feel "weird," you should check your glucose level to make sure it is normal.

- » Being aware of low blood sugar unawareness by preventing and detecting those low blood sugars, even when you do not feel hypoglycemic. Only through regular monitoring may you know that you are having an episode of low blood sugar you might otherwise be completely unaware of.

- » Avoiding hyperosmolar hyperglycemic state (HHS), which is a condition that develops when blood glucose becomes too high (such as above 600 mg/dL or 33.3 mmol/l), causing extreme dehydration and mental status changes. This might not be something that happens in a few hours but instead builds up over time. When you check frequently, you will be able to see when the trend is going in the wrong direction.

- » Evaluating the glucose response to types and amounts of food and physical activity. In that sense, you are an investigator of your own body; only by experimentation and trial-and-error will you know which things to do and which to avoid to have optimal blood sugar control.

- » Determining the appropriate insulin-to-carbohydrate ratios, correction factors (how much insulin is needed to correct your blood glucose level), and basal insulin rates for the intensive management of your insulin-dependent diabetes.

- » Adjusting your treatment strategy by paying attention to changes in lifestyle you need to make or changes in medical treatment/medications you may need to consider.

- » Determining the need for adjustments in insulin dosages during illness. Illness impacts your blood sugars and your need for insulin; anytime you are sick, you need to be more aggressive about checking your sugars so you can regulate your diabetes medications.

Many who take insulin for this disorder need to take it multiple times a day to have tight control over the blood sugars. This all depends on regular self-monitoring of your blood sugars.

You may decide on a schedule that works for you on an everyday basis but find some circumstances change your preset plan. These are the times where you need to consider increasing the frequency of blood sugar checks, so you have optimal control over your sugars in all situations:

- » Identifying and treating low blood sugar if you are on insulin or on agents that can lead to low blood glucose such as glipizide, glyburide, glimepiride.

- » Making decisions concerning food intake or medication adjustment when exercising.

- » Managing intercurrent illness.

- » Managing hypoglycemia (low blood sugar) unawareness.

- » Before performing critical tasks, e.g., driving. It is very important to check blood glucose before starting to drive and every 2 hours while driving.

> » Monitoring recommended glucose control during preconception and pregnancy.

From a practical point of view, the number of blood glucose checks you can realistically perform each day is often based on the number of strips covered by your health insurance plan. The following factors are those I think should be considered when helping my own patients determine their testing frequency and time:

> » For patients with type 2 who are low-risk for developing low blood sugar and in those who do not take insulin or sulfonylurea medications (glipizide, glimepiride, or glyburide), you should test once or less than once per day, depending on your needs and your physician instructions.
>
> » In type 1 diabetes and anyone on a multiple daily insulin regimen, checking the blood glucose levels four or more times per day is an accepted standard. Typically, I recommend that these individuals check their glucose before mealtime insulin dosing. Additionally, postprandial glucose checks (after meals) may be performed to monitor the glucose-raising effects of a meal.
>
> There is little doubt of the value of self-monitoring of the blood glucose levels for individuals who take multiple insulin injections per day, as the self-monitoring of blood glucose results are used to dose insulin or detect hypoglycemia. In fact, more frequent glucose testing is correlated with improved A1c levels.
>
> » Any hypoglycemic (low glucose) symptom also warrants performing a blood glucose check. Some individuals check their glucose levels before bedtime and before driving to ensure their safety. More frequent monitoring is beneficial during insulin dose adjustments, illnesses, pregnancy, periods of heavy exercise or physical activity, and when an oral medication and/or injectable medication or insulin is first prescribed.

» If you are a type 1 diabetic, self-monitoring of blood glucose 6–10 times per day should include: before meals and snacks, occasionally postprandially (after meals), at bedtime, before exercise, when hypoglycemia is suspected, after treating hypoglycemia until normoglycemic, and before critical tasks such as driving.

» For people with type 2 diabetes who are on multiple agents, including insulin, should test at least twice a day up to 6–10 times per day to include: before meals, occasionally post-meal, before exercise or critical tasks such as driving, and at bedtime.

» For people on intensive insulin regimen (taking long and short-acting insulins multiple times a day) should test 6–10 times per day to include: before meals and snacks, occasionally postprandially, at bedtime, before exercise, when hypoglycemia is suspected, after treating hypoglycemia until normoglycemic, and before critical tasks such as driving. On less intensive insulin therapy: more frequent monitoring (e.g., fasting, before/after meals) may be helpful, as increased testing frequency is correlated with improved glycemic control.

» Patients who are on only basal insulin (Toujeo, Lantus, Levemir, Tresiba, or NPH) alone or with additional diabetes medications should test at a minimum: a fasting level and a bedtime level. If you are on basal insulin plus 1 daily mealtime insulin injection or premixed insulin injection, you should test at a minimum: fasting and before taking any pre-prandial (before meals) or premixed insulin. It is also a good idea to periodically check sugars at other times such as before meals, at bedtime, at 3 am (when the sugars can drop), and additional testing before exercise or critical tasks, such as driving.

Once you have reached your A1c goal, less frequent monitoring is acceptable unless you are particularly prone to episodes of hypoglycemia or have some major changes in your lifestyle or medications.

In summary, individuals who are on daily insulin, a sulfonylurea medication, and multiple daily insulin injections should check their sugars more often at between 2and 8 times daily. The same is true during illness or when frequent low blood sugar problems are possible. Your physician will help you decide how often you need to check your sugars. If you know the factors that can affect your blood sugars, your commonsense will tell you when to check your blood sugars more often.

How To Make Glucose Testing Easy With Fingersticks And Get The Most Out Of Limited Data

- *Using an everyday 5- or 7-point blood glucose profile for the week periodically:* This involves doing pre-prandial (before meals) and postprandial (after meals) blood sugar checks plus bedtime blood glucose performed in 1 day. You repeat this every day for 5 to 7 days so you can have better insight as to when some of your blood glucose levels are out of the target range. This kind of spot-checking can be done to find a strategy that you can use (like knowing which foods to avoid in the future and whether or not you need a bedtime snack). You can repeat this strategy periodically.

- *Staggered 2 or 3 blood glucose checks per day for 5 to 7 days:* This is when you do one mealtime check, doing premeal and post-meal blood glucose checks for that meal. You would choose a different meal on another day. This is a good idea for those who have a limited supply of strips. Over a week, you would have two premeal and post-meal blood glucose values for each meal to evaluate during this time. For example, check your blood sugar before and after breakfast on Monday, before and after lunch on Tuesday, before and after dinner on Wednesday, and so on. This will give you a nice scatter plot to see what is going on with your blood sugars during the week after different meals.

- *3-point self-monitoring of blood glucose regimen:* This is when you check your fasting blood sugar, pre-largest-meal blood sugars, and post-largest-meal blood sugars in a single day. This can be very helpful to a newly-diagnosed type 2 diabetic. This regimen provides great information about your glycemic control when fasting and when eating a large meal. For example, you may wake up with a blood sugar of 100 mg/dL (5.5 mmol/l); however, if you do not check any other time, you may not realize that your blood sugars may be going up to 200 mg/dl (11 mmol/l) after dinner.

Ideally, those who find their post-meal blood glucose values out of the target range should work with a registered dietitian who can evaluate the meal composition and corresponding blood glucose results. The goals are to individualize your meal plan and avoid spikes after meals. This approach is in stark contrast to what is often seen in non-insulin-using individuals with type 2 diabetes who are directed to check their blood glucose once a day, first thing in the morning, before eating anything. For individuals with type 2 diabetes whose fasting values are typically in the target range, checking only fasting blood glucose offers little insight into the overall blood glucose control, so it might give you a false sense of your actual glycemic control.

- *An option for people using CGM:* Continuous glucose monitoring CGM) tools such as Dexcom, Freestyle Libre, or Guardian can help you monitor glucose values with less or no finger sticks. These are typically more expensive than a traditional meter and strips. You should check with your insurance provider about the coverage. Libre is relatively inexpensive, but Dexcom is more sophisticated and accurate. I'll talk much more about these later on.

Which Factors Affect Blood Glucose Levels?

You may have a lot of data from blood sugars you measure each day, but these are meaningless if you don't know which things generally raise or lower your blood glucose levels. If you are serious about making sense of the numbers you have, it's a good idea to match the numbers with a brief note about what you ate that day or how much you exercised. Some people use a phone app to keep track of all the information while they are on the go and don't want to keep a notepad or diabetes journal with them. The SugarMDs app is a great way of keeping track of blood sugars and sharing them with your doctor.

Which Factors Affect Blood Sugar The Most?

These things increase Blood Glucose Levels:

- » Inadequate insulin or oral medication dose—this happens when you eat more than the insulin can handle or not correctly counting carbs.
- » Other medications— such as steroids or beta-blockers for high blood pressure. See your doctor about this if you think it is a factor.
- » Stress (usually physical stress like illnesses like colds and other infections, lack of sleep, dehydration, etc.)
- » You have eaten more carbohydrates than you normally do at one time.
- » You are less physically active.

These things may decrease Blood Glucose Levels too low:

- » Physical activity more than is typical for you—you may need to adjust insulin.
- » Too much insulin or oral medications
- » Other medications—talk to your doctor about this if you have started a new medication.
- » Hours after physical activity—some physical activity (depending on the intensity) can lower your glucose significantly up to 24 hours following the actual exercise.
- » You ate fewer carbohydrates than you normally do at that time—this means that people who take a fixed amount of insulin should match their insulin and carb intake correctly. A diabetes coach can help you master this.

Even if you can't make sense of what's happening with everything you've documented regarding your sugars and lifestyle factors, a nutritionist or your endocrinologist may be able to help you. They are trained to spot the things affecting your blood sugar levels you may not be able to pick up on yourself.

Also, keeping a good blood glucose log and keeping an accurate log of what is happening in your life in terms of your diet, physical activity, possible illness, or stress can help your diabetes team to identify where the problem is. The SugarMDs app allows you to track all that.

Do You Really Have To Check Your Blood Sugar 7-10 Times A Day To Know Your Blood Sugar Is Controlled?

I often answer this question with an example like this one: Let's say you have just been diagnosed with diabetes, and you're very nervous about it and the possible complications of not getting the blood sugars well-regulated. You could certainly check your sugars 7-8 times a day but, after a while, you will likely burn out on this regimen. It isn't worth doing it continually because you'll get what you really need by doing it for a week or less.

You could also do the staggered method I talked about earlier, which is easier and cheaper to do. Just make sure you are organized and keep track of which meal was done and what you ate during the meal. When you share this information with your doctor or nutritionist, they will be better able to help you sort out what you need to know.

This is what your table of information might look like either on your paper log or your SugarMDs app:

Day	Fasting Glucose	Meal Chosen	Pre-meal Glucose	Food Intake	Post-meal Glucose	Bed-time Glucose
1	101	Breakf.	101	Toast and butter (2), two eggs, coffee with cream	142	115
2	90	Lunch	110	Ham sandwich, lettuce salad, iced tea, ranch dressing	163	132
3	93	Dinner	114	Porkchop (1), medium baked potato, butter, asparagus, tea	185	124
4		Breakf.				
5		Lunch				
6		Dinner				

It's okay to pick one hour or two hours after each meal, but you should be consistent about it and choose just one hour or two hours. Don't mix them up and document which choice you made so you can show this information to your doctor and have it all make sense. They can then tell you if you need to make any medication changes or if other recommendations are necessary.

Some people say, "Oh, my fasting blood sugar was 180 yesterday and today is 160. Why is that? " I tell them that both levels are still high and that what they eat, how much exercise they do, and what medications they take will affect these numbers greatly.

The bottom line, though, is that they are running high overall, so there is no point in getting hung up on 160 vs. 165 vs. 175. Don't worry about the particular numbers and concentrate on finding the trends. If your fasting blood sugars are always above 140 mg/dL (7.77 mmol/l), try to also check blood sugars before and after meals on different days to see if other blood sugar spikes are happening. This will allow you to see the patterns easier. Pattern recognition will allow you and your doctor to make better decisions to correct the high blood sugars.

Some people think that their 160 mg/dL (8.9 mmol/l) blood sugar sounds okay. They say they can live with that as a fasting level. They don't check any other times of the day. Then, when they check their blood sugar after eating breakfast, they realize that they sometimes go up to 250 mg/dL (13.9 mmol/l). This is something they would not have known unless they actually checked it.

The staggered method we discussed before is usually the best way to do it, especially if you have a limited number of strips, cannot afford strips, or just hate pricking your fingers.

How Many Times Do You Need To Check Your Blood Sugars At The Early Stages Of Diabetes?

If your diabetes is mild and your A1c is less than 7%, you don't have to check them too many times. You can simply check it once a day in the mornings just to keep an eye on your overall blood sugar numbers. You should probably check it after meals occasionally so you can see where your blood sugars are at other times of the day. Still, once a day in the early stages of diabetes is sufficient, especially if your A1c is under fair control.

Let's say you think that you just ate too many carbs, and you want to check on the effect of this. If you check it then, it can help you understand how food affects you depending on what you've eaten. If you are well-controlled overall, for example, and you're waking up with a blood sugar of 100-110 mg/dL (5.5-6.1 mmol/l) each time, you might check it after meals. If you then get a number between 160-170 mg/dL (8.9-9.4 mmol/l) after meals, you are probably doing well.

Can I Stop Taking My Blood Sugars If They Are Consistently Normal?

Some people do that and stop checking their blood sugars altogether. The next thing they know, they're in the 200s again. You don't want to do that either. So try not to be too obsessed, but also don't be too loose or lax about checking your sugars, at least occasionally. Be smart about it. Just find a middle ground. If you're checking it every morning and you get a blood sugar of around 120 mg/dL (6.7 mmol/l) every time, just stop checking it daily for a while and do it a few times a week.

If nothing changes in your diet or exercise levels, maybe check a fasting blood sugar once a week or less. Instead, consider checking it at different times of the day, particularly after a high-carbohydrate or other heavy meal. You will be able to use this kind of information to your advantage when checking a fasting blood sugar is not as helpful.

How Many Times A Day Should I Check My Blood Sugars On Insulin?

If you're on insulin, that's an altogether different story. If you are on basal insulin only, typically given once a day, I would suggest checking the blood sugar before you go to bed and then before you wake up. The reason for this is that it helps make sense of the correct dose to use, especially during the initial titration stage. You don't exactly know how much insulin you will need in the beginning. This means we pick a reasonable number and titrate up or down, depending on the goal and the numbers you get at home.

A lot of people don't understand why we're doing this. The reason is that the long-acting insulin is designed to keep your blood sugar stable overnight and during the day as well. Your liver is constantly making blood sugar, even at night. This is regulated both by insulin and your level of insulin sensitivity or resistance.

When you have diabetes due to insulin resistance, remember that your liver does not realize that there's some insulin present. Your liver will keep making too much sugar because it thinks you need it. To overcome your insulin resistance, diet and exercise will help, but it might not be enough, which is why you need insulin injections.

Basal insulin is a good first choice because you just need to check the morning and evening blood sugars. For those who are not ready to start a basal insulin injection, I sometimes use SugarMD diabetic support supplement for patients who are more naturalistic. It helps in many cases; however, it is not a replacement for basal insulin in all cases, especially not for type 1 diabetics.

If you are on multiple injections of insulin per day, however, it won't be a good idea to simply check your sugars twice a day. You'll need to know more carefully the effects of your meals and your injections on the blood sugars at other times of the day.

So, those individuals taking insulin more than once a day or up to 4 or 5 times a day will need to check their blood sugar at least four times a day up to 7 to 10 times a day. All type 1 diabetics and some advanced type 2 diabetics usually need to take multiple injections a day. This will usually mean taking one injection of basal insulin and three injections of shorter-acting insulin at mealtimes.

Because these individuals need to take multiple injections a day, they really need to know what their blood sugar looks like before they take their insulin injection. Fast-acting insulin types reduce your blood sugar very rapidly. There are two reasons to take this kind of rapid-acting insulin. One is for the correction of high blood sugar immediately, and the second is for the carbohydrates you eat at a meal.

Here's an example: if you're at 200 mg/dL (11.1 mmol/l) before eating, you need to know that level so that you can take a little bit of extra insulin with that meal. The same thing applies if your blood sugars are as low as 70 mg/dL (3.9 mmol/l). You may want to take a couple of units off of your regular dose at that time so that you avoid low blood sugar. You'll also want to make sure you eat.

Also, monitoring your blood sugar also helps you understand how you are doing overall. Let's say you check your blood sugar before breakfast and then check it before lunch. If your blood sugar goes up quite a bit every time you eat breakfast and it's still in the range of 160-170 mg/dL (8.0-9.4 mmol/l) by lunchtime, you know that you need to take more insulin for breakfast every morning. Checking blood sugars before meals on insulin helps you adjust your insulin; it also gives your doctor some important data to help them understand what's going on with your blood sugars.

How To Check Your Blood Sugar Accurately With Minimal Pain And Effort

- » Wash your fingers with warm water when you can and shake your hand below your waist before the fingerstick to increase the circulation. This may help with the pain because you will have to prick your finger deeper when your fingers are cold.

- » Make sure to get a fresh lancet (pricker) each time. Reusing lancets will make the needle dull, causing the puncture to be more painful.

- » Always use a lancing device to adjust the depth of the lancet (the prick). Lancing too deep will hurt.

- » You can gently milk your finger after lancing. Do not do it forcefully, which can cause false results.

- » Always stick the lancet on the side of the finger because the sides of the fingers have fewer nerve endings than the middle of the fingertips.

- » Rotating fingertips after each fingerstick will also reduce injury to the skin, thus reducing pain overall.

Which Glucose Meter To Choose From?

Most of the time, the glucose meter you choose boils down to your insurance coverage. On the other hand, glucose meter companies continuously improve their meters. In my opinion, you should pay more attention to the frequent monitoring of your blood sugars rather than the accuracy of the glucose meter.

Given that the best glucose monitor will naturally have a 5 to 10% error and the worst meter has a 20% error rate, I am unsure if paying the $50 difference per month is worth it. Concentrating more on pattern recognition and less on the exact numbers may give you better results. I am not saying you should go out and buy the worst meter on the market, however. It is just that this is not the most important factor in helping you manage your blood sugars.

If you can get a very accurate glucose meter, that would be great. If you cannot get the best glucose meter, it is still okay. If you can get a continuous monitoring system, that is even better. Then you will not have to do any fingersticks and have access to your blood sugars at any time during the day.

How To Record Blood Sugars Accurately And Quickly

The best way to record your blood sugars, in my opinion, is to use a meter that has Bluetooth technology and a phone application that can collect your blood sugars automatically. On the other hand, these may not provide enough information for you and your doctor. Your diet, your exercise, and stress levels all matter. As a result, we have developed an app called "SugarMDs" that helps to include these important factors.

For patients who are not technology savvy, you should consider a structured glucose logbook that is kept nice and neat so that it is presentable and legible. It should include information besides just your blood sugar levels.

The more information you include, the better will your endocrinologist be able to interpret your blood sugar values. Ideally, you need to record the blood sugar level in the first column, carbohydrates consumed in the next, medication taken next, and so on. See the example below. Unusual events should be noted, such as excessive physical activity, stress, anxiety, and medications that can affect blood sugar, such as steroids.

Date	Time	Blood Sugar	Fasting Y/N	Carbs Eaten	Medications Taken	Unusual Events
10/20	8 am	122	Y		10 U Reg insulin	
	8:30 am			39		
	10 am	169	N			Stressful day, anxiety
	Noon	150	N		15 U Reg Insulin	
	12:20 pm			45		
	2 pm	155	N			
	5 pm	137	N	41	15 U Reg Insulin	Worked out before dinner
	7 pm	141	N			
	9 pm	155	N		Basal Insulin taken	Bedtime early, tired
10/21	8 am	100	Y		10 U Reg Insulin	
	8:30 am			27		

Common Factors Affecting The Accuracy Of Blood Glucose Results

» If the sensor strip is not fully inserted into the meter, this can cause a falsely low blood sugar. Always be sure the strip is fully inserted into the meter.

» When the fingertip is contaminated with a sugary substance, the results clearly will be higher. This makes sense, right? Please wash your hands before checking your blood sugar or clean them with an alcohol wipe.

» When there is not enough blood on the strip, you may get a falsely low result. Warming your finger or rubbing the finger to bring blood to the fingertip can avoid this problem. Also, make sure to have the lancet device set at an appropriate depth.

» A commonly neglected problem is that the batteries are too low, giving error codes. Be aware of the battery level. Error messages do not always mean that your meter stopped working or is broken.

» Pay attention to the expiration date of your strips; obtain new test strips/solutions and store them according to the directions.

» Dehydrated individuals may have a falsely high blood sugar result.

» Do not squeeze the fingertip too hard to squeeze blood out if the blood is not flowing. This can lead to a falsely low blood sugar.

» Results from other sites such as the forearm or palm will not match blood sugar results from the fingertips. No matter where you measure your blood sugar, try to be consistent.

» Anemic individuals may measure a falsely high blood sugar than is actual. On the other hand, if you are diagnosed with polycythemia/increased hematocrit, you may find yourself seeing falsely low levels.

» Make sure your strips are still in good condition. Defective test strips can give inaccurate results. If you are not getting accurate results without any other explanation, try a new batch of strips.

Blood Sugar Monitoring Tips To Help Control Your Diabetes:

1. *Be regular about checking your sugars.* Checking your blood sugar levels regularly gives you very important information about your diabetic self-management. It also helps you know when your blood sugar levels are on target and when they are not. You will also be able to make more appropriate food and activity adjustments so that your body can perform at its best.

2. *Checking blood sugar should not be a chore.* Remember that monitoring helps to control your diabetes. Monitoring helps you

understand how different foods affect your blood sugar, and when the optimal timing is for adding activity. The timing of your exercise will impact your blood sugars in ways you need to discover through trial and error. It will also help you know if your diabetic medications are working.

3. *Look for trends in your daily blood sugars.* This will help you identify things like oncoming illness or times when you can predict that your sugars will be low. When you find these trends, you can modify your behaviors (like eating, medications, and exercise) so you don't have an episode of low or high blood sugar you can completely avoid.

4. *Check other things besides blood sugar.* Managing your diabetes means more than just monitoring blood sugar levels. You need to keep close track of your blood pressure, weight, cholesterol levels, heart health, sleep, mood, medications, and eye, kidney, and foot health at appropriate intervals recommended by your endocrinologist.

Trending Now: CGM (Continuous Glucose Monitoring Systems)

We will talk more in-depth about CGM systems in the last chapter, but I think it is reasonable to touch on this topic here while we are talking about glucose monitoring.

Continuous Glucose Monitoring (CGM) is a medical method that uses a device similar to an insulin pump. It is self-inserted into the skin non-surgically. The system then generates real-time readings of your glucose levels.

Traditional finger prick-testing of blood glucose levels give readings of your blood sugar level at a single point in time. It can't tell you what your blood sugar will be in an hour, and it can't tell you if your sugars are trending upward or downward. CGM (both Dexcom and the Freestyle Libre) allows users to see blood sugar trends anytime. Some CGMs do not even require finger-sticks for calibrations anymore. Dexcom and the Freestyle Libre do not require any calibrations or fingersticks.
CGM systems are easy to use. These monitoring systems are perfect for personal

use and are often recommended by endocrinologists because they are so simple and easy to use. People who live with diabetes can check their glucose levels with real-time readings anytime without fingersticks. CGM systems can be used with an insulin pump or independently just to track your sugars. Additionally, these readings can also be generated on a real-time basis or collected over a short time period.

Are Fingersticks Necessary On Dexcom G6 Or Freestyle Libre CGM?

While the companies that sell CGM devices say you don't have to do any fingersticks, this is only partially true. There will be times when you will still need to use this method of checking your blood sugars.

Here's what happens if you're using a CGM device: Any CGM is somewhat delayed when the blood sugars are changing rapidly. If you check a fingerstick instead, you will see that when your blood sugars are changing rapidly, your Dexcom will not give you an accurate number.

For example, when the Dexcom G6 says your blood sugar is low, this is usually an accurate assessment. So if you eat something for the low blood sugar reading, the Dexcom will keep saying your blood sugar is too low due to a delay in blood sugar measurement. If you keep eating to "fix the number, you'll soon see a blood sugar above 300 mg/dL (16.6 mmol/l).

The reason for this is there is a delay in the Dexcom reading, so you can't really rely on your CGM reading in the example above. Instead, you should eat something with 15-20 grams of carbohydrates in it. Then recheck your number in 15-20 minutes using a fingerstick measurement. Hopefully, you will get a number around 120 mg/dL (6.7 mmol/l), which is a good response.

Your Dexcom may still say your blood sugar is 75 mg/dL (4,2 mmol/l), but it should also show that it is trending upward, which is exactly what you've demonstrated with your fingerstick measurement. This is one reason why you should still have a glucose meter, even if you have a CGM device.

Is CGM The Right Option For Me?

Later I will talk in-depth about all CGM systems to help you understand them and help you make better decisions should you intend to buy one of these devices. For now, I will give you a quick summary.

Some people love the Dexcom G6, while others are perfectly okay with the Freestyle Libre system. When I ask patients' opinions on Dexcom versus Freestyle Libre, they have very little idea why they like one over the other.

Some people are already using an insulin pump to manage their glucose levels. They might believe that using a CGM system is not a necessity. However, CGM systems like the Dexcom G6 or Freestyle Libre are vital tools for managing diabetes. When used in conjunction with insulin pumps or even multiple daily injections, they can improve the quality of diabetes care. Both Dexcom G6 and Freestyle Libre have proven themselves to be accurate in making treatment decisions based on the readings you get.

If you identify with the following issues, then getting a CGM system such as Dexcom G6 or Freestyle Libre is the best option for you:

- » If you are unable to meet and maintain the optimal levels of your A1C results
- » You frequently experience low glucose levels
- » You are mostly unaware of your blood sugar level
- » You want to lower your A1C targets safely without triggering or causing a higher risk for hypoglycemia
- » Your blood sugar levels fluctuate frequently

Before you get a CGM system, remember to consult with your endocrinologist or seek help from a knowledgeable specialist who understands these systems.

The Benefits Of CGM Systems

Using a CGM system can make it easier for you to manage your diabetic condition and also live your life with more freedom. The following are the major ones:

1. *Lower your A1C levels*

   As an out-patient device, CGM systems such as Dexcom G6 or Freestyle Libre are the most effective in helping people maintain and lower their A1C levels safely. It's hailed as the best method for glycemic management for outpatient use!

2. *Detect lows and highs*

   With constant readings being offered, the CGM system can give fairly accurate readings about your glucose levels. We will talk about why I say fairly, since there are some problems associated with any CGM system in terms of correctness in certain conditions. The data gathered can alert you about your highs and lows before they occur. It can prevent people from experiencing hypoglycemia (low blood sugar) or hyperglycemia.

4. Taking Medications

In this section, I am going to talk about the medications and other treatments you might need as part of the management of your diabetes. Most diabetics will need some type of medical treatment to manage their blood sugars, even if they live a healthy lifestyle. There's nothing wrong with that. You just need to know the risks and benefits of each treatment and medication you are taking.

You will see how much research has been done in the past 50 years to help diabetics have better glucose control at all times. I will talk about all the drugs and treatments available—the good and the bad. As always, you should trust your endocrinologist to help you decide the treatment options that fit for you.

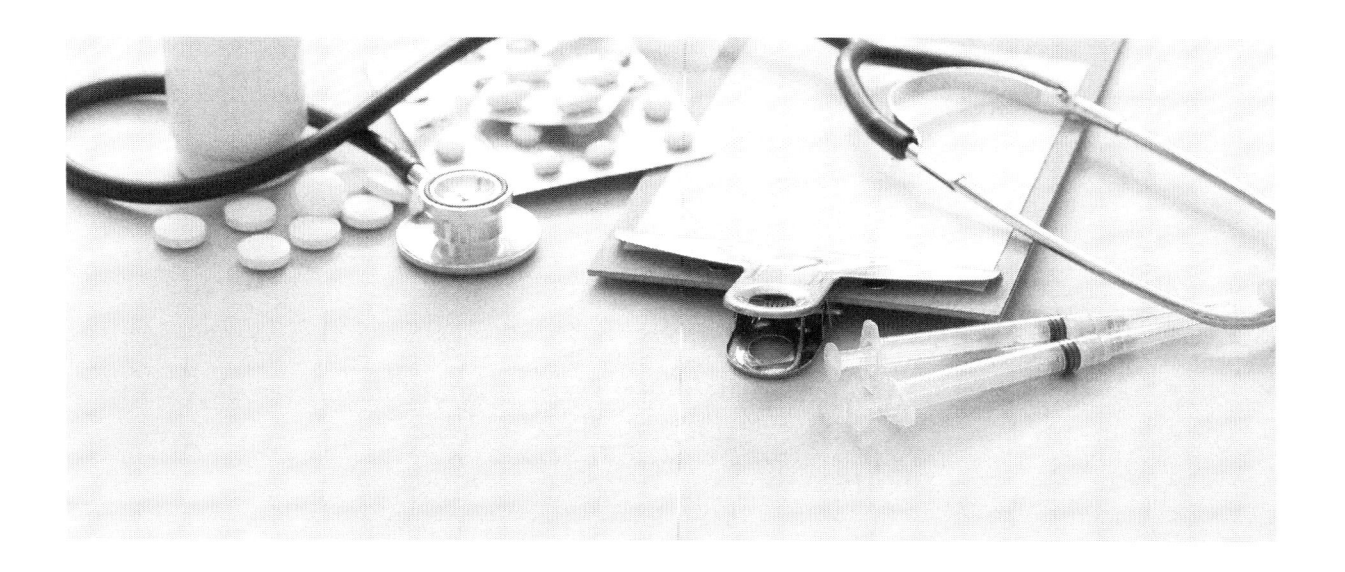

🖅 Fast Fact

The term "insulin" wasn't even invented until 1910, and treatment for diabetes has only been available since 1922 when the first person in the world received insulin for their diabetes. The first oral drugs for type 2 diabetes were invented in 1942 and were widely available by the 1960s. These were the sulfonylurea drugs; I will talk about them, too, even though many other drugs are available now.

Tips You'Ll Need To Optimize Your Medication Management:

- ***Know which pills you really need to take and why.*** There are several types of medications that are often recommended for people with diabetes. You might need pills, injections for lowering your blood sugar, medicines for blood pressure reduction, and pills for lowering cholesterol. Many of these are used to prevent diabetes complications like kidney failure, blindness, strokes, and heart attacks.

- ***All medications will have risks and benefits.*** It is a good idea to discuss the benefits and risks of any medications you are taking with your endocrinologist. You also need to remember that diabetes is progressive and that there is no shame in taking medications; most people need them. Many of these medications will mean the difference in your risk of adverse outcomes of diabetes (blindness, kidney failure, heart attacks, and stroke).

- ***Keep track of side effects and tell your doctor about them.*** Nearly all medications will have side effects, but many are not dangerous. Tell your doctor about all the side effects that you are having; he or she will tell you if you need to stop your medication or how you can avoid these side effects. Again, it's all about risk versus benefit. There are usually alternative medications you can use if you have a side effect you can't tolerate.

- ***Try to learn how your medications work.*** Every medication is different and, once you know how your medications work, you'll see the tangible effect they have on your body. You'll also know if a medication isn't working like it's supposed to. When you are dealing with a chronic disease like diabetes, you are your own advocate. Knowledge is power when dealing with diabetes and the medications used to treat it.

- *Ask for help.* Diabetes is expensive to manage. If you are having trouble affording your medications, do not hesitate to ask for help. If it is too hard for you to keep up with costs, there are programs to help make medications more affordable. Ask for help before you decide to ration your diabetic medications. Also, tell your doctor if you are taking herbal medications or medications you get over the counter.

Medications That Affect Blood Sugars

This is a brief summary of the different drugs that act to reduce blood sugars in diabetic patients:

Overview of Diebetes Drugs

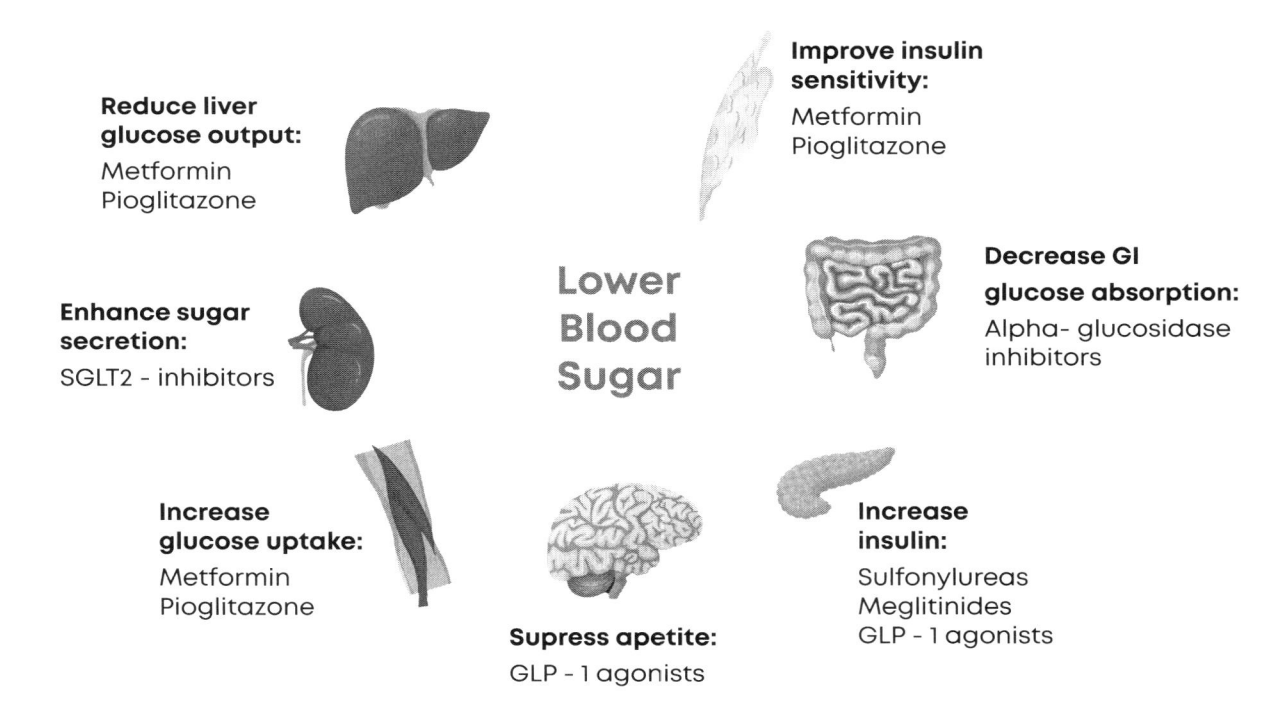

Reduce liver glucose output:
Metformin
Pioglitazone

Improve insulin sensitivity:
Metformin
Pioglitazone

Enhance sugar secretion:
SGLT2 - inhibitors

Decrease GI glucose absorption:
Alpha- glucosidase inhibitors

Increase glucose uptake:
Metformin
Pioglitazone

Increase insulin:
Sulfonylureas
Meglitinides
GLP - 1 agonists

Supress apetite:
GLP - 1 agonists

Lower Blood Sugar

Generic Drugs For Diabetes

There are few classes of medications on the market today that are generic. Some of them are very useful, while others have a lot of problems associated with them. Branded drugs are certainly not free of problems, but I think research and development in recent years have helped us dramatically improve the quality of diabetes care.

It's a lot like cars. Cars in the 1960s can be compared to the cars of today. Both have four tires and a steering wheel but, even though they seem to be doing the same job, your experience in driving these two types of cars will be totally different.

I will try to educate you and eliminate some of the misconceptions you may have about these drugs from hearing or seeing different things from the internet or media.

Sulfonylureas And Meglitinides: Why You Shouldn'T Use Them As First-Line Agents

Some of the most commonly prescribed medications historically for diabetes have been the sulfonylureas (glipizide, glimepiride, glyburide) and meglitinides (repaglinide, nateglinide). They are generally taken once or twice a day, 30 minutes before a meal. You can take sulfonylureas on their own or alongside other diabetes drugs such as metformin.

How Do The Sulfonylureas Work?

Sulfonylureas and meglitinides directly stimulate the release of insulin from the pancreas, reducing blood sugar levels. Because they work by stimulating insulin secretion, they are useful only in patients with some remaining pancreatic function.

Since insulin production becomes continuous and is not based on the glucose levels, the person has to eat in order to prevent low blood sugars after taking the drug. They work by stimulating your pancreas to make insulin in a non-glucose dependent manner. This means the pancreas puts out insulin regardless of your blood sugar values. As a result, one of the main side effects of sulfonylureas is low blood sugar (below 70 mg/dL or 3.9 mmol/l). This is the opposite of what we want in diabetes management. People are supposed to restrict carbs, but with these drugs, the appetite increases, so the individual puts on weight.

Due to the continuous insulin production by the pancreas, the main side effects of these sulfonylurea drugs are low blood sugar and weight gain. This is because insulin promotes the storage of the fuel/nutrients you eat. There are many other long term side effects of these sulfonylurea drugs I will talk about in this section.

I don't think the sulfonylurea drugs are necessarily the best medications for diabetes, especially now. They have been on the market for a long time, and there are many other options for you other than these. The side effects and problems associated with sulfonylureas have become more and more clear over time. The most common side effects of any medications of this class are weight gain and hypoglycemia (low blood sugar), beta-cell failure, and possible heart-related complications.

Why Do Sulfonylureas Have Such A Bad Reputation?

In addition to the weight gain and low blood sugar seen as side effects of these drugs, there is some scientific evidence out there that makes them less popular. Here are a few examples:

1. Beta cells are the main insulin-producing cells in the pancreas. Sulfonylureas may speed up this pancreatic beta-cell failure.

   Pancreatic beta-cell cell death is a key feature in the progression of diabetes and poor long-term diabetes outcomes. As the pancreas loses the ability to secrete insulin due to beta-cell exhaustion, patients end up needing insulin earlier rather than later. This is exactly what the sulfonylureas do; they exhaust the pancreas. Within 1 to 2 years, sulfonylureas begin to lose their effectiveness in some patients.

2. Some studies suggest that treatment with sulfonylureas may be associated with side effects and poorer outcomes in patients who have a heart attack as well. This is especially true for glyburide. All of the drugs of this class have been linked to more heart attacks and a higher rate of premature death.

Sulfonylureas And Low Blood Sugars

If you are on glipizide, glimepiride, or glyburide, you have to be careful about those situations in which hypoglycemia (low blood sugar) is most likely to occur. They are as follows:

- » After exercise or if you miss a meal.

- » When the medication dose is too high (if you have frequent low blood sugars, you should reduce the dose of these drugs).

- » With the use of longer-acting drugs like glyburide or extended-release forms of these drugs. Glyburide has the highest risk of low blood sugar among the sulfonylureas.

- » If you are undernourished or have alcohol intoxication.

- » Should you have impaired kidney or heart function or gastrointestinal disease, you also be careful using drugs.

- » With other drugs at the same time, such as salicylates, sulfonamides, fibric acid derivatives (such as gemfibrozil), and warfarin. These drugs make it harder to get rid of the sulfonylureas in your system.

- » After being in the hospital. Your medication needs may change after hospital admission.

On the other hand, people with certain subtypes of MODY are the only perfect candidates for sulfonylurea medications. Others with diabetes benefit far more from other classes of drugs and not necessarily from this drug class.

Now I will talk about the many other types of diabetes medications that do not cause weight gain, including those that can actually lead to significant weight loss. Also, many other diabetic medications do not have low blood sugar as a side effect either. Since we can choose medications that can lead to weight loss and without the risk of low blood sugar, most endocrinologists agree that there is more benefit from using sulfonylurea drugs.

Metformin: Advantages And Disadvantages

Metformin is a "first-line" medication for type 2 diabetes mellitus. This means it is one of the first drugs doctors prescribe for diabetes. It is also used for prediabetes, gestational diabetes, and polycystic ovarian syndrome. It works by reducing glucose production in the liver, increasing glucose uptake by the cells, and decreasing glucose absorption by the GI tract. As a result, the overall insulin secretion by the pancreas is less, which is beneficial in reducing insulin resistance.

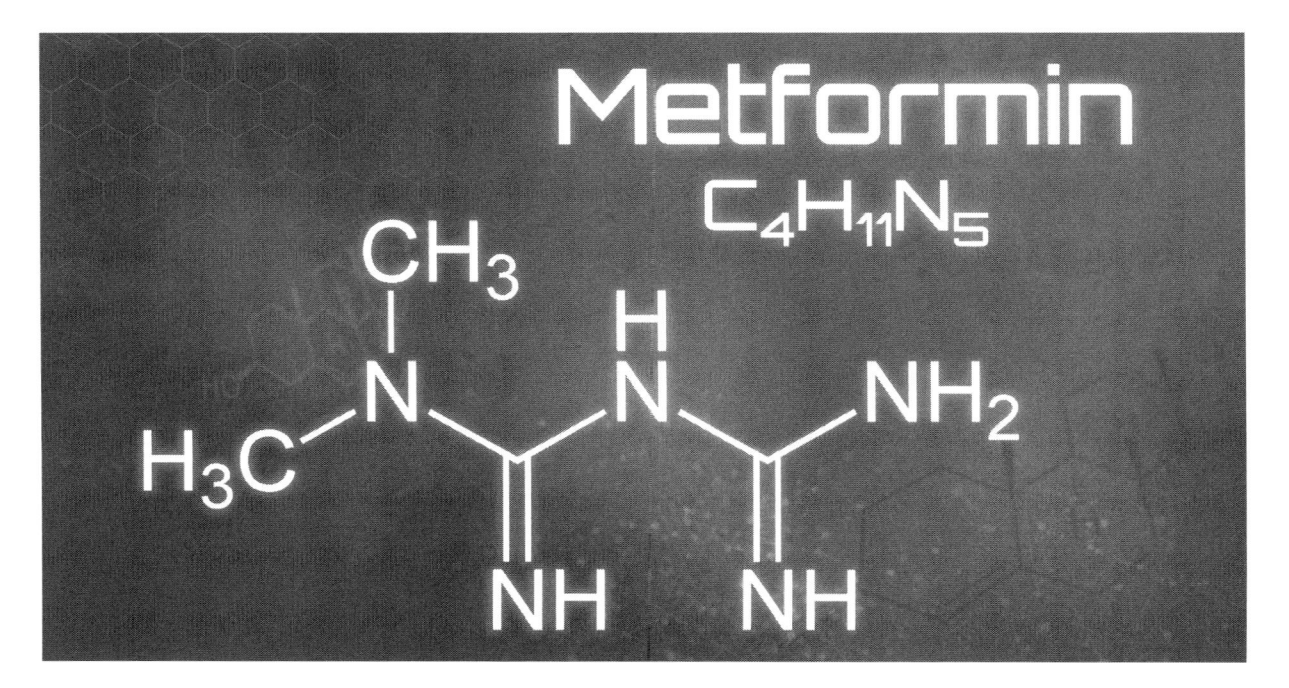

While metformin is a commonly used drug for diabetes and prediabetes, there are many *misconceptions* about using it. Some of these falsehoods include the following:

- *Metformin can damage your kidneys and liver*—the truth is that metformin can be used even if you have advanced kidney disease (stage 3 or better) as part of your diabetes.

- *Metformin can cause dementia*—the truth is that even people with dementia can safely take metformin.

- *Metformin is harmful during pregnancy*—while metformin does reach the baby through the placenta, there is no known risk of birth defects or pregnancy complications if this medication is taken in pregnancy.

- *You cannot use metformin if you have heart disease*—in truth, metformin taken for diabetes actually reduces the risk of heart attacks, especially if started early in the disease process. It is only avoided in those with sudden heart failure who are in the hospital.

- *Metformin can increase cholesterol levels*—the truth is that the LDL (bad) cholesterol drops after starting metformin. The triglyceride level levels and HDL (good) cholesterol levels increase. These are advantages of taking metformin that help reduce the chances of stroke and heart attacks.

- *Metformin can increase the cancer risk*—actually, metformin has been found to reduce the risk of many types of cancer.

- *Metformin can damage the pancreas*—metformin doesn't damage the pancreas and will reduce the chances of getting pancreatic cancer.

When Should Metformin Be Avoided?

There are situations where you should avoid taking metformin. If you have severely impaired renal function should not take metformin. If your kidney function (as measured by the glomerular filtration rate or GFR) is below 30 (stage IV kidney disease), you should stop taking metformin or not start it at all.

Active or progressive liver disease can be a problem as well if you are taking metformin. Uncontrolled or active liver disease can cause metformin to build up in the bloodstream. On the other hand, if you just have abnormal liver tests from fatty liver, you can take this medication. Chronic liver disease that is stable also not a reason to stop taking metformin.

Active alcohol abuse is another reason to avoid taking metformin. This is because acute liver failure can happen at any time when you abuse alcohol. You can still drink socially, but if you have a problem with excessive alcohol use, you should tell your doctor about this.

If you've ever suffered from lactic acidosis (low pH in the blood)) during metformin treatment, you should not take this medication as it can come back when you take it again.

Metformin Side Effects

Metformin can cause a metallic taste in the mouth, mild reduction in appetite, nausea, abdominal discomfort, and diarrhea. On the bright side, most of these gastrointestinal side effects are temporary, lasting anywhere from 1 to 3 weeks in most people who take it. There are some, however, who will have lasting side effects when taking this medication. Talk to your doctor if you have severe or lasting symptoms.

These are a few things you need to do to avoid problems when taking this drug:

- ***Check your B12 levels.*** Because metformin can reduce your vitamin B12 levels, you should have these checked periodically. Low B12 levels can cause neuropathy or numbness in your feet and legs. Have this level checked every year or if you have new symptoms of neuropathy.

- ***Be aware of the chances of lactic acidosis.*** This is an uncommon side effect of metformin but might happen if you have acute kidney failure, sudden liver failure, or active heart failure and also take metformin.

- ***Rare side effects of metformin.*** These include chest pain, flushing, rash, headache, stuffy nose, cold-like symptoms, or excessive sweating. Call your doctor if you have any of these symptoms and you think it's from taking metformin.

There are things you can do to reduce these side effects. You should always start slow, especially if you are concerned about side effects. Some people take doses as low as 500 milligrams once weekly before gradually increasing the dose to 1 gram (1000 milligrams) twice a day, which is a common target amount to take. Here are some other tips for reducing the side effects of the drug:

  » Start taking no more than 500 mg a day.

  » Start taking metformin always with meals.

  » The evening meal is the best time to start taking metformin.

- » If you are taking instant release tablets, swallow them whole. Do not try to chew, crush, or break the tablet.

- » If you have a swallowing problem, talk to your endocrinologist. A suspension for metformin is also available. For the suspension, you will need to shake it well before using it.

- » Only titrate the metformin dose upward after side effects subside

- » You can increase the metformin to 500 mg twice a day with meals only if metformin 500 mg is tolerated with the evening meal.

- » If twice a day is tolerated with 500 mg tablets, you can increase it to 2 tablets twice a day for maximum efficacy.

- » More than 2000 mg of metformin will not be any more effective than taking 2000 mg per day of the drug.

- » Sometimes giving a break to taking metformin for a few weeks may help reduce your diarrhea. Restarting metformin may not give diarrhea again after his break.

- » If diarrhea happens or you are throwing up, call your doctor. You will need to drink more fluids to keep from losing too much fluid.

- » If you are 65 or older, use this drug with care. You could have more side effects.

You can also take metformin with meals or use the extended-release form of the drug. These changes will make a big difference in the side effects you experience when taking metformin. The extended-release form is still cheap and better tolerated than the regular formulation of this medication. Look for the name "ER" after the drug name on your bottle. If you don't see that, talk to the pharmacist or your doctor about changing the prescription.

Metformin And Weight Loss

Weight loss when taking metformin is definitely possible, but it varies from person to person. Insulin-resistant people who take it for six months and are overweight can lose up to 12 pounds of body weight, although most diabetics will typically lose just 1-2 pounds after six months of use. It also seems to depend on how insulin-resistant you are. The more insulin-resistance, the more effective is the weight loss seen with this drug.

There are a couple of reasons why metformin helps with weight loss in diabetes. Because it helps reduce the blood sugar level using non-insulin mechanisms, it reduces the amount of insulin you need to make; fewer glucose molecules get turned into stored fat as a result. The abdominal fat cells see less insulin in your body, so they don't fill up with fat as easily when you take metformin.

Another positive effect of metformin that promotes weight loss is a reduction in your appetite. Up to about 5 percent of your body weight is possible, depending on your situation.

Metformin And Diarrhea

One of the most common side effects of metformin is diarrhea, although it will usually be temporary, and there are things you can do to avoid this side effect. Up to 25 percent of people taking metformin will have some GI side effects, and up to 10 percent of people can't tolerate the medication at all. No one knows why some people do well on metformin and others don't, but it could be a hereditary thing we cannot control.

Metformin decreases glucose uptake by the intestines. It means that lactic acid can build up in the GI tract, causing it to be irritated. Metformin increases the production of incretin hormones, which can also lead to diarrhea. Bile acids increase as well, which can affect your stools. The bacteria in your gut change; this would normally be helpful, but in this case, it leads to a higher chance of diarrhea. Lastly, metformin activates the receptors in the GI tract that respond to serotonin. More serotonin is released so that you'll have a chance of diarrhea, nausea, and vomiting.

Other gastrointestinal side effects are nausea, vomiting, and increased gas. Some people will have chest discomfort unrelated to a heart or lung problem. As mentioned, you might rarely see palpitations or flushing. About 6 percent of people will have headaches, and 10 percent of people notice a change in their ability to taste food.

The Bottom Line On Metformin

Metformin has been used effectively to treat diabetes for many years. Doctors have lots of experience taking it, and there is a lot of medical research showing it is safe and effective for gestational diabetes and prediabetes as well as type 2 diabetes. It is inexpensive and often the first medication used for the treatment of diabetes, partly because it also reduces the risk of many cancers and heart disease.

Slight weight loss is often seen among people who take it. There is also good evidence to suggest it will prolong your life. It's for these reasons that I don't hesitate to prescribe this medication for those who need it.

My approach to prescribing this drug is to use a limited dose of metformin (up to 1000 milligrams per day) if you have a GFR of between 30 and 44 (and no active kidney disease). If the GFR is less than 30, I stop the medication. I also stop metformin if a person needs to take intravenous contrast dye for an x-ray procedure. This is because kidney failure can happen in those who need to have contrast dye; it helps if the person isn't already taking metformin should this happen.

I monitor all my patients on metformin by measuring their A1c every 3-6 months and the kidney function and B12 levels annually. B12 deficiency is more common among those who've taken the drug for a long period of time (at least five years), people who've had bariatric surgery, and individuals who eat a vegetarian or vegan diet.

Because of the side effects of metformin, I use SugarMD Advanced Glucose Support for my patients who do not want to deal with these side effects. Everyone is different, and my role is to respect and accommodate each of my patients based on their individual needs and wishes.

Pioglitazone - Good Or Bad?

Pioglitazone goes by the brand name of Actos. It was approved by the FDA in 1999 for the treatment of type 2 diabetes. It belongs to a class of drugs called thiazolidinediones. Rosiglitazone was once used commonly but fell out of favor after some conflicting data following an aftermarket study. These drugs increase insulin sensitivity by acting on fat and muscle tissue to increase their uptake of glucose. This reduces the available glucose in the bloodstream. It also decreases the production of glucose by the liver (a minor effect).

Generally, pioglitazone and rosiglitazone are not prescribed as initial therapy in people who have type 2 diabetes. It is definitely not indicated for patients with type 1 diabetes because they need to have insulin as their only therapy. On the other hand, pioglitazone may still offer an advantage in severe insulin resistance for people who've had nonalcoholic fatty liver disease (NASH) or those with a history of a recent stroke.

People who should not take pioglitazone include:

- » People who have heart failure or any evidence of fluid overload
- » Diabetics with a history of fracture or at high risk for fracture (more common in women)
- » People with diabetes who have active liver disease (liver enzymes > 2.5 times above the upper reference limit)
- » Anybody with an active or history of bladder cancer
- » Type 1 diabetics
- » Diabetes during pregnancy

I typically start at 15 mg daily if, after a few weeks, there is inadequate control based upon fasting blood glucose values, I increase the daily dose by 15 mg up to the maximum dose of 45 mg daily. However, the side effects of weight gain and edema likely to happen at higher doses.

Most Common Adverse Reactions From Pioglitazone (Actos)

You can expect the following adverse reactions from pioglitazone (Actos):

- » Swelling, mostly around the ankles
- » Low blood sugar if combined with a sulfonylurea or insulin. You should increase the frequency of blood sugar checks every time you start any antidiabetic medication.
- » Increased risk of catching a cold, upper respiratory infection, etc.
- » Increases risk of heart failure if taken together with insulin.
- » Headaches may increase. The reason for increased headaches is unknown.
- » Potential increased risk of bone fractures, especially in postmenopausal women
- » Potential weight gain if used by itself or combined with insulin or sulfonylureas

Other common risks include weight gain, heart failure, and possibly a small increase in the risk of bladder cancer. This means you need to fully understand the risks and benefits of taking this class of medications.

Lower doses should be used when possible to minimize potential adverse effects, especially when it comes to weight gain and edema. As a general principle, I try to individualize the choices and doses I recommend for those with type 2 diabetes mellitus.

On the other hand, nowadays, we use rosiglitazone only rarely because of the concern about research showing a possible increased risk for cardiovascular events.

Is Pioglitazone Effective And Are There Risks To Worry About?

When thiazolidinediones like pioglitazone are used as the only therapy for a person's diabetes, the expected decrease in A1C is approximately 0.5 to 1.4 percent. In some cases, that can be even more than 2% if the initial A1c level is more than 10%. Both pioglitazone and rosiglitazone increase the risk of heart failure, especially when used with insulin.

People with type 2 diabetes mellitus and biopsy-proven nonalcoholic fatty liver disease (NASH) can improve the inflammation in the liver after using pioglitazone. Remember that fatty livers are usually the result of excessive abdominal weight gain.

Pioglitazone improves blood glucose primarily by increasing insulin sensitivity. This means that it is much less likely to cause low blood sugar (hypoglycemia) when used alone compared to sulfonylureas or insulin.

On the other hand, there is significant evidence that pioglitazone can reduce bone density and increase the risk of fractures, particularly in older women. The real risk for each person, however, is small. This means you are not guaranteed at all to have a fracture because you're taking this medication. I do not use it in women who have known low bone density or other risks for fractures.

There are some concerns about the association between bladder cancer and pioglitazone (Actos), although at best, this association is controversial, and studies on the issue have shown conflicting results. As a reasonable precaution, I do not use pioglitazone in patients with active bladder cancer. One study showed a link between the use of this drug and bladder cancer among those who took it for an average of only two years.

The Bottom Line

To summarize, although pioglitazone is not the first therapy used in treating type 2 diabetes, it is still beneficial in patients with significant insulin resistance and nonalcoholic fatty liver disease. I use pioglitazone very carefully, if at all, on female patients who are postmenopausal due to the potential increased risk of bone fractures.

I do not use this medicine on patients who have a history of bladder cancer or active bladder cancer due to the possible increased risk of using it in these people. Individuals who take pioglitazone (Actos) should be very careful about the increased risk of fluid retention, edema, and an increased risk of heart failure, especially when combined with insulin.

Name-Brand Drugs For Diabetes

Let's talk about name-brand medications for diabetes. We have over 80 name-brand diabetic medications today, and choosing among them or understanding how each one works can be a complicated task. I will try to make it easy for you and help you understand the benefits and risks of each class.

DPP-IV Inhibitors (Januvia, Tradjenta, Saxagliptin, Alogliptin, And Others)

DPP-IV inhibitors or dipeptidyl peptidase IV inhibitors are drugs that increase the activity of the incretin hormones. The incretins, called GLP-1 and GIP, increase insulin secretion and decrease glucagon secretion. These hormones have the effect of decreasing glucose production by the liver.

Common drugs of this class are Januvia, Janumet, Tradjenta, and several others. It works by increasing the availability of the incretin hormones in the GI tract. They help you make insulin right after you eat. Diabetics tend to be fairly resistant to these hormones. By boosting these gastrointestinal hormones, you will be able to make more insulin when you eat. Unfortunately, it is only a mild to moderately effective drug that can reduce the A1c anywhere from 0.6-2%, depending on the starting A1c level.

The only generic DPP-4 as of 2021 is Alogliptin.

What Are The Side Effects Of DPP-4 Inhibitors?

- » The most common side effect is low blood sugar only if used with insulin or sulfonylurea agents, like glipizide, glyburide, and glimepiride.

- » If these medications are used in combination with metformin or by themselves, it is not a high-risk medication for causing low blood sugar.

- » Sinusitis or pharyngitis are also relatively common. In my experience, sinus problems are the most common side effects.

- » Some people may report nausea or diarrhea.

- » There are rare cases of acute pancreatitis, anaphylaxis, joint pains, back pain, constipation, and headache.

- » Some other side effects are limb pain, muscle pains, mouth ulcers, kidney failure, and skin rash.

- » Sometimes severe joint pains can happen with Januvia. These joint pains may start within a day but also can happen years after treatment starts.

- » Hypersensitivity reactions, such as severe skin rash or anaphylactic shock, can happen.

- » It has not been well-studied in pregnancy, so I do not recommend it.

DPP-4 Inhibitors And Pancreatic Disease

There have been reports of Januvia being linked to acute pancreatitis. Whether Januvia causes pancreatitis directly is not known. In my experience, this is a very rare side effect. Some of the pancreatitis cases led to the patient being very sick or dying. Again, this is a rare side effect.

The Bottom Line

In my diabetes practice, I do not prescribe Januvia too often. I have a bias, as I generally see patients with uncontrolled diabetes. Most of my patients will need more intensive or more effective therapies than you'll get with these drugs. Januvia or Tradjenta, or Alogliptin may be a good option for a newly diagnosed diabetic who has a significant fear of needles.

Unfortunately, these drugs also do not have a weight loss effect or any cardiovascular benefit, while some other branded antidiabetic medications for type 2 diabetes have proven cardiovascular benefit and a chance for weight loss. Due to these issues, Januvia is at a disadvantage in my practice of diabetes management. My goal is not only to control blood sugars but also to reduce cardiovascular disease and help patients lose weight.

This class can be handy in elderly patients who may not tolerate medications that can cause weight loss or dehydration. It can also be a very effective medication for patients on dialysis. Elderly nursing home patients generally respond well to Januvia, especially if they were diagnosed with diabetes later in life.

Every patient is unique. I choose medications if they are necessary, based on the specific patient's needs. This requires a detailed clinical understanding of the patient and an understanding of all the other diabetic medications in the market. This helps me determine what is best for the patient.

GLP-1-Smart Insulin Secretion- Why Are They So Popular Now?

Individuals who still can make insulin because they have functional beta cells can utilize this advantage by taking GLP-1 agonist agents. GLP-1 agonists allow your beta cells to work only when needed and keep them from overworking. This effect preserves the life of your remaining beta cells. They also help your body regulate blood sugars in many different ways. Here are some:

> » GLP-1 delays food absorption from the intestines, allowing time for insulin response to better match digestion and lower post-meal readings.
>
> » They stimulate the release of insulin from the beta cells proportionately based on the glucose level.
>
> » These agents can improve the size and number of beta cells. This often restores insulin secretion and increases the amount of insulin produced to prevent the glucose from rising after meals.
>
> » Also, in the pancreas, GLP-1 agonists reduce the inappropriate and excessive release of glucagon after meals. Glucagon is a hormone that typically raises blood sugar levels. In diabetics, the level of this hormone increases inappropriately after meals. As a result, it is less likely to have glucose spikes after meals.
>
> » In the brain, GLP-1 suppresses the appetite. As a result, you are less likely to eat; this is an effect that lasts for an extended period of time in many people.

Common GLP-1 Medications: Ozempic, Rybelsus, Victoza, Trulicity, Bydureon, And Byetta

These medications are the most commonly used drugs in this class. They are all medications that mimic the GLP-1 hormone in that they activate the GLP-1 receptor found in the pancreas and brain. They act then just like glucagon-like peptide-1 (decreasing liver production of glucose, increasing glucose uptake by the cells, and increasing insulin production with meals). They have some differences that set them apart. I will talk about each of these differences in this section.

GLP-1 Agonists Effects

Side effects from taking these medications are common. They are not, however, always severe. They are only approved as medications for type 2 diabetes. Most people can tolerate these drugs. Common side effects include these:

- *GI Side Effects:* Up to 10 to 20% of patients will report nausea, vomiting, diarrhea, or constipation. These are the most common side effects reported. Other commonly reported side effects are gastroesophageal reflux disease, bloating, or abdominal pain.

- *Heart-related side effects*: GLP-1 agonists can occasionally increase your heart rate or cause minor rhythm problems, especially in those with underlying heart rhythm issues. These are far less common issues than those related to the GI tract.

- *Fatigue:* Although most patients will feel better and more energetic after taking these medications, sometimes a patient can report fatigue.

- *Low Blood Sugars:* Low blood sugars below 70 mg/dL (3.9 mmol/l) may occur only when these drugs are taken together with insulin or sulfonylurea agents. GLP-1 agonists alone should not cause low blood sugars.

Rarely Reported Problems With GLP-1 Agonists

These issues are not at all common with GLP-1 agonists, but you should know about them anyway:

> » Acute kidney failure, which typically happens if the medication reduces your appetite too much, and you do not drink enough. Dehydration can cause kidney failure. It isn't the medication but the dehydration that causes kidney failure.

- » Chronic or worsening kidney failure only happens if you are chronically dehydrated. Try to stay hydrated as much as possible.

- » Anaphylaxis, angioedema, and hypersensitivity reactions can happen with these medications, just as they can with any drug.

- » Pancreatitis is rarely reported in patients taking GLP-1 agonists. However, no data is suggesting that they directly cause pancreatitis.

When it comes to pancreatitis, you should be aware of the signs and symptoms of this complication. The symptoms typically include severe abdominal pain radiating to the back. The abdominal pain is generally severe and is commonly associated with nausea and vomiting.

Avoiding Side Effects With GLP-Agonists

How can you reduce the side effects of these medications? The good news is that most side effects of the GLP-1 agonist drugs will go away within 2 to 3 weeks. If the side effects are not unbearable and your sugars are significantly improving, I would suggest staying on any of these medications for 2 to 3 weeks before making a decision.

Some people prefer switching to another GLP-1 agonist instead. For example, Ozempic has an easier titration schedule that makes it easier to tolerate this medication.

To reduce the side effect of nausea, there are a couple of things you can do:

- » Eating smaller portions and eat frequently!
- » Avoid fatty foods, such as fried food.
- » Avoid spicy food.
- » Try to use ginger as a spice in your diet, or try ginger tea. Ginger is natural antinausea food.

- » If the nausea is too much, you can ask your endocrinologist to give you an antinausea medication as well.

- » Reduce your dose if not already on the smallest dose.

- » Avoid other medications that can also cause nausea.

Stay in touch with your endocrinologist to remedy the problems you are having and act on the issues immediately.

Who Should Not Take A GLP-1 Agonist Drug?

There are several clear-cut reasons why you might not be a good candidate for these medications. Some of these are listed:

- » If you have had a history of severe hypersensitivity to the drug
- » Allergy to any component of the formulation of the GLP-1 agonist drug
- » Allergy to one GLP-1 medication does not mean you will be allergic to another brand in that class.
- » Personal or family history of medullary thyroid carcinoma (MTC).
- » Patients with multiple endocrine neoplasia syndrome type 2 (MEN2).

If you have had an allergic reaction to this or any drug, do not hesitate to report this to your primary care doctor or endocrinologist. Go to the emergency department immediately.

About Thyroid Cancer And GLP-1 Agonists

It is unknown if any GLP-1 agonist drug causes thyroid C-cell tumors (medullary thyroid carcinoma (MTC) in humans. The warning is there because of the increased risk of this cancer in laboratory rats given the drug. You do not need to have routine monitoring of your blood or thyroid (using an ultrasound), as there is no proof that it would make a difference. This is a rare cancer, usually seen as part of a hereditary disease called MEN2 (multiple endocrine neoplasia 2). Only about 1 in 30,000 people has this disorder.

If you have a history of medullary thyroid cancer or pancreatitis in your family, make sure you inform your doctor before you start a GLP-1 agonist. More than likely, you will not be a candidate for any of these drugs if that is the case. Always report to your doctor if you have symptoms such as a neck mass, swallowing difficulty, shortness of breath, or persistent hoarseness. If you have thyroid nodules, you should discuss this with your endocrinologist before starting a GLP-1 agonist drug.

Disorders Which Might Impact Side Effects From A GLP-1 Agonist

- *Bariatric surgery:* If you have had bariatric surgery recently, you may have problems staying hydrated. If you get dehydrated, your kidneys may be injured, which will worsen if you are on a GLP-1 agonist medication. Your endocrinologist should carefully monitor you to prevent dehydration.

  You should drink at least 60 ounces of water per day to avoid dehydration. If you are in a hot environment and sweating a lot, I would recommend drinking at least 100 ounces of water per day. That is around 3 liters of water. Also, after gastric bypass surgery, the GLP-1 hormones similar to GLP-1 agonists increase. This situation can cause overexposure to these hormonal agents if you are also taking a GLP-1 agonist.

- *Gastrointestinal disease:* If you have Crohn's disease, ulcerative colitis, severe gastroparesis, or any other severe gastrointestinal disease, you should not be using any GLP-1 agonist drug. In the same way, if you have moderate to severe liver disease, your endocrinologist will need to pay special attention to monitoring you because you could have an increased risk of low blood sugars.

- ***Kidney problems/kidney failure:*** As I discussed, dehydration may happen due to appetite reduction. If you have underlying kidney impairment, this can rapidly get worse if you are dehydrated. To avoid that, please pay attention to your hydration status. Make sure you drink enough water to keep your urine a light yellow color. If you are having diarrhea and vomiting, you can quickly get dehydrated from this as well.

How To Take A GLP-1 Agonist Drug

You inject these medications directly into the skin, which is called the subcutaneous route. They come in an autoinjector, which means you do not need to pinch your skin or try to angle the pen.

You should never try to inject a GLP-1 agonist drug intravenously or intramuscularly. You can inject them into a variety of body parts. Most of my patients will use the abdomen; however, you can also use the back of the upper arm or thigh. When using these medications weekly, it is a good idea to rotate the injection site. Please use a different part of your abdomen or thigh every time you inject an injectable diabetes drug.

You can take your injectable GLP-1 agonist on the same day of the week, but the timing does not have to be an exact match. If you are taking the medication every Sunday, for example, you can take it on Sunday in the morning, in the afternoon, or in the evening. You can also take it regardless of meals. You can also take it with or without insulin. However, you cannot mix any of these GLP-1 agonists with any insulin, meaning you have to do separate injections if you take both a GLP-1 agonist and insulin injections.

Using A GLP-1 Agonist During Pregnancy And Breastfeeding

None of the GLP-1 agonists are recommended during pregnancy. Metformin and insulin are the most common agents used during pregnancy if needed. We do not know if these medications show up in the breastmilk; however, I would not recommend my patients to use them while breastfeeding.

Positive Effects Of Taking A GLP-1 Agonist Drug

One of the side effects of these medications is appetite reduction, which can lead to significant weight loss. This is one of the reasons they are so popular among type 2 diabetics. In my experience in our diabetes care center, people who use a GLP-1 agonist can lose up to 30 to 40 pounds. Unfortunately, this side effect may not apply to everyone. Some patients may not even lose a pound.

Summary Of GLP-1 Agonist Pros And Cons

Pros	Cons
• Strong A1c reduction • Significant weight loss • Heart benefits (reduced heart attacks) • Convenient: Taken once a week.	• Gastrointestinal side effects such as nausea and diarrhea • Expensive • Injectable except for Rybelsus • Potential(not proven) increased risk of rare cancers • Potential increased risk of diabetic eye disease

SGLT2 Inhibitors: Jardiance, Farxiga, Invokana, And Steglatro

SGLT2 inhibitors (sodium-glucose transporter 2 inhibitors) prevent the kidneys from taking glucose back into the bloodstream after it is filtered into the urine. The end result is that you will excrete or lose this glucose by the kidneys. You essentially lose those calories because your kidneys get rid of them.

As I mentioned, normal kidneys reabsorb all of the glucose they filter into the urine. SGLT2 inhibitors make it easier to urinate excessive blood sugars through the kidneys. Spilling of glucose into the urine happens at much lower blood sugar ranges than normal; this means that the kidneys can excrete glucose even though your blood sugars aren't high.

When it comes to blood sugar control, the SGLT2 inhibitors can be as effective as Glipizide or Januvia. They have similar strengths when compared with one another. The main benefit of these medications comes from their ability to reduce the incidence of heart failure and heart attacks. This makes them better choices than many other drugs, including Glipizide and Januvia.

If your A1c is around 8%, it will decrease by about 0.8%. The higher your A1c, the more the SGLT2 inhibitor will reduce this level. This is great if your A1c is 10%; it means that these drugs can reduce your A1c by about 1.5%.

In my opinion, medications in the GLP-1 class are more effective than the SGLT2 inhibitors. For example, Ozempic is more effective than any of the SGLT2 inhibitors for things like the amount of weight loss you can achieve and the degree of blood sugar control.

Pros And Cons Of SGLT2 Inhibitors

As with any diabetes drug, there will be pros and cons to using them. The SGLT2 inhibitors are no exception. Let's look at what we know about the good and bad aspects of these medications:

Pros

- *Weight loss.* SGLT2 inhibitors can definitely help you lose weight. You can lose up to 70 g of sugar per day. That is about 280 calories lost each day. If you are on insulin or a sulfonylurea, however, this effect might be limited. If you combine an SGLT2 inhibitor with Ozempic and/or metformin, on the other hand, you can lose a great deal of weight. This is a great option, but it is very expensive to actually do without a good insurance plan. I always encourage my patients to take advantage of coupon savings available at doctor's offices or websites of these medications.

- ***Prevention of heart failure.*** When you excrete excessive blood sugar, your body also excretes water along with the sugar. When there is less excess water in the body, your heart struggles less to pump your blood volume. This is likely why these medications have been shown to reduce the risk of heart failure and the risk of dying from a heart attack.

- ***Reduction in blood pressure.*** SGLT2 inhibitors can also reduce your blood pressure. They work as I just described; a loss of water in your body means a reduction in blood pressure. This is also part of the reason why it helps reduce your risk of heart attacks and heart failure. If your blood pressure is high, an SGLT2 inhibitor drug might be the drug for you.

- ***Prevention of kidney disease.*** This reduction in blood volume actually helps you take the pressure off your kidneys unless you become dehydrated. This is the reason why it reduces the progression of chronic kidney disease progression in most people. The key here, however, is that you must remain hydrated at all times.

Cons

- ***SGLT2 Inhibitors are expensive.*** They can be an expensive medication to take without coupons or insurance coverage to help you. Talk to your doctor or the manufacturer about any discounts or coupons you can use to make it easier and cheaper to take these medications.

- ***Increased appetite and thirst.*** The SGLT2 inhibitors may increase your appetite because of the sugar lost in the urine. If you increase the intake of carbohydrates due to this side effect, you may not lose as much weight as you would otherwise expect. You can be thirstier as a result of fluid loss in urine. You need to pay attention to staying hydrated.

- ***Increased genital infections.*** SGLT2 inhibitors can lead to yeast infections in the genitals because of the high sugar content. . It is more common among diabetic women but is seen in men as well. Bacterial urinary tract infections can also happen for the same reason. The worst-case scenario is called Fournier's gangrene, which is a deadly but rare genital infection. I have never seen a case of this myself after treating thousands of patients.

- *Risk of diabetic ketoacidosis.* Very rarely, some patients may develop diabetic ketoacidosis. As a result, these medications are not indicated for patients with type 1 diabetes.

- *Risk of dehydration.* If you are on a diuretic (water pill) for high blood pressure along with an SGLT2 inhibitor, you have a higher than average risk for dehydration.

Avoid SGLT2 Inhibitors Under These Circumstances:

» You are prone to frequent urinary tract infections or yeast infections.

» You have a history of diabetic ketoacidosis.

» You are at high risk for dehydration.

» You have a prior history of foot ulcers or a current diabetic foot ulcer.

» You have low bone density and a high risk of fractures.

» You have advanced chronic kidney disease (GFR< 45).

There are some other rare but serious side effects of the SGLT2 inhibitor drugs you should know about:

» Mood changes, confusion, muscle pain, or weakness.

» A rapid heartbeat that does not feel normal.

» Dizziness or passing out.

» Seizures.

» Feeling very tired or weak and not hungry.

> » Unable to pass urine.

> » Fast breathing; very bad stomach pain or throwing up; feeling very sleepy; shortness of breath; feeling very tired or weak. This can indicate diabetic ketoacidosis.

Insulins

While you will want to help manage your type 2 diabetes with diet, exercise, and oral medications, insulin is sometimes an absolute necessity when everything else fails to achieve good diabetic control.

Certainly, healthy food choices and physical activity can greatly impact your diabetes outcome. It might, however, not be enough to maintain good blood sugar control. If it is determined you need insulin, the reason for taking it is to help you better manage your disease.

Your endocrinologist should carefully evaluate your situation and decide if you need it; remember that many non-insulin options can still help you. Most of the time, basal insulin is the type of insulin you will use as a first step.

The Type And Duration Of Diabetes Determine Whether You Need Insulin Or Not!

If you have type 1 diabetes, you will certainly need to take insulin. There is no pill or non-insulin injection that will help you produce insulin without functional beta cells. Because insulin is a protein, it cannot easily be put into an actual pill you can take. Instead, it almost always must be injected.

On the other hand, if you have type 2 diabetes, you can often manage it in the beginning by making healthy food choices and increasing your physical activity. You must be asking, why would you ever need insulin then. The key point here is that lifestyle changes work best in the beginning stages of diabetes; insulin is more commonly needed later when all other choices have been exhausted. For patients careful with their diabetes and food choices, I do not expect insulin use before 20 years of diabetes. On the other hand, when diabetes is uncontrolled, you may need insulin less than 10 to 15 years after the diagnosis.

I've talked about a few of the medications used to treat type 2 diabetes when it becomes bad enough that diet and lifestyle do not work. There are more than 80 of these medications to choose from. I base the choices I make on the patient's individual situation, such as the desire for weight loss, the need for excellent blood sugar control, and even medication costs.

Most of the time, these drugs can help delay the start of insulin for a long time. Over time, however, you may need more than one medication at a time to help control your blood glucose on a regular basis.

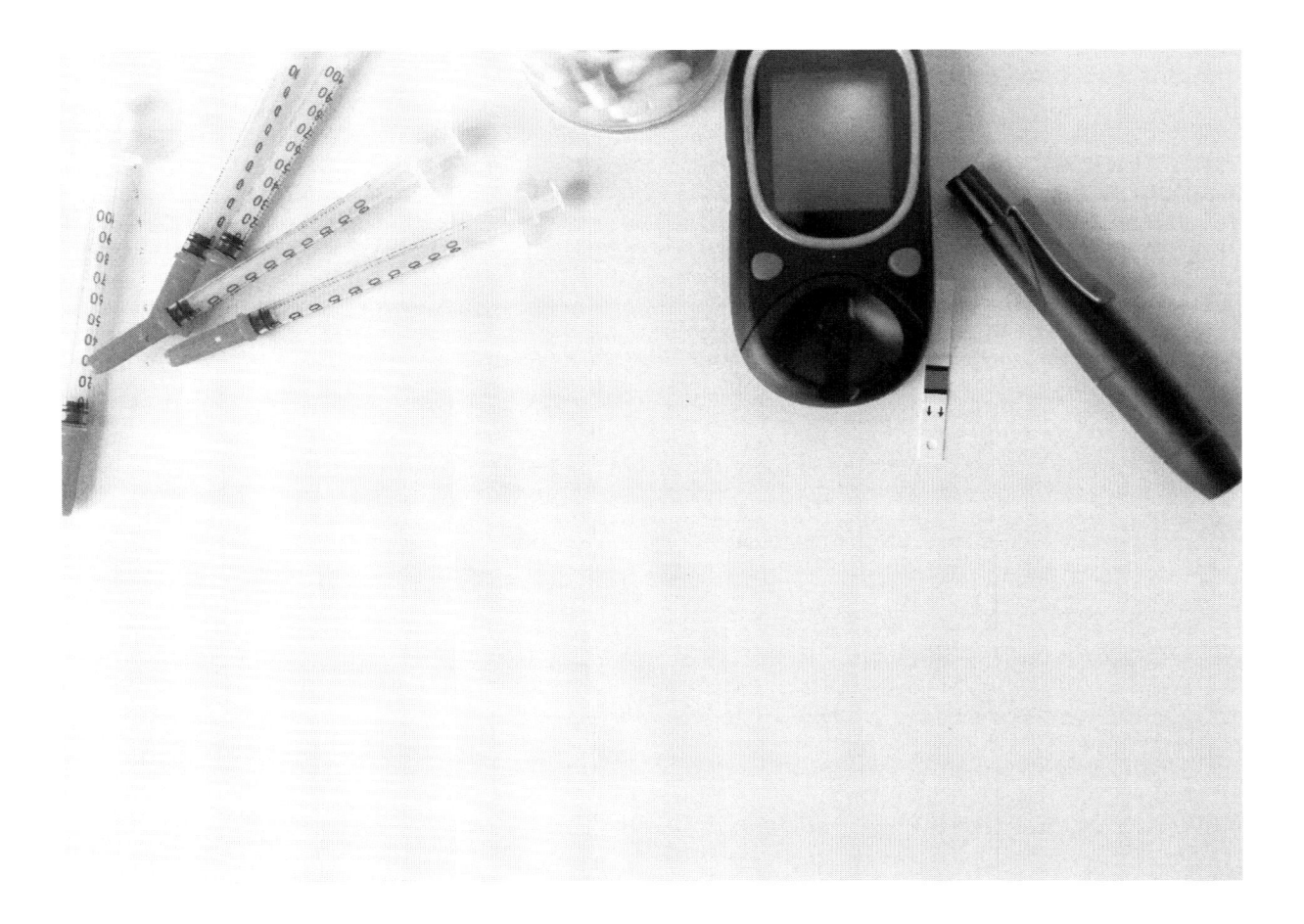

If you do not need insulin on a routine basis, you may still require insulin therapy at specific times throughout your life. Some examples are situations that stress your body, like pregnancy, when steroids are prescribed, or if you are sick in the hospital.

What Types Of Insulins Are Available?

There are many types of insulin. What sets them apart is how quickly they work, when they peak in your blood, and how long they last in your system. _It is very important to know this information about the specific kind of insulin you are taking._ With this knowledge, you can manage your diabetes much better.

There are also insulins available in different strengths; the most common strength is U-100. This simply means that there are 100 units of insulin per 1 mL of the constituted drug in suspension. U-500 is also available. It is used in patients who are more insulin resistant and is more concentrated. It is prescribed almost always by endocrinologists.

There are also U–200 (Tresiba and Humalog) and U-300 (Toujeo) insulins. Unlike U-500 U insulin, these do not show effects much different than their U-100 counterparts of the same brand. When insulin is more concentrated, the volume goes down, which helps deliver the injections under the skin. Syringes and "mixing" insulin are a thing of the past. Nowadays, we all use insulin pens.

Pay Attention To These 3 Important Features:

- » The "Onset" is the length of time before insulin reaches the bloodstream and begins lowering your blood sugar.
- » "Peak-time" is the time during which insulin is at maximum strength in terms of lowering your blood sugar.
- » "Duration" is how long insulin continues to lower your blood glucose.

Common Insulins On The Market And Their Features:

As you can see, there are a lot of types of insulin out there. You need to know what type of insulin you are taking and the exact onset time, peak time, and duration of your brand of insulin. They can be divided into rapid-acting, regular (short-acting), intermediate-acting, and long-acting types. There is even inhaled insulin to consider. These are the basics:

- *Rapid-acting insulins:* They begin to work about 15 minutes after injection and peak in about an hour. They continue to work for 2 to 4 hours. There are several branded and generic names for these rapid/fast-acting forms: Insulin glulisine (Apidra), insulin lispro (Admelog, Humalog), and insulin aspart (Fiasp, NovoLog). These fast-acting insulins are the most popular options used before mealtimes. This is because onset time is short, so they are convenient to use before meals and wear off after meals.

- *Regular or short-acting insulins:* These usually reach the bloodstream within 30 minutes after injection. They peak anywhere from 2 to 3 hours after injection and are effective for approximately 3 to 6 hours. The major brand and generic names for this type are Human Regular, Humulin R, and Novolin R. These are generally very cheap but are more likely to cause low blood sugar. This is because the duration of action is too long if used for mealtime. Since the onset of action is longer, they are less convenient to take. You need to take these at least 30 minutes before a meal. Also, you will have to use syringes. Pens are not available for these insulins.

- *Intermediate-acting insulins:* These generally reach the bloodstream about 2 to 4 hours after injection. They peak about 4 to 12 hours later and are effective for about 12 to 18 hours. The brand and generic names for these insulins are NPH, Humulin N, and Novolin N. Humulin and Novolin. There are also cheaper insulins. If you are willing to take two injections a day, I sometimes use this insulin as long-acting insulin instead of more expensive insulins such as Lantus, Levemir, Toujeo, and Tresiba. Yet, with Humulin and Novolin, there is more potential for low blood sugars and weight gain.

- *Long-acting insulins:* These reach the bloodstream several hours after injection and tend to lower glucose levels up to 20-hours later or longer. The brand and generic names are degludec (Tresiba), detemir (Levemir), and glargine (Basaglar, Lantus, and Toujeo). These are used as basal insulin to prevent spikes, mainly during the night. Since these insulins have more stable insulin release into your blood after the injection, the potential for low blood sugar is less than intermediate-acting insulin we discussed above. I typically prefer long-acting insulins over intermediate-acting insulins unless there is a cost concern.

- *Inhaled insulin:* This begins working within 12 to 15 minutes, peaks by 30 minutes, and is out of your system in 180 minutes. The brand name is Afrezza (Technosphere insulin-inhalation system). Insurance approval for this insulin remains difficult.

- *Combination insulin/GLP-1 Types:* The brand and generic names are Insulin degludec and liraglutide (Xultophy) and insulin glargine and lixisenatide (Soliqua).

- *Premixed insulin:* People who cannot afford insulin pens or prefer fewer injections may benefit from premixed forms of insulin. They have significant limitations. Because they are mixtures of long and short-acting insulins, it is harder and more complex to make small adjustments in the individual components of the medicines. It may work for people who have a very stable meal schedule and routine. The selection of who might most benefit from these combination drugs without risk is important. The brand and generic names are NovoLog 70/30, Humalog 50/50, Humalog 75/25, Novolin 70/30, and Humulin 70/30.

How Do I Take Insulin?

How you take insulin depends on many factors, such as your lifestyle, insurance coverage, and individual preferences. If needles aren't for you, you may decide on a different method. Your doctor can discuss the various options and help decide what's best for you.

Insulin Pen Priming

Insulin pens are prefilled with insulin and are disposable. Other pens have a cartridge you can insert and replace after each use. They look similar to an actual pen, except they have a needle at the tip. Pens are convenient and easier to use but are costlier than needles and syringes. The cost to you varies based on your insurance coverage. Also, some insulins aren't available in vials and syringes, but most of them are available in pen form.

You will need to prime your pen to remove any air bubbles from the needle or cartridge that can collect during and between uses. This also ensures that the pen is working correctly. You prime the pen by squirting a unit or so of insulin into the air. Without priming before each use, you may be at risk of getting too much or too little medication.

If you have a problem with your vision, you can position the needle tip over your hand so that when the priming dose is expelled out, you can feel it on your skin. For people with diabetic neuropathy, you can touch your hand to your lips and take a sniff. The distinct smell of insulin will assure you that it is being delivered properly.

NOTE: *Priming your pen is recommended before use and after changing the needle, but it's important to follow the manufacturer's instructions.*

Injecting Insulin

Using a small pen needle and/or syringe, you can inject insulin under your skin. If using a vial and syringe, you must first draw up your dose from the bottle into a syringe. Prepare the injection site by cleansing with alcohol (this is optional if the skin is clean), gently pinching the skin to create a two- to three-inch skinfold ("only" if you are too skinny or have a needle longer than 6 mm, otherwise pinching the skin is not necessary), and quickly inserting the needle at a 90-degree angle (straight up and down).

Insulin works fastest when you inject it into your legs. You should rotate injection sites to include your belly, thigh, buttocks, or the back part of the upper arm. Avoid the 2 inches around the belly button. People on insulin may require one to four injections per day to reach blood glucose target levels, while others may only require a single injection.

INSULIN INJECTION AREAS

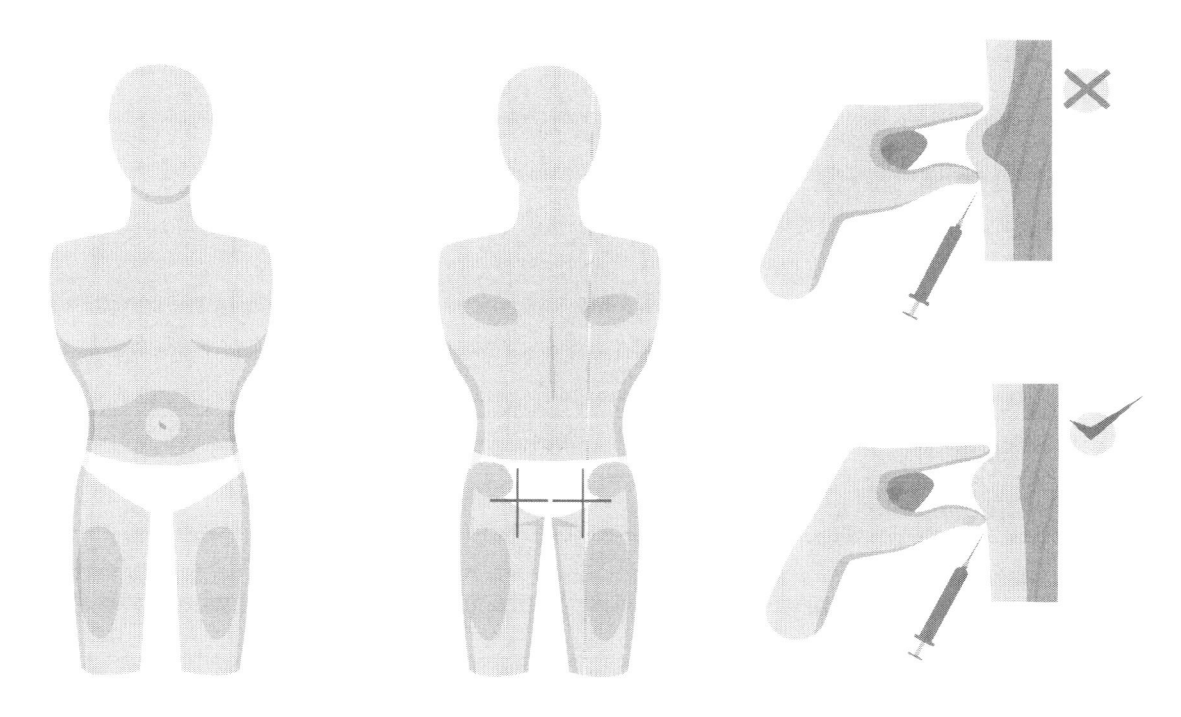

🛩 Fast Fact

What is inhaled insulin, and why isn't everyone using it? Inhaled insulin is breathed into your body in a powdered form from a device into your mouth. The insulin then goes into your lungs and migrates into your bloodstream. Only adults with type 1 and type 2 diabetes can use it. It's been around since 2006 in various forms, but it is expensive to use, no better than injected insulin, and has failed to gain much popularity because its use is so limited. Yet, some patients with type 1 diabetes have success with it when they have early blood sugar spikes or late low blood sugars with injectable insulins.

More About Long-Acting Insulins

I often prescribe a long-acting type of insulin for patients needing basal insulin. It is delivered over an extended period of time. For example, if you take 24 units of Lantus, 1 unit of insulin will be released to your bloodstream every hour in the next 24 hours. It has several mechanisms of action:

- » The target organs for long-acting insulin include the liver, skeletal muscle, and adipose tissue.
- » Long-acting insulin helps the liver pick up glucose so it can be stored as glycogen.
- » Also, within the liver, it prevents glucose from going into the bloodstream.
- » It helps glucose uptake in the skeletal muscle and adipose tissue as well, so these tissues can use it.

Because it keeps the liver from putting out glucose over time, it helps reduce the problem of blood sugars rising during the night.

I prescribe basal insulins such as Lantus pen, Basaglar pen, Levemir, Tresiba, or Toujeo if you cannot maintain adequate blood sugar control after a step-wise trial of other medications like metformin, other oral anti-diabetic medications, or non-insulin injectable drugs, such as GLP-1 analogs.

On the other hand, basal insulin may be needed earlier than later under these circumstances (You need to meet all three conditions for insulin to be a must; otherwise, I manage high blood sugars without insulin first):

- » If your A1c is greater than 10%
- » Your blood glucose is greater than 300 mg/dL (16.6 mmol/l)
- » You are symptomatic

If you have any diabetes symptoms (excessive urination or excessive thirst) or the other criteria mentioned, you might need to take long-acting insulin as initial therapy.

For people with type 1 diabetes, long-acting insulins must be used along with rapid- or short-acting insulins. I call this taking multiple daily injection regimens. Typically, the basal insulin requirement for insulins like Lantus is between 30 and 40% of the total daily dose for patients with type 1 diabetes. Severe side effects can occur with inappropriate use.

The dosage requirement will change from person to person. The normal dose for Lantus given maximally is between 0.4 to 0.5 units/kg/day. However, I sometimes consider using a more conservative initial dose of between 0.1 to 0.2 units/kg/day to avoid the potential for hypoglycemia (low blood sugar). It is given once a day most of the time.

Higher initial doses may be necessary for my patients who are obese or sedentary. To avoid side effects, please discuss the proper dosage you might need with your endocrinologist.

The dosage must be titrated to achieve glucose control and avoid hypoglycemia (low blood sugar). I adjust the dose to maintain premeal and bedtime glucose within the target range. Since combinations of agents are frequently used, dosage adjustment must address the specific individual. To minimize the risk of hypoglycemia, I titrate the basal insulin dose once or twice weekly. Very slow titration, such as 1 unit of change per day, is also appropriate for certain people.

What Happens If You Have Low Blood Sugar On Long-Acting Insulin?

If low blood sugar happens with long-acting insulin, and you have no clear reason for the problem (such as exercise or fasting), I recommend decreasing the dose by 10% to 20%. If you have severely low blood sugar, I reduce the dose by 20% to 40%. Severely low blood sugar means you needed assistance from another person to recover or had a blood glucose of less than 40 mg/dL (2.2 mmol/l).

Practical Information On Taking A Long-Acting Insulin

If you are on NPH insulin, converting from once-daily NPH insulin to a long-acting insulin is easy; the dose for Lantus, for example, is exactly the same. However, if you are on twice-daily NPH insulin when you change to a Lantus pen, your once-a-day initial dose should be 80% of the total daily dose of NPH. If you are changing from Toujeo to the Lantus Solostar pen or Basaglar, you should also consider a 20% reduction in your insulin dose.

If you are changing from once-a-day Lantus to once-daily Toujeo or once-daily Basaglar, the initial dose should be the same; however, generally, my patients need a higher daily dosage of Toujeo to achieve the same level of glycemic control as with Lantus. If you are changing from the Lantus Solostar pen to Tresiba, no dose adjustment is necessary.

The manufacturer says you do not need to change the dose for liver disease or kidney disease, but I have seen a decreased need for Lantus among my patients with both of these problems. Children may use Lantus without much difficulty.

You should be aware of the fact that all the basal insulins can increase your blood volume and cause swelling of your feet and slight weight gain. Rarely, low blood potassium (hypokalemia) is seen because insulin puts potassium into the cells.

Certainly, you can use long-acting insulin with other diabetic medications (except with pioglitazone in heart failure patients) if you are well-monitored for signs of low blood sugar. You can also use it in pregnancy, even though it isn't FDA-approved for this use as long as you are working with an endocrinologist to guide you. If you have bariatric surgery, you may not need this type of basal insulin anymore.

Diabetic Medications And Alcohol Use

You need to know that there is a direct correlation between alcohol intake, poor diabetes control, and high HbA1c levels. Why is this? Part of the problem is that many diabetic patients who consume alcohol frequently actually have less food consumption. Those who drink alcohol while taking metformin also may not adhere to dietary and medication recommendations. This could be due to alcohol's effects on one's judgment.

Drinking alcohol can take you away from exercise and glucose self-monitoring. Remember too, that alcohol can cause low blood sugars. As a result, most people are hesitant to take their medications (including insulin and metformin) while they are drinking.

This problem with adherence happens even with moderate drinkers who often show similar patterns of nonadherence with exercise, diet, and taking their diabetic drugs. These things also contribute to poor outcomes among those with diabetes.

Very small amounts of alcohol (such as a glass of wine) may not have an immediate effect on your blood sugars. On the other hand, if you are a diabetic taking insulin in addition to metformin, your risk for complications is higher. Moderate to heavy alcohol consumption (> 2-3 drinks per day) will definitely increase your risk of low blood sugars. Low blood sugars can happen even 24 hours after you drink alcohol. Your risk is greater, depending on how much alcohol you consume.

If you are taking metformin and a sulfonylurea drug, your own risk of having low blood sugars with alcohol dramatically increases. Another reason to limit alcohol is that taking metformin and alcohol together can lead to lactic acidosis. I would recommend alcohol intake to less than two drinks a day.

Diabetic Medications, Alcohol Use, And Lactic Acidosis

Many medications can increase lactic acid levels. The more medications you are on for diabetes, the higher is your risk of elevated lactic acid levels. Alcohol is practically a drug in that sense. Since both alcohol and metformin can increase the chances of lactic acidosis, your risk of lactic acidosis significantly increases. This is even more commonly seen if you already have chronic kidney disease.

What Are The Symptoms Of Lactic Acidosis When Taking Your Diabetic Medications And Alcohol?

As said, the risk of lactic acidosis with your diabetic medications is minimal. If you are on a diabetic medication and drink alcohol, however, watch out for the following symptoms. This is more commonly seen if you have consumed a moderate to heavy amount of alcohol:

- » Abdominal pain
- » Excessive tiredness
- » Rapid heart rate
- » Confusion and changes in mental status
- » Nausea with or without vomiting
- » Fast breathing
- » Shortness of breath

If You Drink Alcohol, Should You Stop Taking Metformin Or Other Diabetic Medications?

Stopping your diabetic medication for any reason without discussing it with your doctor may not be a wise idea. It is a better idea to reduce or stop drinking alcohol altogether. This is true, regardless of what you take for your diabetes, although certain medications, as you know, will worsen the effect of alcohol on your body. These are the same ones that most contribute to the risk of lactic acidosis.

Diabetes Drugs That Cause Weight Gain Or Weight Loss

Excessive weight gain and not being able to lose weight is a really common problem with type 2 diabetes. Many want to know why they have gained so much weight and how best to try and lose it. I often talk to them about medications they can take to lose at least the recommended 5% of body weight needed to improve diabetic control. Let's look at weight gain in diabetes and how you can best manage this common problem.

Common Reasons For Weight Gain In Diabetes:

1. *Insulin resistance:* The most common reason for gaining weight with diabetes is insulin resistance. I've talked about this in detail in chapter two. To summarize, when you have insulin resistance, your body creates a lot of insulin. Since insulin itself is a hormone that causes weight gain, insulin resistance creates a vicious cycle that makes it harder to lose weight.

2. *Insulin treatments* (such as Lantus, Levemir, NovoLog, Humalog, Apidra, Toujeo, Tresiba, Basaglar, Novolin, and Humulin): Diabetics on insulin therapy are at a higher risk for weight gain. If you are on Lantus, Levemir, Humalog, NovoLog, Apidra, Fiasp, Novolin, or Humulin, then you are on insulin. The job of insulin is to transfer glucose from the blood into the tissues. The tissues that need glucose the most are fat and muscle. Typically fat cells are faster than muscle cells in picking up glucose. So far, sounds good, right? So why do we gain weight on insulin?

   If you are a normal person, your body makes insulin when you eat, yet insulin taken from outside sources causes much more weight gain than insulin made by the pancreas. Why is that?

   This is because your body makes only enough insulin to get the job done; the insulin levels go down right after the blood sugar starts coming down. However, when you are taking insulin for diabetes, the insulin levels in your body do not automatically go down. Instead, you have injected a specific amount of insulin into your body that might not match your carbohydrate intake.

Insulin has a certain half-life and duration before it can be eliminated from your system. Unless you perfectly match the insulin with the food you eat, your blood glucose will continue to go down, and your body will be in a "hunger" state.

If you give just the right amount of insulin for the food, weight gain may not be a problem. The problem is that most people inaccurately estimate the insulin that they need or do not take insulin consistently to achieve an optimal insulin-to-food ratio. As a result, most people end up overeating to avoid low blood sugar, which leads to weight gain.

Also, insulin is a hormone that causes water retention. As a result, weight gain can be in the form of water retention more than fat in the beginning. Talk to your endocrinologist for alternative medications to insulin.

3. *Sulfonylurea treatments (such as glipizide, glyburide, glimepiride):* These medications work in a way that makes you prone to low blood sugars and weight gain. These agents essentially whip up your pancreas to make more insulin at a steady rate.

In reality, you only need extra insulin after you eat. In between meals, you do not need as much insulin. The problem is that when you are on a sulfonylurea drug, your body constantly makes insulin. The constantly elevated insulin levels continue to reduce your blood sugars. As a result, you start feeling hungrier than usual. Moreover, if you miss a meal, you may have low blood sugar, which makes you eat even more.

What then is the solution? Avoid sulfonylureas if you can. There are alternative medications to sulfonylureas that do not have weight gain as a side effect. Most of the time, primary care physicians will prescribe sulfonylureas because they are generic, easy to obtain, and reduce blood sugars quickly. Unfortunately, you will pay the price with weight gain and frequent low blood sugars.

Diabetes Medications That Cause Weight Loss

The diabetes drugs most associated with weight loss are metformin, the GLP-1 agonist agents, and the SGLT2 inhibitors. The GLP-1 agonist agents include Ozempic, Rybelsus, Trulicity, and Bydureon. The SGLT2 inhibitors include Jardiance, Invokana, Farxiga, and Steglatro.

Metformin

I've already said that metformin can cause weight loss. It is the only generic drug that will do this. The weight loss is not significant in most people; it is only about 1-2% of your total body weight. It isn't much, but it is better than gaining the weight you'll see with the sulfonylureas or insulin. No one knows how it works for weight loss, but the metallic taste in the mouth and diarrhea some people get might play a small role.

Ozempic, Trulicity, Rybelsus, And Bydureon

Ozempic, Trulicity, Bydureon, and Rybelsus directly affect the hypothalamus at the "appetite center." This means that cravings become less, and half of what you normally eat can make you feel full. If weight loss is difficult for you with diabetes, talk to your endocrinologist about something like these for weight loss. Your ability to lose weight will definitely be a lot easier if you take these medications. These drugs are pricey, so your insurance company might be reluctant to cover for them.

In research studies, Ozempic appears to be the most effective medication for weight loss. In my diabetes practice, I find that injectable GLP-1 agonists and Rybelsus appear to be similarly effective. The GLP-1 agonists are easier to use overall; I often recommend these medications in my patients with dexterity problems or for those who have never given themselves an injection or are hesitant to start using them.

Rybelsus is the only oral GLP-1 agent as of 2020. For people who object to the idea of an injection, Rybelsus comes in handy. It is a medication that you will have to take on an empty stomach with 4 ounces of water. You will have to wait 30 minutes after taking the medication to eat. This can be somewhat inconvenient for many people. On the other hand, Ozempic, Trulicity, and Bydureon are once-a-week injections. Mostly it boils down to the individual patient preference and insurance coverage.

What About An SGLT2 Inhibitor Like Invokana, Farxiga, Or Steglatro And Weight Loss?

The diabetic medications that cause weight loss include those of the SGLT-2 class, which includes Jardiance, Invokana, Farxiga, and Steglatro.

These medications work by helping sugar get excreted from the body. Normally, the kidneys do not allow excretion of blood sugar until the sugar level in the blood is greater than 220 mg/dL (12.3mmol/l). This is how people with very uncontrolled diabetes lose weight without any medication. It is not a healthy way to lose weight, so I definitely do not recommend this. Some young people with type I diabetic discover this and stop using their insulin in order to lose weight. This is very dangerous and nearly suicidal because many end up with diabetic ketoacidosis, which can be fatal.

On the other hand, losing weight while controlling diabetes is not a bad idea. By using these medications, people with diabetes will be able to excrete excessive amounts of glucose with blood sugars between 100-200 mg/dL (5.5-11.1 mg/dL). This is where most diabetic patients maintain blood sugars, so this is a nice way for them to lose weight.

Without these medications lowering the threshold for spilling sugar into the urine, losing sugar in the urine is not possible unless your diabetes is very uncontrolled. Up to 300 calories per day can be lost in the urine just by taking Invokana, Jardiance, Steglatro, or Farxiga. Due to the excretion of sugar in the urine, the risk of a bladder or kidney infection will be higher when using these medications. This is something you and your doctor will have to watch out for.

The Bottom Line

As you can see, several diabetic medications can help you lose weight, especially if you participate in the lifestyle changes you already know how to do. Each of these drugs—Ozempic, Rybelsus, Trulicity, Bydureon, Jardiance, Farxiga, Invokana, and Steglatro—can be used on selected individuals in order to help with diabetes control as well as weight loss.

Each person is unique, and the choice of medication depends on you and your situation. Getting a consult from an endocrinologist is a very important step in deciding what's best for you. If any of these is effective, you might lose enough weight to have better diabetic control.

5. Problem-Solving And Healthy Coping

Most people think that diabetes is all about blood sugar. Just eat right, monitor your blood sugars, and exercise, then it's all good after that. In reality, diabetes is so much more than that. It's a chronic disease with serious implications if you don't take care of it. The problem is that taking care of your health with diabetes is very stressful, which often leads to a greater risk of anxiety and depression.

Everyone will have problems with something related to their diabetes care. Problems are part of life. You can't foresee and plan for every situation you may encounter. Yet, there are many problem-solving skills that can help you prepare for unforeseen situations.

Start by identifying the problem. Then look for possible solutions. If you do not have an immediate solution yourself, you can ask your family, your endocrinologist, or your diabetes coach for suggestions. These are people who have seen all kinds of diabetes issues and their solutions, so they are great resources for you.

CHAPTER 4 - DIABETES MANAGEMENT

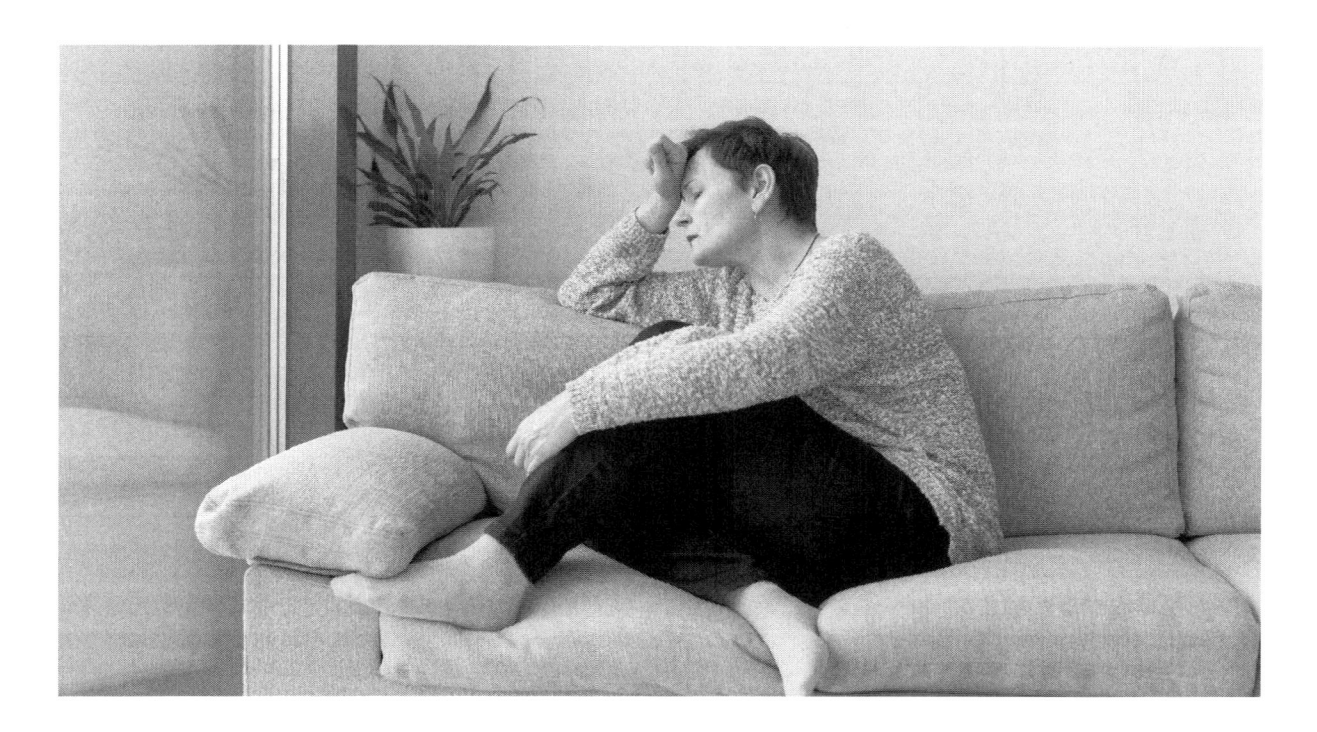

There can be many difficult problems related to diabetes you'll need to overcome. For example, diabetes is expensive—too expensive for many to get the care they deserve. This can put a huge financial strain on families that only gets worse if the diabetic gets sick and is unable to work. Socially, it can be difficult to explain your "injections" at the restaurant table or the bag of supplies you need to carry with you to check your sugars or manage blood pressure lows.

There is also a sense of loss and of a reduced quality of life (which is real and not imagined). What do you choose for Christmas dinner, for example, when there is a table full of mostly carbs to select from?

A select few people will stick religiously to dietary recommendations but, realistically, these are rare people. There are many diabetic rebels out there who have too many days where they just don't care and decide to eat out at an all-you-can-eat pasta restaurant. It's such a natural response and yet, for your diabetes, the cumulative effect of doing this too often can mean the difference between getting complications or not later on.

Let's look at some common and realistic problems faced by the diabetic and his or her family. When you can manage these aspects of your life, your quality of life will improve, and so will your outlook. As with any chronic disease, your attitude counts for a lot.

Stress And Depression

Living with diabetes can take an acute physical toll on your body, which often leads to depression. You might think that depression is purely psychological, but so much of it has to do with your physical state of health.

As I mentioned, diabetes is not just a physical disease. It can also emotionally wreck a person and severely upset the natural balance of their hormones. As the disease begins to take root inside the body, it causes all kinds of mental health problems like depression, anxiety, and hopelessness. People often feel like they have lost control over their health, which can make them feel incompetent, lonely, and abandoned.
Both type 1 and Type 2 diabetics run the risk of developing severe depression. Clinical evidence suggests that diabetic patients have a greater tendency to develop depression during the early stages of the disease process. Coping with a life-altering disease like diabetes can be very traumatic and damaging to both a person's physical and mental health. There is a deep stigma attached to mental illnesses; this often prevents the person from reaching out and seeking help.

Diabetic symptoms can cause the person to feel lonely, isolated, and increasingly frustrated. They often feel like they're the only ones fighting the kind physical and mental battle they are enduring.

Because of reduced levels of 'happy hormones,' the diabetic patient with depression tends to experience low energy levels. Due to this, they might not even indulge in proper self-care as prescribed by their doctor.

Depression "Stats" In Diabetes And How To Seek Help

If you or someone you know is currently experiencing diabetes with depression and have diabetes, then the first step is to acquaint yourself with its symptoms. As I just mentioned, depression can often go undiagnosed because of the profound stigma tied to it. This means you need to be aware of what it looks like and do something as soon as you notice any symptoms.

If you haven't been able to step out of bed for the past few days or are unable to think beyond your disease, then it's time to seek mental care. There are many places you can go for help.

Alarming Symptoms Of Depression In Diabetic Patients

Understanding the symptoms and reporting them to a counselor or therapist is extremely important. Here are the most alarming signs of depression that you must watch out for. Ideally, these signs should last for more than two weeks at a stretch to be positively diagnosed with depression.

1. *Insomnia and Depression*

    Like depressed individuals, diabetics may experience mild to severe insomnia. They wake up earlier than usual and have difficulty going back to sleep. Alternatively, their sleep cycles can also worsen and lead to too much sleep. Anything that is out of the ordinary definitely qualifies as a depressive symptom.

2. *Morning Blues*

    Experiencing angst or general sadness upon waking up is a common depressive sign in diabetics and any depressed person. They have trouble getting out of bed and checking their morning blood glucose levels. If you're feeling sad, blue, or lonely for no particular reason for a prolonged period, then you might have depression.

3. *Fluctuations in Appetite in Depression and Diabetes*

   Diabetics are supposed to consume a low-sugar, low-fat, and high-fiber diet. This means a person who used to devour desserts, fast food, and other delicacies will have to cut back dramatically. On top of this restricted lifestyle, changes inside the body can also cause sudden weight gain or weight loss. All of this can influence appetite and may even cause a reduction in weight over time.

4. *Sudden Loss of Pleasure in Depression*

   You might not feel like indulging in your hobbies and interests as much as you used to. As mental health slows down and fatigue kicks in, the motivation to fulfill daily goals can drop. Loss of pleasure in things that used to give you some enjoyment is a classic sign of depression, so you shouldn't ignore this.

5. *Suicidal Thoughts or Thoughts of Self-Harm*

   Experiencing suicidal thoughts is the last and final stage of depression with diabetes. Having no glimmer of hope and feeling worthless despite favorable things happening around you can quickly escalate to suicidal tendencies.

   Thinking that you deserve to die or hurt yourself is a common final sign that requires urgent mental health assistance. It often starts with feeling guilty about irrational things that can cause your mind to talk down to yourself. "You will never be happy," "You never do anything right," or "You're such a burden to everyone around you" are commonly occurring thoughts that should be addressed immediately.

What You Can Do About Diabetes And Depression

Diabetes is certainly not the end of the world. It may be a life-changing disease that can push you into a deep sense of trauma, but with the right lifestyle and mindful choices, you can quickly come out of it as well. Diabetes can be self-managed with a healthy lifestyle, mental health help, and emotional support from loved ones. Depression does not have to be the fate of every diabetic.

CHAPTER 4 - DIABETES MANAGEMENT

It's time to take control of your life and health. Don't let this disease get the better of you or your mental health. You are far more than diabetes, and it doesn't define your potential and ability to heal. Here are some ways through which you can successfully come out of depression and manage your diabetes well.

1. *Always Record Your Blood Glucose Readings*

   Your body will respond best when it sticks to a routine. If you are diabetic, you need to be more vigilant about what you're eating. Therefore, always take your glucose readings in the morning, before, and after a meal to keep track. This will give you a greater sense of control over your body and will help you get rid of hopelessness and depressive feelings during diabetes management.

2. *Start Eating Healthy*

   The power of nature is indispensable. It's time to ditch all those sugary, greasy foods that are slowing down your body's metabolism. Make healthy food a habit. And no, this doesn't mean that you need to follow a military diet.

   Eating healthy means you include fresh and wholesome foods like fruits, vegetables, seeds, and high-fiber foods in your diet. However, the key to eating healthy is starting small. Replace a full-fried egg with a boiled one, start having a green smoothie in the morning, or simply replace your usual white bread with brown, multi-grain bread.

   Keep the changes small and consistent, and you'll be amazed at the results in a few months. When you start eating healthy, you will be in a better place to take control of your body and mind. Eating better can improve your mood and eliminate depression with diabetes.

3. *Drink Lots of Water*

   Water is the secret to life. It hydrates and purifies our bodies. By drinking at least 7-8 glasses of water, you will allow your body to flush out all those nasty toxins and gunk from medications and saturated foods. If you don't think you can drink plain water, try fruit-flavored water with no sweeteners in it at all.

4. *Try Intermittent Fasting*

    Many diabetic patients have reported positive changes in their blood sugar levels after fasting at the intervals I discussed earlier. By doing so, the body launches into a self-healing process where it eliminates toxins and recharges itself. It is especially helpful for Type 2 diabetes as it helps you maintain a healthy weight and increases your sense of self-control.

5. *Sweat It Out*

    Exercise can boost the happy hormones inside your body. Dedicate at least 30 minutes of your time to a bit of cardio and strength training. You will be amazed at how drastically it improves your mood and increases your motivation to manage your disease. It will also help you maintain a healthy weight and eliminate depression during diabetes.

6. *Practice Mindfulness*

    Just like exercise, mindful practices like yoga and deep diaphragmatic breathing can do wonders to put your mind at peace. Every morning, step out in the sun or sit in a comfy spot and practice deep breathing. Train your mind to exhale out the bad energy and take in the fresh spirits of the morning sun. This is part of cognitive therapy for depression with diabetes.

7. *Seek Diabetes Care*

    If you're having a hard time, seek mental help from a professional to help you understand your disease and find out how you can combat it successfully. Don't shy away from accepting your depression. If you're feeling low or sad without any reason, talk to a loved one.

8. ***Break the Stigma Around Depression and Diabetes***

    Take your health into your hands and break the stigma around depression. Reach out to professionals available to you on a 24/7 basis. Options to consider include the National Suicide Prevention Line at 800-273-TALK (8255) or the NAMI Text Helpline: Just text NAMI to 741-741. Both of these are 24/7 free services.

Diabetes, depression, and anxiety seem to go hand in hand for reasons that are probably both psychological and physical. Don't try to power through when you feel like you need some genuine and compassionate help to deal with your problems. Things that seem overwhelming one day are often much less overwhelming when time passes and when you get the help you need.

Your Social Life With Diabetes

Diabetes may have several effects on your social life. You can learn to manage your diabetes so that it has little effect on your ability to eat out or go to social gatherings. Most people do well as long as they have smaller portions and are a little more careful to avoid processed carbs and sauces.

If you only eat out occasionally, your diabetes will be easier to manage. I would recommend trying to eat more often at home. This will give you more power over eating healthily and help you make better food choices.

You also need to limit your alcohol intake. Avoiding alcohol can be difficult, especially when you go out with friends. Like everything in your life, being responsible and accountable for your health will keep you from consuming excessive amounts of carbs and alcohol when you are eating out.

Your family and friends are essential in helping you manage your diabetes. You will need to keep them in the loop. You will need to also teach them why healthy foods are also better for them. All of your family members carry similar genes, which makes them susceptible to develop diabetes if they do not have it already. When everyone in the family eats healthy food, the health of each family member is greatly improved.

You can take your spouse or your children with you for diabetes education sessions, or you can watch my **SugarMD YouTube videos** together with them to educate the entire family. You can ask for support from your family to help remind you to take your medications and be mindful about what you are eating.

Common Financial Problems With Diabetes

Diabetes management can be very expensive. The average cost of health care for a person with diabetes is $17,000 a year. With co-pays and high deductibles in today's environment, patients end up paying thousands of dollars out-of-pocket as well. That is another reason I have developed **Dr. Ergin's SugarMD Advanced Glucose Support**. On the other hand, many of you might still need other medications as time goes on.

Most people who have diabetes will need help paying for their medications and medical bills at some point. You can seek financial aid through pharmaceutical companies' patient assistance programs, which can be very generous for many people. You can also look for help from the government or private healthcare plans and local/state programs. Any of these may help you pay for your diabetic medications and supplies.

Just go to the website of the medication you are taking and look for the patient assistance tab. You can also Google the words "patient assistance" and the company name. For example, if you Google "patient assistance Novo Nordisk," "patient assistance Eli Lilly," or "patient assistance Florida State," you can find a lot of helpful information. They typically disclose the criteria you need to be eligible for patient assistance. For example, most pharmaceutical companies will assist you if your total income is below 400% of the federal poverty level.

Sick Day Management Of Diabetes

Like everyone else, if you are diabetic, you may get sick. When you are sick, it may be a little more difficult to manage your diabetes. When my patients are sick, I recommend they monitor their blood sugars more often and make smart decisions about their health.

Although I know that monitoring your blood sugar more often is the last thing you want to do when you are sick, but not monitoring your blood sugars can cost you because you could have a much more prolonged and complicated course of your sickness. As you know, uncontrolled blood sugars will make the healing process a lot slower and more complicated.

Interestingly, when you are sick, your body is under increased stress; it means you will need either more medications or more insulin during that time. This may not always be true if your illness is making you throw up or limiting your fluid intake significantly. Even then, it is important to ensure that your blood sugars are not rising too much or going too low.

For example, take the case of someone who takes basal insulin, such as Lantus, Levemir, Toujeo, or Tresiba. They will still need to take basal insulin while sick, but they may need to take a little less or a little more of their basal dose, depending on how their blood sugars are running during the illness. Some patients will need a greater bolus of insulin before meals if they normally take it. Type 1 diabetic patients are at risk of developing diabetic ketoacidosis when they are sick, which can be very dangerous and can lead to death if not managed appropriately. If you are not able to keep food down, are getting dehydrated, feeling short of breath, or experiencing abdominal pain and vomiting, you will need to report to the emergency department immediately.

If your symptoms are not severe, you can manage your high blood sugars using a sliding-scale insulin schedule and by staying hydrated if this is possible. You need to keep taking some insulin so you can keep your blood sugars and ketones under control. Anytime you detect a moderate or large amount of ketones in your urine, you will need to report to the emergency room.

Follow These Additional Steps When You're Sick Even If Your Blood Sugar Is Within Good Range:

» Continue taking your insulin and diabetes pills as usual, unless there is a drastic decrease in your food intake.

» Test your blood sugar every 4 hours and keep track of the results. If your blood sugars are rising, correct these high blood sugars using a sliding-scale insulin schedule. If you do not have fast-acting insulin, you will need guidance from your doctor.

» Try to stay hydrated and drink zero-calorie liquids. Try to eat if you can.

» If you feel warm, remember to check your temperature. A fever may be a sign of infection. If you have a fever above 101 F (38.5 C), go to the emergency room.

» Drinking 6 to 8 ounces every hour can help prevent dehydration. You may sometimes need to drink beverages with sugar if you cannot eat carbohydrates from other food choices due to excessive nausea. Drink small portions of these sweet beverages to keep your blood sugar from getting too high.

Eating Out

More Americans than ever are eating out at least once a week nowadays. Many more eat out nearly every day. As you cannot control how the food is prepared at restaurants, you need to plan ahead and be ready to ask questions about the food you are eating. Here are some tips to help you:

» Check the menu before you go. Make sure there is food that will taste good and also be good for you and your diabetes. If there are too many tempting food items, you may want to choose another place to eat. With practice and good monitoring skills, you will also know which foods are good and which ones are not healthy for you. Many restaurants post the nutritional content of their menu items online.

- » Portion control can be difficult at a restaurant. Ordering one plate and sharing with someone is a great way to practice portion control and prevent waste.

- » Drinking a good-sized glass of water when you arrive at the restaurant can fill you up and keep you from overeating.

- » Eating a small, healthy snack, such as nuts or a carbohydrate with a lot of fiber, can help you care of your appetite before you go out. This will reduce the risk of binge eating or overindulgence.

- » As you know, the fat content in the food you eat raises your blood sugar more than just the carbohydrates alone. Avoid fatty foods if possible.

- » When you order proteins, make sure you order them grilled or baked instead of fried.

- » Always ask for healthy sides such as veggies instead of rice or potatoes.

- » Ordering sauces on the side can help you control the calories and carbs that are typically added on top of the dish.

It is possible to eat out when you have diabetes. You need to be vigilant about choosing healthy foods for you, and you need to avoid eating out more than a few times per month.

Vacations And Holidays

Whether you celebrate Christmas, Ramadan, Hanukkah, or Kwanzaa, food is undoubtedly the star of the celebration. During those special times of the year, your life should be filled with joy, traditions, family, friends, and calories too. Unfortunately, many of your holiday favorites do stack up when you have diabetes. This may lead you to ask if diabetes holds you back from enjoying the many wonderful foods available during this delightful time.

Holiday favorites need to be limited in the quantities you eat or drink. Think about making more reasonable choices limiting portion sizes. Also, remember to consult with your doctor if you have any concerns about what to eat or whether to go out to eat. Holiday drinks like eggnog and hot chocolate can be modified to be healthier, or you can drink things like vanilla chai tea for the holidays instead.

Special holiday treats like gingerbread cookies, fruitcakes, and candy (candy canes and peppermint bark) are best eaten in small portions. The same is true for holiday pies like pecan pie and pumpkin pie. Most cookies (chocolate chip and sugar cookies) should be limited if possible; holiday table favorites like macaroni and cheese, dinner rolls, and potato latke are high in carbs, so fewer of these items are a good choice. If you like wine with your meal, select dry wines, which have fewer carbs in them. Portion sizing is hard at any time but is much more difficult around the holidays.

Traveling For Diabetics

Traveling is stressful anytime. It is more stressful when you have diabetes and need to think about irregular eating schedules while traveling, changes in sleep patterns due to time zone changes, and an increased risk for exposure to diseases from being in large groups (including large family groups). Traveling during flu season or to foreign countries carry added risks. In foreign countries, you may not have access to excellent healthcare you might need if you get sick.

Many people travel long distances to be with family and friends during special times in their lives. Others travel for enjoyment. There is no reason a person with diabetes cannot do these things with reasonable safety measures in place; infectious diseases in the US and abroad are always going to be a concern you need to think about.

As you know, diabetes and other chronic diseases are significant risk factors increasing the risk of death from many infectious diseases. Diabetics tend to be sicker longer; this means you should try hard not to get sick in the first place.

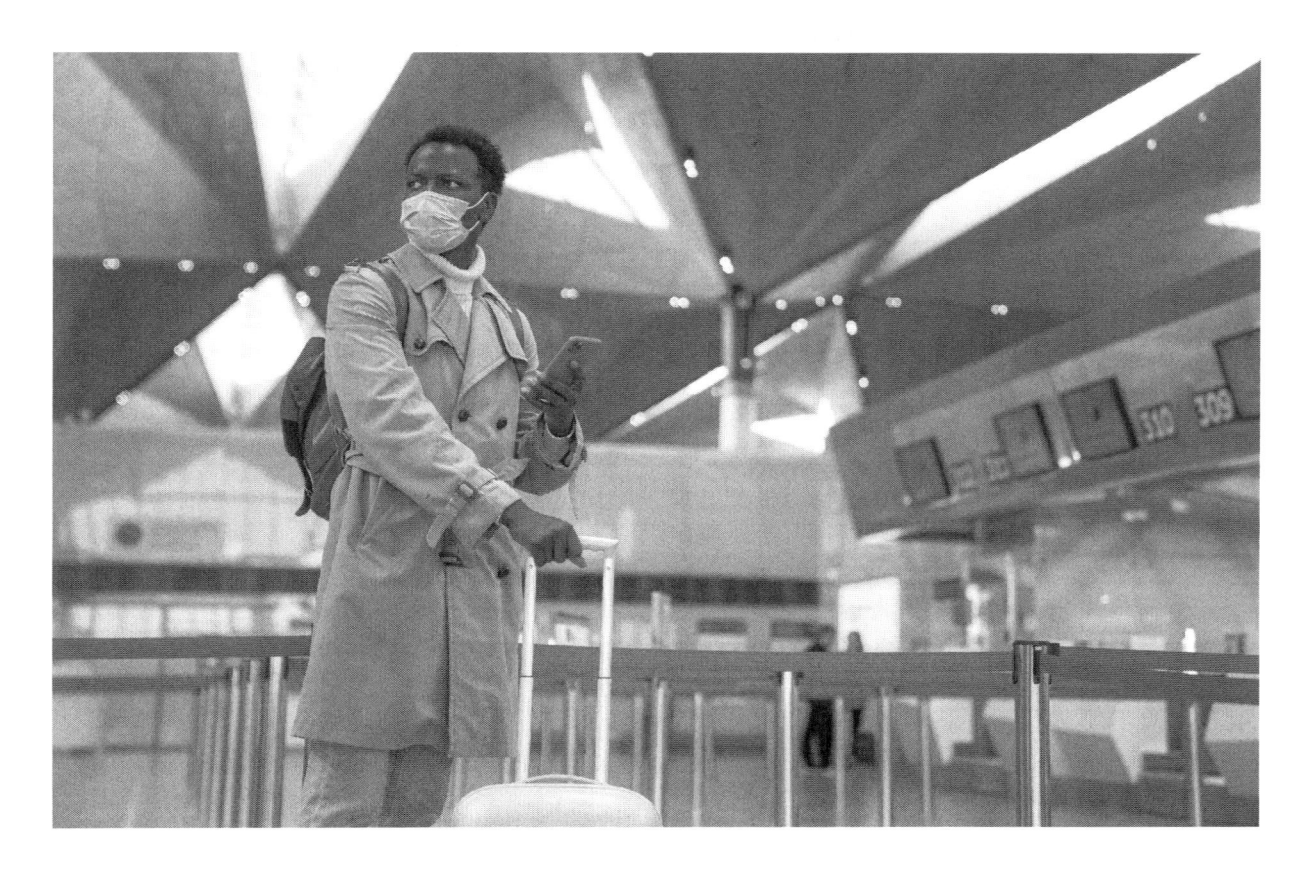

For these reasons, I tell my diabetic patients to take extra measures to protect themselves from all sorts of infectious diseases.

Traveling does increase the risk of getting sick for many reasons. There is a risk anytime you travel to a new place, meet in large groups, or suffer the stress of having your routine disrupted. These are my tips for safely traveling and meeting in large groups when there is an infectious disease epidemic such as influenza or COVID-19:

» Consider wearing a mask in enclosed places If you are very high risk for infectious diseases. Make sure your mouth and nose are covered when in public spaces.

» Maintain a social distancing from people not in your immediate household.

- » Wash your hands and use hand sanitizer frequently.

- » Try not to touch your face.

- » After your gathering, take extra precautions to make sure you watch for the development of a disease you may have caught while traveling.

- » Disinfect areas where a lot of people are gathered.

- » See your doctor if you don't feel well and let him or her know from where you have returned after traveling.

Keep checking your sugars, and remember to continue to watch carbs and take your medications. If you are in doubt about how to take your medications while traveling, talk to your endocrinologist about how you should do this. Traveling to different time zones is the most challenging, as medications are often time-dependent.

Playing Sports With Diabetes

Patients with diabetes can play sports, just like anyone else. They just need to pay attention to a few things as they play so they can avoid low blood sugars (hypoglycemia) and high blood sugars (hyperglycemia) during and after playing sports.
Mild to moderate-intensity exercise tends to reduce blood sugar slowly; on the other hand, intense exercise can spike your blood sugars temporarily during the exercise. This is especially true in insulin-deficient type 1 diabetic individuals. Both moderate and intense exercise can cause low blood sugars as much as 24 hours after the exercise took place.

Here are a couple of precautions to take so you can avoid problems while playing sports or exercising:

- » Test your blood sugar before being active, during the activity, and every 4-6 hours in the hours following exercise. If you are doing this activity repeatedly, you will know your body's response, and you won't have to check too many times before knowing what to do to avoid blood glucose excursions.

» You may have to adjust your insulin on the days you are playing sports or exercising more than usual. For example, you may have to reduce your basal insulin anywhere from 20% up to 50%, depending on the activity level and your body's response.

» If you are on mealtime insulin, you may prefer to skip the mealtime insulin before you start exercise unless your blood sugar is very high to begin with (greater than 250 mg/dL or 13.9 mmol/l). If your blood sugars are this high, you may want to correct your high blood sugar with an adequate amount of insulin. Otherwise, your blood sugar may continue to rise, especially with the kind of intense activity that often happens while playing sports. If you are not playing sports, you can try to reduce your high blood sugars by participating in activities like brisk walking.

» If you are on sulfonylurea agents such as glipizide, glyburide, and glimepiride, or if you already have taken a bolus of mealtime insulin AND your blood sugars are below 150 mg/dL (8.3 mmol/l), you may want to have a snack before starting exercise. Having a carb snack with a low fat content can help raise your blood sugar when you feel or detect that it is too low.

» Having a continuous glucose monitoring device such as Dexcom or Freestyle Libre can be very helpful to continuously monitor blood sugars during the activity. You need to understand how to interpret and analyze your glucose using these monitoring systems.

» For individuals who are wearing insulin pumps, you may need to suspend or reduce insulin delivery by 50% or more during the exercise. You may also need to reduce the basal insulin delivery in the device by 20 to 30% up to 24 hours following the activity.

Like anything, the more you know how your body responds to exercise, and the more you learn how to manage your sugars on the days you are playing sports, the better able you will be to perform like any other athlete without difficulty.

6. Reducing Your Risk Of Complications

Once you realize that diabetes has many complications, you also know the job you need to do to avoid them. The list is long and frightening, but most are preventable if you understand ways to prevent them:

- » Heart attacks
- » Strokes
- » Kidney failure
- » Amputations
- » Sleep apnea
- » Dental problems
- » Higher risk of severe infections
- » Vision loss
- » Hearing problems

In addition to keeping your blood glucose under control, the steps you need to take also include these:

- » Control your blood pressure
- » Manage your cholesterol
- » See an eye doctor regularly
- » See your dentist regularly

» See a podiatrist regularly

» Quit smoking

» Get professional mental health management for stress and depression

Your endocrinologist will be the main quarterback for you in managing your diabetes in every aspect. Make sure you choose an endocrinologist who will partner with you and your health first.

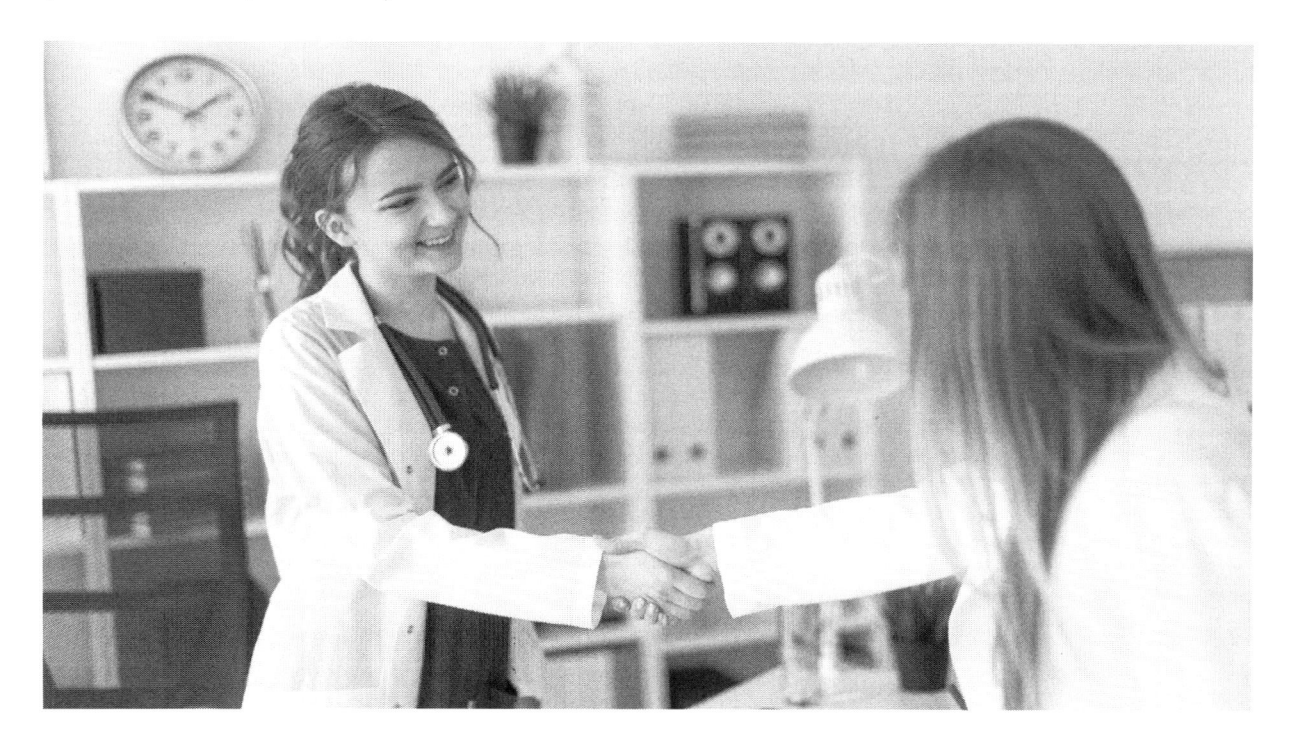

The Legacy Effect

As a result, controlling diabetes at the early stages is extremely important. This is called the **Legacy Effect**. The Legacy Effect means that if your blood sugars are poorly controlled in the very early stages of this process, the complications you get from having diabetes are much more likely in the future, even if blood sugar control is consistently controlled later in life. It is also the case if the diabetes is controlled early but later loses that control. In this scenario, your risks for complications are less. This is why early control of diabetes is so crucial.

This is also why it's important to work on the problem as soon as the blood sugar defect is identified. Even if a total cure is not possible for your diabetes, staying in remission and not letting diabetes dominate your life and cause complications are possible.

As I mentioned, managing the legacy effect in diabetes involves the early aggressive treatment and control of diabetes, which can leave a positive legacy in the long-term. Here is how it works;

When a person is diagnosed with diabetes, if they take it seriously and are aggressive and dedicated to controlling diabetes in the first ten years, the chances of complications are much lower, even if they lose control after the first ten years. But, if that same person is in denial or negligent concerning their diabetes care in the first ten years, the complications will settle in early on.

If, after ten years of uncontrolled diabetes, the person then decides to be careful and control their sugars, the overall outcomes are not going to be nearly as good as would be the case in the first person's example (who has done well in the first ten years). So my recommendation is…do not wait to take control of your diabetes. The time to take action is today and not tomorrow.

How Do You Know If Your Diabetes Is Under Control In The First Ten Years?

Most commonly, it's the A1c that many physicians use as a benchmark for blood sugar control. As long as the individual does not have many episodes of low blood sugars, an A1c of less than 7% is a reasonable goal for many patients, although achieving an A1c below 6.5% is more desirable. If you just got diagnosed with diabetes, you can easily get your A1c to less than 6.5% or even less than 6%.

In the early stages of diabetes, lifestyle changes will have a very significant effect on your blood sugars. Simple interventions, such as quitting regular Coke or juice, or stopping eating white bread, may lead to a great improvement in blood sugars. On the other hand, in the later stages of the disease, these simple lifestyle changes may not have a significant effect at all because the pancreatic beta cells are already damaged permanently.

Even medications work much better early on. For example, if you start taking metformin when you are first diagnosed with diabetes, you can bring your blood sugars down twice as easily in the early stages. It is hared to do this in the latter stages of the disease (10 to 15 years after the initial diagnosis).

The choice of medication is also very important. Although metformin is the most commonly prescribed medication, it may not be the best choice for you. Every medication also has different side effects and merits. A well-thought-out plan in the beginning is very important.

Many of my patients use Dr. Ergin's SugarMD Advanced Glucose Support diabetes supplement to help support their healthy blood glucose levels. In my experience, this practice has helped my patients achieve their goals with fewer medications. Also, keep that in mind that if you are not responding to a medicine or supplement, you may simply need a dose increase or a change to another agent.

Diabetes is fraught with complications, especially if you have uncontrolled disease. Because of the Legacy Effect, if you don't manage your diabetes in its earliest stages or don't know you have it until it is advanced already, the risk of complications might still be there—even if you are the perfect diabetic with the best possible control now.

Let's look at the possible complications you can expect and how you can prevent and treat them. Many of the complications require you to see other specialists, such as an ophthalmologist for eye disease and kidney specialists (nephrologists) for kidney disease.

Reducing Your Risks Of Heart Disease And Stroke

I am going to get serious now about diabetes because I think you need to know a few truths about this disease. My intention is not to scare you or worry you but to give you the incentive you need to do what it takes to get your diabetes into remission. If you are still in the prediabetes stage, this advice is even more important; this is because you have an even better chance of avoiding becoming diabetic altogether and having a long and healthy life.

Diabetes Is The Most Common Reason For Heart Attacks And Strokes.

<u>Insulin resistance is the primary reason for cardiovascular disease.</u> Insulin resistance involves high insulin levels, elevated lipids, and cholesterol in the bloodstream. This is the perfect recipe for the development of clogged arteries. Clogged arteries are the main cause of both heart attacks and strokes. Ironically, this happens very early on in the early stages of diabetes.

The Biggest Risk: Heart Disease And Stroke

The American Heart Association says that at least 68 percent of people aged 65 or older who also have diabetes die from heart attacks/heart disease, and 16 percent die from a stroke. Diabetes remains at the seventh leading cause of death, usually from some type of diabetes complication. Diabetes is the underlying cause of death, with 80,000 people per year dying of the disease and its complications in the US.

The most common complication and a major cause of death among diabetics is cardiovascular disease, which includes heart attacks, strokes, and peripheral vascular disease. Diabetics are 2-3 times more likely to die from heart disease than non-diabetics. Research shows that patients who are in their early 40s with a history of all three of the related diseases (diabetes, stroke, and heart attack) could have around 23 years of lost life.

STAGES OF ATHEROSCLEROSIS

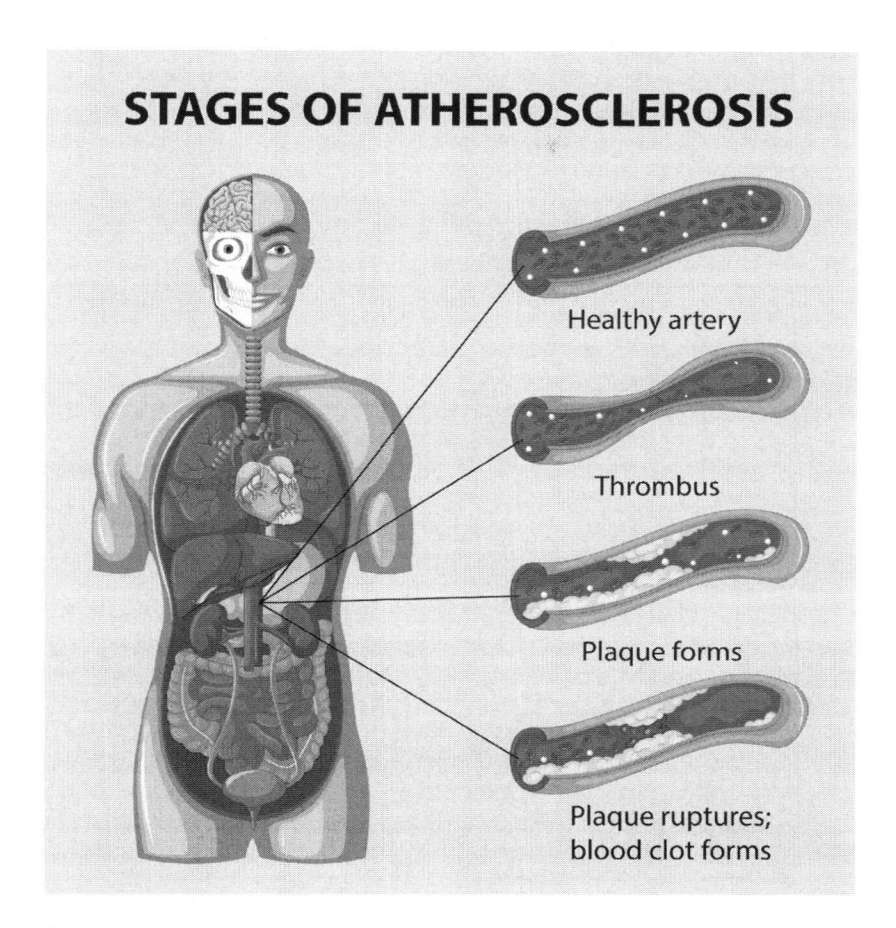

- Healthy artery
- Thrombus
- Plaque forms
- Plaque ruptures; blood clot forms

While these three diseases seem different, they are mostly due to the same thing. As you know, insulin resistance leads to clogged arteries or atherosclerosis. Each of these areas, the brain, the heart, and your limbs, depends on an open circulatory system to function. If the blood vessels are clogged to each of these body parts, you will have tissue damage. That's all these diseases are—tissue damage to the heart, brain, or legs (sometimes the arms too) and complications from this lack of circulation.

Because the main cause of clogged arteries is insulin resistance, your best option is to have this managed as soon as you can. You would benefit most from seeing an endocrinologist or diabetes care center that will address insulin resistance as soon as you know you have it.

Is Diabetes-Related Heart Disease Preventable?

The American Heart Association considers diabetes to be one of the seven major preventable or controllable risk factors for cardiovascular disease. To understand how to prevent heart disease, you have to understand what causes heart disease to begin with. There are many risk factors either related to diabetes or often seen in diabetics that cause heart disease. These are:

- » High blood pressure
- » High cholesterol
- » Smoking
- » Diabetes/insulin resistance
- » Obesity
- » Lack of activity
- » Family history
- » Ethnic background

Other risk factors include:

- » Older age
- » Male gender
- » Poor diet
- » Excessive alcohol use

Not all of these things are modifiable; you can't change your gender or ethnicity, for example. But you can see there are many things you can change. You can quit smoking, lose weight, eat healthier, and exercise. Not easy, you're thinking? This is where you can get a lot of help from your endocrinologist or diabetes coach, and of course, empowering yourself with knowledge, which is what I am trying to achieve for you via this book.

CHAPTER 4 - DIABETES MANAGEMENT

The good news is that with good diabetes care that includes blood sugar control along with cholesterol and blood pressure control, you can make a difference and help prevent heart attacks and strokes in your future.

As an endocrinologist who treats diabetics daily, I don't just look at blood sugar numbers without thinking of the other risk factors that could be changed or modified. I recognize that in the US, only 20% of Americans with diabetes have their diabetes, cholesterol, and blood pressure controlled all at the same time. In my practice, I aim for this number to be 90% or more.

You need to know that diabetes, high blood pressure, and high cholesterol are each one leg of a tripod. If one leg is weak or broken, the tripod cannot stand. If your LDL is above 100, if your blood pressure is above 140/90, and if your diabetes control is not adequate, please get a consultation with an endocrinologist who will manage all of these things together.

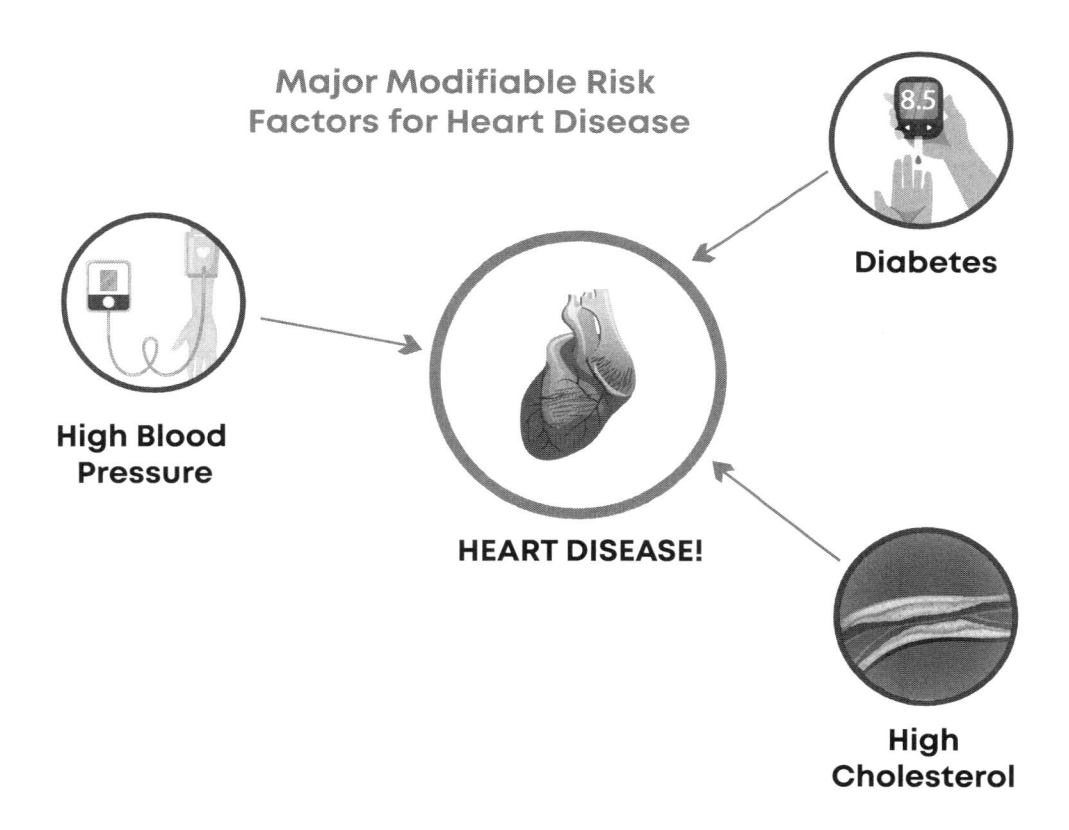

Major Modifiable Risk Factors for Heart Disease

High Blood Pressure

Diabetes

HEART DISEASE!

High Cholesterol

There are medications and lifestyle changes you can do to reduce the chances that high cholesterol or high blood pressure will contribute to developing heart disease. In my practice, I focus on using lifestyle and medications to maximize blood sugar control so that diabetes won't also be such a huge risk factor in getting heart disease.

What Does It Mean To Have Each Of These Risk Factors Controlled In A Diabetic?

When tackling each leg of this tripod in developing heart disease, I look at these things:

- *Blood sugar control*—Controlled blood sugar is defined as an A1c of less than 7% in most people. Getting to less than a 7% A1c may not be easy in elderly individuals who have multiple other medical problems. The younger you are, the lower your A1c you should aim for. The American Association of Clinical Endocrinologists recommends an A1c of less than 6.5% in relatively healthy individuals. I aim for my patients to have the lowest A1c reasonably achievable for their diabetes care plan.

- *Blood pressure control*—A blood pressure less than 140/90 is the minimum requirement. Less than 130/80 is more desirable, if possible. Most of the time, this goal is achievable with dietary changes, such as reducing the salt content in your diet. You can easily do that by avoiding canned food, packaged food, and frozen food. Instead, you should eat fresh food, which is healthier for you. If medications are necessary, do not be afraid to discuss your options with your endocrinologist.

- *Cholesterol control*—In general, I want you to keep your LDL-cholesterol less than 100 mg/dL. For people who've already had a heart attack, I want to keep it less than 70 mg/dL. Medications can help reduce your LDL. Your LDL is somewhat responsive to dietary changes, but most of the time, you'll need medications to achieve such low LDL goals.

Your HDL-cholesterol (good cholesterol) also plays a role. A number greater than 50 mg/dL in men and greater than 60 mg/dL in women is what I'm looking for. Your HDL-cholesterol is very responsive to exercise and not so responsive to medications. The triglyceride goal is less than 150 mg/dL. Some medications can reduce your triglyceride levels, but dietary changes are the most helpful. Try to reduce your intake of processed carbs and animal fat.

How Can I Stop Insulin Resistance, Prevent The Progression Of Diabetes, And Lessen The Chances Of Developing Heart Attacks And Strokes?

Unfortunately, some people are destined to have insulin resistance because of their genetic background. Even so, you can change your destiny. You may be at a disadvantage because of your genetic inheritance, but defeating insulin resistance is very possible if you begin the right kinds of lifestyle changes and take the recommended medications and/or diabetic supplements, such as SugarMD Advanced Glucose Support, when or if you need this. You can do this!

After you make these changes (including exercise, dietary changes, and weight loss), your insulin resistance will surely improve. When there is less insulin resistance, it may never be necessary to take insulin or any other medications later in life. As a result, further progression to diabetes and its complications also will not happen.

Your endocrinologist will be the best person to give you the right advice. Along with the support of a diabetes education specialist and your endocrinologist, you can gain control over your health.

Diabetic Neuropathy

Diabetic neuropathy is a type of nerve damage due to diabetes. As a diabetes specialist, I commonly hear about neuropathy from my type 1 and type 2 diabetes patients. Diabetic neuropathy is so common that up to 26% of people already have diabetic neuropathy at the time they are diagnosed with diabetes.

Most of my patients have a generalized type of neuropathy. This usually means the feet are the most affected. There are many non-medicinal and medicinal options for this type of neuropathy, such as gabapentin/Neurontin, Cymbalta, and Lyrica (which is not a first-line medication). They relieve symptoms only and do not reverse the disease process.

Let's look at the signs and symptoms of neuropathy, the risk factors, and the treatment options available.

Signs Of Diabetic Neuropathy

The most common symptoms of diabetic neuropathy are loss of sensation, numbness, tingling, and/or burning pain in the feet. These symptoms tend to be worst at rest, at night, and during sleep; they improve with activity, such as walking. Some people will initially have very painful feet, while others have numbness or no symptoms at all, even if the nerve damage has started.

Diabetic neuropathy commonly affects both sides of the body in the same way. If the symptoms are not present on both sides, I will typically look for other causes of neuropathy. Most people have their first indication of neuropathy in their toes. As the disease progresses, the numbness and pain will gradually move up the legs. The hands are not affected until the symptoms in the legs reach above the mid-calf.

In time, the ability to sense pain will be lost, which significantly increases the risk of injury. Unfortunately, these injuries are the often initial culprit in the development of a diabetic ulcer that can lead to an amputation if not taken care of properly.

Different Types Of Diabetic Neuropathy

Nerve damage can be of different types based on the areas of your body involved and the kinds of nerves it affects in the body. Based on these features, neuropathy is usually divided into different types. You might experience any of the following kinds of neuropathy:

1. ***Polyneuropathy or Peripheral Neuropathy:*** This is considered to be the most common type of nerve damage. It causes damage to the nerves in the feet, hands, legs, and arms. It usually starts from the feet but, if left unchecked, it will progress to involve areas higher up on the legs. The most significant sign of peripheral neuropathy caused by diabetes is that it affects both feet at the same time.

    Other common symptoms are:

    » Tingling in the feet, even during the night

    » Extreme sensitivity to pain or actual pain in feet

    » Numbness and loss of feeling in the feet, even when injured

    » Weak muscles in the legs and difficulty in walking

    If you have any of these problems, please remember to mention them to your endocrinologist ASAP.

2. ***Autonomic Neuropathy:*** This type of nerve damage affects the nerves of your autonomic system in the body. This includes your digestive system, sex organs, urinary tract, sweat glands, cardiovascular system, and eyes. Some of the most common signs of autonomic neuropathy are:

    » Bladder paralysis – nerve damage in the bladder, which causes urine to be retained in the bladder and urinary tract infections (UTI)

    » ED or Erectile dysfunction– nerve damage to the pudendal nerve, which goes to the penis in men

    » Diarrhea or constipation – caused by nerve damage in the intestines

    » Digestive issues – Bloating, vomiting, and poor or fast absorption of food, leading to gastroparesis, which is another form of neuropathy affecting the stomach.

3. ***Charcot's Joint:*** This is diabetic neuropathy affecting a joint. It can lead to the breakdown of the joint. It largely affects the foot and can cause complete loss of sensation of the area. It can affect your ability to sense your joint position. The leg muscles can start to weaken, which means that the joint is not properly supported. The joint may be swollen and inflamed.

4. ***Cranial Neuropathy:*** This diabetic neuropathy affects all 12 nerves, which control your eye movement, hearing, sight, and taste. It can be dangerous as it can cause paralysis in the eye muscles. The eye muscles are the first areas affected by cranial neuropathy.

    Other symptoms include:

    » Pain around the affected eye – usually on one side of your face

    » Double vision

5. ***Compression Mononeuropathy:*** This condition occurs when only one nerve is damaged; it is fairly common among diabetics. There are two scenarios where it commonly occurs. One is when damage happens to a blood vessel restricting blood flow to the nerve. The second is when nerves are damaged in areas where they must pass over bone or a connective tissue nerve tunnel (usually in the wrists or fingers).

    Common symptoms for this condition are:

    » Numbness in fingers

    » Swelling of fingers

    » Prickling feeling in the fingers

    » Pain or difficulty in tasks such as knitting or driving

6. ***Femoral Diabetic Neuropathy:*** This type of diabetic neuropathy commonly occurs in type 2 diabetics. You will usually have pain on one thigh, followed by muscle weakness and eventually muscle wasting in the thigh. Another form of femoral neuropathy is called diabetic

amyotrophy. This causes weakness on both sides of the thighs but often no pain. The type of nerve damage is due to diseased small blood vessels.

7. *Focal Diabetic Neuropathy:* This nerve damage is similar to cranial neuropathy because it can cause eye damage. However, it usually affects many different nerves, causing pain and weakness throughout the body.

    Common symptoms for focal neuropathy include:

    » Double vision

    » Bell's Palsy – Paralysis of one side of the face

    » Pain in the thigh

    » Pain in other parts of the body

8. *Thoracic/Lumbar Radiculopathy:* Similar to femoral diabetic neuropathy, thoracic or lumbar radiculopathy is a form of mononeuropathy (meaning one nerve is involved); it is relatively common. It doesn't affect the thighs but the torso of a person. It affects the abdominal wall muscles or the chest muscles on one or both sides. It is also seen more commonly in type 2 diabetics. Pain and weakness can happen in areas supplied by other affected nerves.

9. *Unilateral Foot Drop due to Neuropathy in Diabetes:* This type of nerve damage affects the foot and makes it impossible for you to walk or stand. You can't pick up your foot, and it might not respond if touched or stimulated. It is usually due to damage of the peroneal nerve in the leg, either because of compression of the nerve or from blood vessel damage near the nerve.

Detecting Diabetic Neuropathy

Most of the time, the diagnosis is clear based on your history; however, some examination findings can also help detect diabetic neuropathy. Some of the signs could be:

- » An inability to say if your toe is moved by the doctor up or down because you can't feel it well enough to say

- » An inability to feel the vibration of a tuning fork placed on the skin of the foot

- » An inability to feel light touch sensations

- » A reduction in your Achille's tendon reflexes

More extensive testing can be done if the diagnosis is in doubt. These include nerve conduction studies, nerve biopsies, and imaging tests. However, these types of exhaustive tests are not usually needed to diagnose diabetic neuropathy.

If there is a suspicion of nerve damage, but it isn't clear, you may have to undergo an electromyogram or nerve conduction study. These tests are designed to read the response from your nerves and see how the nerves affect the muscles. Nerve damage leads to abnormal testing of these areas.

Based on your condition, the tests you have might be different. In some cases, the nerve damage might be so pronounced that a physical exam might be enough to determine it.

Some Diabetic Foot Ulcers Are Due To Diabetic Neuropathy

Unfortunately, when you cannot feel pain, heat, or cold in your feet, the risk of unnoticed injury goes up. Injuries that would typically cause pain in normal individuals, such as stepping on a nail or splinter or wearing unfit shoes, do not necessarily cause pain if you have neuropathy. This is why it is very important to check the bottoms of your feet daily; otherwise, a small sore can develop into a large ulcer.

By the time you notice the injury, it may be too late. If there is an infection that goes into the bone, doctors may not be able to save the limb. Although your doctor may check the bottoms of your feet and your sensation in the office, you should be the one primarily responsible for checking your own feet daily or at least a few times a week. If you see something, report it to your endocrinologist immediately.

Risk Factors/Causes Of Diabetic Neuropathy

The biggest risk factor in patients with diabetic neuropathy is uncontrolled high blood sugars. Your endocrinologist should help you early on to find ways to control high blood sugars so you can prevent or slow the progression of diabetic neuropathy.

Other factors can further increase the risk of developing diabetic neuropathy, including:

- Coronary heart disease
- Elevated triglyceride levels
- Being overweight (a body mass index >25)
- High blood pressure
- Smoking

Treatment Of Diabetic Neuropathy

Treatment of diabetic neuropathy is possible and includes several levels of care. These treatments are control of blood glucose levels, prevention of injury, and management of painful symptoms. I like to emphasize three main facts with my patients to help improve their symptoms of diabetic neuropathy:

1. You should follow your endocrinologist's instructions for tight control of blood sugar levels.
2. You should be attentive in the care of your feet to prevent an ulcer.
3. Your doctor may prescribe you medications to reduce the pain caused by diabetic neuropathy.

Although diabetic neuropathy may not be reversible, preventing the progression of the disease is important. On the other hand, improving diabetes can also improve your diabetic neuropathy in months, if not within weeks.

One caveat to this that diabetics should be aware of is that when blood sugars rapidly improve, the underlying diabetic neuropathy can temporarily or paradoxically worsen for a few weeks or more. The neuropathy symptoms dramatically improve if you can maintain steady control over your blood sugars. You should seek help from your endocrinologist on a daily, weekly, or monthly basis, instead of every 3 to 6 months. If your diabetes is currently not controlled and the medications you are given are not helping.

If you have type 1 diabetes, you may need an insulin pump and a continuous glucose monitoring device or remote glucose monitoring to control your blood sugars more strictly. For those with type 2 diabetes, although insulin pumps and continuous glucose monitoring are still good options, you may have other medical or nonmedical options to try before you need these.

Diabetic neuropathy pain can be very disturbing, especially at night. If it is advanced, it may be very difficult to control. Thankfully, only a small percentage of people with diabetic neuropathy experience severe pain. Most of these have had longstanding uncontrolled diabetes.

In general, sensitivity to neuropathy pain varies from patient to patient, and some may feel more pain than others. This pain can be temporary if it is new and has happened from a recent health change such as significant weight loss, diabetic ketoacidosis, or a rapid control of blood sugars.

When my patient has pain, I typically start with medications that have been approved by the FDA, such as Lyrica, Cymbalta, gabapentin, and alpha-lipoic acid. Some of these medications are not necessarily designed for diabetic neuropathy; instead, they are used for the treatment of depression or seizures. The dose used for the treatment of diabetic neuropathy is typically much less than the doses we use for the treatment of depression.

Most of the time, I start medications taken at night as this is the time that the pain is most severe. Also, some of these medications may have side effects such as drowsiness. As a result, taking these medications at nighttime is the best option for many patients.

Sometimes I combine medications, like amitriptyline plus gabapentin/Neurontin. I do not combine Cymbalta with amitriptyline since these are both antidepressant medications. Gabapentin and Lyrica can also be combined if necessary.

These are the most commonly used drugs for diabetic neuropathy:

1. *Duloxetine/Cymbalta* – this can be taken once or twice a day with food. You should not be taking Cymbalta if you are on other antidepressant medications. The most common side effects include nausea, sleepiness, dizziness, decreased appetite, and constipation.

2. *Neurontin/gabapentin* — this medication is most commonly used for seizure prevention. For diabetic neuropathy, it is usually taken by mouth three times per day. The most common side effects are dizziness, drowsiness, and confusion. Gabapentin can be taken with amitriptyline and Cymbalta but not with Lyrica. Most of the time, I give Neurontin/gabapentin at night to prevent pain during sleep.

3. *Lyrica/pregabalin* — Lyrica/pregabalin is also a seizure medication, just like gabapentin/Neurontin. On the other hand, clinically appears to be much more effective than Neurontin. I also give Lyrica at nighttime using a low dose to start, gradually increasing the dose within weeks until symptoms are better. The most common side are dizziness, sleepiness, confusion, swelling in the feet and ankles, and weight gain. It is a controlled substance due to the potential for addiction. It can be taken with duloxetine, amitriptyline, or nortriptyline, but not with gabapentin.

4. *Alpha-lipoic acid* – this can also potentially be helpful as an antioxidant medication. Although there are no long-term studies, some short-term studies proved helpful for diabetic neuropathy.

If these oral agents fail, I may prescribe a compounded topical medication that can include gabapentin and lidocaine, plus other medications that can help with pain control. I typically recommend these topical creams be applied twice a day.

Diabetic Foot Care

The American Diabetes Association recommends that diabetic patients should have a foot examination once per year. Personally, I say you should be looking carefully at all parts of your feet at least twice a week yourself, especially the area between the toes every few days or every day. Look for blisters, ulcers, broken skin, ulcers, and areas of increased redness or warmth.

You should also pay close attention to changes in callus formation. Calluses are the areas with diminished sensation, which will naturally lead to ulcer formation under certain conditions. Let your endocrinologist know if you notice if any of these changes or have any concerns about your feet.

If you cannot easily examine your own feet, you can ask your partner or use a mirror to examine your feet. If you make this a routine, it will be a part of your life that should not be a cumbersome task. Some other important tips:

1. You should also avoid activities that could damage your feet.
2. Avoid soaking your feet for a long time or wearing wet or sweaty socks.
3. Try to avoid using hot water and test the temperature of the water with your hand first before putting your feet into hot water.
4. Do not pop blisters.
5. Never cut the cuticles or let anyone cut your cuticles.
6. Trim the toenails carefully. If you think you will need help, ask help from a podiatrist for this task.

7. Keep your feet clean by washing your feet daily; however, make sure you dry them well and never keep them wet. Use moisturizing cream and lotion to prevent breaks in the skin due to dryness.

8. If you have diabetic neuropathy, seeing a podiatrist at least one time may be a good idea to see if you will need a fitted shoe to prevent calluses and blisters.

Preventing Diabetic Neuropathy

Prevention of nerve damage is usually the best option because treatment after the fact can be lengthy, difficult, and often painful. Some types of nerve damage will go away on their own. In such cases, pain medication is the only thing you need. In other cases, the best way to prevent diabetic neuropathy is to have the best diabetes control you can. In other words, keep your A1c as low as possible. Prevention of neuropathy should be your major focus early in the course of your diabetes. The following are some of the ways you can prevent nerve damage:

1. *Maintain Healthy Glucose Levels:* Monitor your glucose levels and keep them down. This is because nerve damage mainly occurs from high blood sugar levels. Most endocrinologists recommend that you use a CGM (continuous glucose monitor) such as Dexcom G6 or Freestyle Libre to track your sugars. You should also have an A1C test at least twice a year to understand your average blood sugar levels. In some instances, more frequent A1c testing is justified.

2. *Be Attentive to Your Feet:* Always be attentive to your feet and pay attention to any numbness, sensitivity, and tingling you have or evidence of sores, lesions, or signs of infections on your feet. Always keep your feet properly cleaned and disinfected to control any infections. If left unchecked, you could need an amputation; your neuropathy will make it difficult for the infection to heal.

3. *Exercise and Dietary Changes:* Exercising and meal control are necessities, but you should be careful when you are exercising. If you get injured during exercise, it can be difficult for your injury to heal.

B12 is an important supplement in the diet you should take to keep your nerves healthy. Stay away from food with a high glycemic index.

Diabetic neuropathy is common yet preventable. Treatment is also available. You do not have to suffer from the pain due to diabetic neuropathy. Prevention is always preferable to having to treat your symptoms after they have begun.

Peripheral Vascular Disease

Vascular disease in diabetes is also sometimes called peripheral vascular disease or peripheral arterial disease because it mainly affects the arteries of the periphery of your body (your limbs). Because your legs are longer and further from your heart, these are the body parts most affected by the poor blood flow you'd get if your small-sized arteries are partially or completely blocked.

The same thing that causes heart attacks leads to vascular disease of the legs (atherosclerosis). While you might need an amputation if the blood flow to your legs is severe enough, most amputations happen from diabetic neuropathy and poor healing of any sores you get; you need good blood flow to heal foot sores.

How Do Diabetic Foot Ulcers And Gangrene Begin?

With vascular disease, diabetic foot sores become ulcers that then get infected. Poor circulation also means antibiotics for infection have a harder time getting to the site. This is where severe infections and gangrene can happen.

Remember that when your blood sugars are increased and when you're insulin resistant, these things will have a significant impact on the narrowing of your blood vessels, especially the small arteries, which are those that supply blood to your hands or your feet.

What happens is that these blood vessels start getting clogged up over time, often in the early stages of diabetes. The nerves that need nourishment from those blood vessels or arteries begin to die off.

It's a combination of multiple factors that lead to infected ulcers and gangrene. The nerve damage causes a loss of sensation under your feet and, if you walk barefoot, you can step on things and might not notice the injury. You can also get sores by wearing ill-fitting shoes that rub too much on vulnerable spots in your feet. Your feet aren't the cleanest part of your body, so it's easy to have a break in the skin become infected.

Anytime you have an opening in the skin, you make the tissue in that area vulnerable to having the bacteria on your skin get inside and set up an infection. It can even happen if you clean your feet regularly and wear shoes and socks. High blood sugars in your blood and tissues allow the bacteria to thrive better. This is the optimal situation for the start of an infection of your foot tissues. Untreated infections lead to foot ulcers.

The infection often gets deeper and deeper and can sometimes reach the bone. These deep infections are very difficult to heal on your own, so you often need antibiotics to help them heal. If the infected sore is not healing, we turn to surgeons to remove some of the dead and dying tissue without performing an actual amputation. This is sometimes enough to help the remaining healthier tissue to heal.

Unfortunately, gangrene can set in. Gangrene is often a combination of infection and a lot of dead tissue. This dead tissue cannot regenerate itself and, if your life is at risk because you have so much decomposing tissue on your foot or leg, the surgeon must remove the toe, foot, or even part of the leg to save your life. Most people who need to have an amputation will lose part of their foot, their foot at the level of the ankle, or the leg above or just below the knee.

Bone infections are an especially difficult problem to treat because it's almost impossible to get the infection out of it. If the infection is cured at all, it will often take weeks or months to be successful in doing this. If you add the problem of high blood sugars that feed the infection and the weak immune system seen in many diabetics, getting rid of the infection is extremely difficult.

Remember that diabetic wound care management involves a lot of teamwork. If you have your primary care doctor giving you an antibiotic for a diabetic foot ulcer and your infection is not getting better, you need to see your podiatrist. If you don't have one, go immediately to the emergency department.

Some hospitals will have wound care centers with podiatrists or orthopedic surgeons trained to treat complex wound infections. Diabetic foot ulcers should be very carefully observed until they heal completely to prevent needing an amputation. Your doctor may also talk to a vascular surgeon if something can be done to open your arteries and improve your leg circulation.

Most of the time, your podiatrist, endocrinologist, vascular surgeon, wound care nurses, and sometimes an infectious disease specialist will work together to get rid of your infection and save the limb. You are part of the team when you practice foot self-exams to prevent infections from starting in the first place.

Kidney Disease

Kidney disease in diabetics is called diabetic nephropathy. It leads to CKD or "chronic kidney disease." Most people do not realize that diabetes-related chronic kidney disease is extremely common. Many diabetics don't even know that they have it. Only 10 percent of diabetics with stage 3 diabetic kidney disease are even aware of their diagnosis.

This unawareness is also common among people with stage 4 kidney disease; less than 60 percent of these individuals are aware of their disease. Stage 5 kidney disease means you need dialysis. More than 50,000 people with end-stage kidney disease from diabetes are on dialysis in the US.

Realistically, how can you prevent a problem you aren't even aware of? Let's look at this common diabetic complication and explore ways you can prevent and manage it, so you never need dialysis or a kidney transplant.

Stages of Chronic Kidney Disease		GFR*	% of Kidney Function
Stage 1	Kidney damage with **normal** kidney function	90 or higher	90-100%
Stage 2	Kidney damage with **mild loss of** kidney function	89-60	89-60%
Stage 3a	**Mild to moderate** loss of kidney function	59-45	59-45%
Stage 3b	**Moderate to severe** loss of kidney function	44-30	44-30%
Stage 4	**Severe** loss of kidney function	29-15	29-15%
Stage 5	Kidney **failure**	less than 15	<15%

Your GFR number tells you how much kidney function you have. As kidney disease gets worse, the GFR number goes down.

How Does Diabetic Kidney Disease Develop?

High blood sugars in your bloodstream cause your blood cells to become sticky. They tend to stick to one another and along the sides of the blood vessels. The blood vessels become inflamed, which attracts inflammation chemicals to the area. This makes the inflammation even worse.

Remember how I said insulin resistance was also a major culprit in causing this problem? It means you start having these blood vessel changes even before you have true diabetes. When this happens in the small arteries within the kidneys, they become larger, and blood flow increases to the kidney filtering system. This lasts only a short while before the kidneys begin to burn out. This is when you start having chronic kidney disease.

Because healthy cells in the kidney die off in early diabetic kidney disease, the blood flow starts to drop. We measure the blood flow through the kidneys using the GFR or *glomerular filtration rate*. You can find your GFR on your lab tests where the kidney testing (creatinine and BUN) are located. There will often be two values listed, one for African Americans and one for all others. Find the one that fits for you and look it up on the image to find your stage.

Another important thing that happens in the diabetic kidney is that glucose absorption increases. It means that even if glucose is filtered in the urine, it gets absorbed easily back into your bloodstream. This causes the blood sugar to remain high.

Remember that the class of diabetic drugs, including Jardiance, Invokana, Steglatro, and Farxiga, work by decreasing glucose absorption. These drugs help reduce the glucose load in the blood by allowing your kidneys to excrete more sugar in the urine. Some of these drugs, such as Invokana and Jardiance, have also been shown to reduce the progression of chronic kidney disease. They do this by reducing the stress on the kidneys.

Other drugs used for diabetes do not improve kidney function. Metformin, for example, does not dramatically damage the kidney but should not be used in those with severe CKD. Metformin doesn't clear out of the body as well in severe kidney disease, so it tends to accumulate in the blood. This buildup of metformin can lead to excess acid in the body, which can be dangerous. Your endocrinologist will tell you when it's time to stop metformin if your kidneys are damaged. I rarely stop metformin until my patient has stage 4 CKD(GFR<30). Yet, I do not start someone on metformin if GFR is below 60. The FDA also recommends this practice.

What Are The Risk Factors For Diabetic Kidney Disease?

All diabetics have a risk for kidney disease, but there are some risk factors you should be aware of:

» Increasing age and longer duration of diabetes play a role.

» Race and ethnicity is a risk factor; if you are an African-American, Latino, or American Indian, your risk for CKD is higher.

» CKD from diabetes is more common in women than in men.

» Low socioeconomic status increases the risk of CKD because of decreased access to healthcare and fewer opportunities to prevent the disease from occurring.

» Obesity is an independent risk factor, even without diabetes.

» Smoking is a huge risk factor independent of diabetes. When combined with diabetes, smoking can be very detrimental to kidney function.

» Having persistently high blood sugar levels/out of control diabetes.

» High blood pressure is also an important risk factor in the progression of kidney disease.

» Genetic factors also contribute to the development of kidney disease from diabetes.

» Acute kidney injury, on top of chronic kidney disease, is also more likely in patients with diabetes. Dehydration especially can trigger acute on top of chronic kidney disease.

Doctors can often detect kidney diseases relatively early by finding protein in a urine sample. This is called *microalbuminuria*. Your GFR might even be normal at this stage. If the amount of protein is greater than 30 mg/gram of urine, we call that *microalbuminuria* and, If the amount of proteins is greater than 300 mg/gram of urine, this is called *macroalbuminuria*. Protein in the urine isn't seen in every case, but if there is a large amount of it, it can increase the rate of worsening of your kidney disease.

Signs And Symptoms Of Chronic Kidney Disease

You probably won't notice you have CKD until it is relatively advanced (stage 4 and 5 mostly). If you have symptoms, you'll most likely see these only in advanced kidney disease. They include fluid overload (swelling in the legs, excessive urination at night), high potassium levels in the blood, low CO2 level in the blood, high blood pressure, and worsening high blood pressure, anemia, and osteoporosis (fragile bones).

By the time you need dialysis, you could easily have signs of uremia. These include lack of appetite, nausea, vomiting, fluid around the heart, neuropathy, poor concentration, lethargy, and seizures.

How Is Diabetic Kidney Disease Prevented And Managed?

Even though CKD from diabetes is often seen before you know you have diabetes or when the disease is in its early stages, there are things you can do to keep it from getting worse. There is no reason to expect to have dialysis in your future if you can help participate in these management strategies:

- ***Control your blood pressure:*** Strict blood pressure control is extremely important in addition to blood sugar control in managing your CKD. Blood pressure control not only reduces the progression of kidney disease but also reduces your risk of dying from heart disease. CKD is a risk factor for heart attacks and stroke by itself, so if you can improve your blood pressure, it has a major impact on your health. The sad fact is that most diabetics die of heart disease before they need dialysis from chronic kidney disease, so managing blood pressure crucial in decreasing mortality. The most common agents we use for blood pressure control in patients with diabetes are called ACE inhibitors or angiotensin receptor blockers.

- ***Control your blood sugars:*** You need to strive to keep your blood sugar as close to normal as possible without causing significantly low blood sugars (hypoglycemia). Keeping your A1c less than 7 (and less than 6.5 if possible) is the ultimate goal for most patients not at risk for low blood sugars. For older patients (80 years or above) or for those who have too many problems with a high risk of low blood sugar, the optimal A1c goal is sometimes higher. Continuous glucose monitoring systems such as Dexcom and Freestyle Libre are extremely helpful to help prevent low blood sugars as well as high blood sugars.

- *Manage obesity:* Controlling obesity is another important factor in preventing kidney disease. We try to use medications that can help with weight loss, such as Byetta, Bydureon, Trulicity, Ozempic, Jardiance, Invokana, or Farxiga. These agents not only help with weight loss; they also reduce the progression of kidney disease. The only problem with these agents is that they are very expensive. I work with insurance companies and patients to try to get them the most affordable and effective medications.

- *Manage your cholesterol:* Reducing cholesterol levels (especially your LDL-cholesterol) is extremely important. There are safe and effective medications you can take if diet alone is ineffective in helping normalize your lipid profile/cholesterol levels.

Many people ask me about restricting protein in chronic kidney disease. It isn't known if it will make a difference to keep your protein intake very low. My recommendation is to avoid eating excessive amounts of protein and instead stick to about 50-60 grams per day.

You should have your kidney-related blood work (including the GFR) every 3-6 months when you have diabetes-induced chronic kidney disease. Your blood pressure and medications should be reviewed by your endocrinologist at every visit. Your A1c is also checked along with your cholesterol levels at regular intervals.

You should know that not everyone with diabetes and chronic kidney disease will need dialysis. Some will progress rapidly and need dialysis relatively quickly, while others have stable disease and will never need dialysis. If you can continue to reduce your risk factors for kidney disease progression, you will be more likely to have stable rather than progressive disease.

Diabetic Retinopathy

Diabetic retinopathy can lead to blindness if not managed as soon as problems develop. You may not know yourself that you have early eye disease or retinopathy, which is why you need regular eye exams with an eye doctor/ophthalmologist who will dilate your eye and look at the retina, which is the back of the eye containing the cells that take your visual signals and send them back to the brain. You would not be able to see at all without healthy retinal cells.

The risk factors you should know about for diabetic eye disease include:

- *A long duration of diabetes:* The longer you have diabetes, and the higher your blood sugars, the faster the progression of diabetic retinopathy. Both type 1 and type 2 diabetics can develop diabetic retinopathy early on in their disease. Exactly who will develop diabetic retinopathy remains uncertain. Sometimes it develops even before diabetes is diagnosed; at other times, it takes more than five years with uncontrolled diabetes to have eye disease. It appears that some people are more susceptible to eye damage from high blood sugars than others.

- *Poor diabetes/glucose control:* Even a small decrease in A1C can be beneficial in reducing diabetic eye disease. For example, each 1 percent decrease in A1C reduces the diabetic retinopathy risk by approximately 20-30 percent. Remember the Legacy Effect and the fact that early diabetes control will have a tremendous impact in the long-term. Many diabetic medications, especially if you take them as soon as your endocrinologist recommends them, can help control the risk of diabetic eye disease.

- *Hypertension:* High blood pressure definitely affects the blood vessels, just like high blood sugar does. This means that controlling your blood pressure elevations may be equally important as controlling blood sugars.

- *Having other diabetes-related complications:* People who have diabetic nephropathy are more likely to develop diabetic retinopathy as well. Having diabetic neuropathy also means you need to watch your eyes more carefully for evidence of disease.

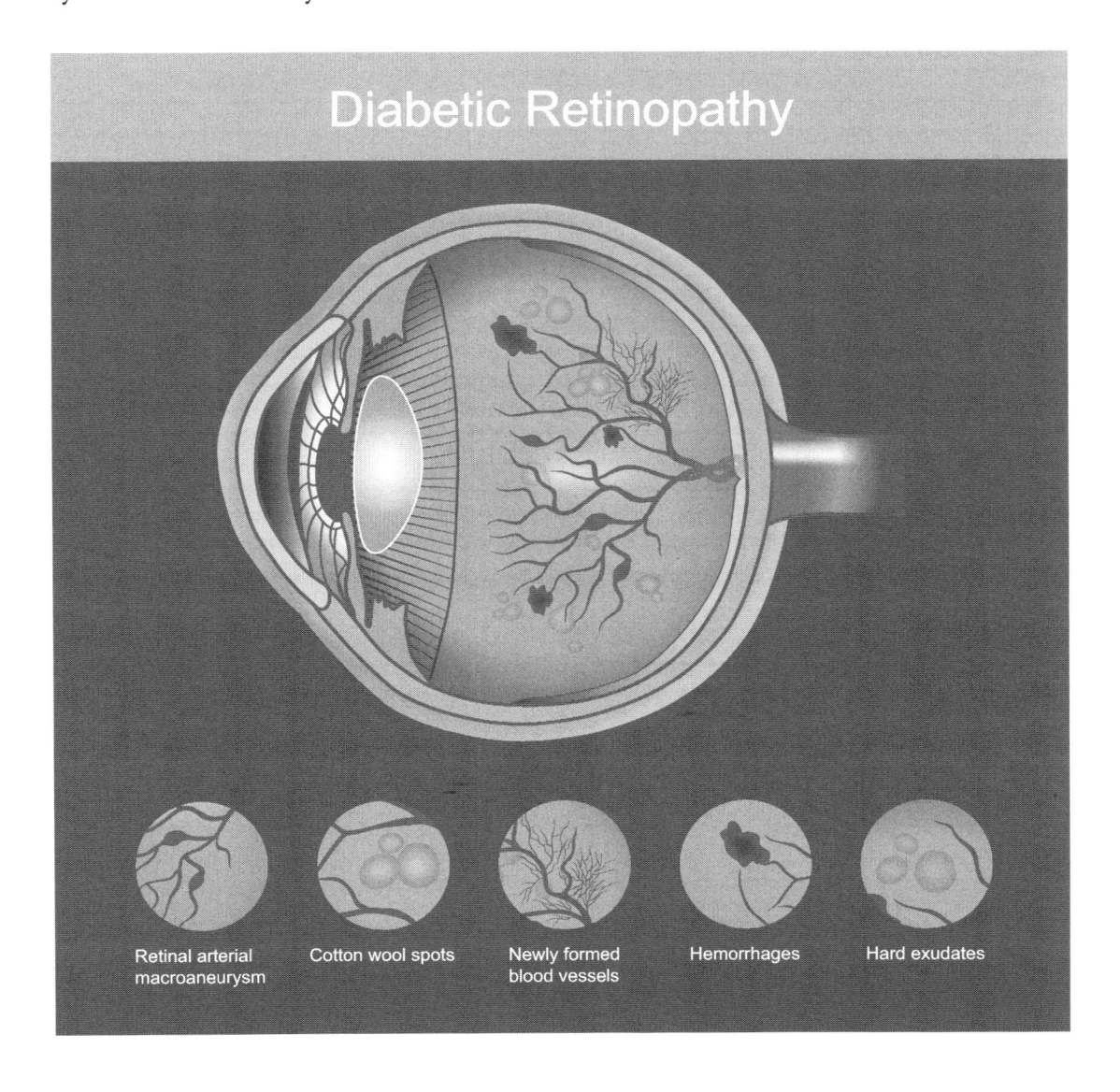

Diabetic Retinopathy

- Retinal arterial macroaneurysm
- Cotton wool spots
- Newly formed blood vessels
- Hemorrhages
- Hard exudates

- ***High cholesterol:*** High cholesterol is certainly a high-risk situation for the development of diabetic retinopathy. High cholesterol is just as bad for your blood vessels as is high blood sugar.

- ***Pregnancy:*** Pregnancy transiently increases the risk for progression of diabetic retinopathy. I counsel my pregnant patients for the potential increase in the risk of retinopathy while they are pregnant. I recommend more frequent retinal evaluations during pregnancy and for one year afterward.

Symptoms Of Diabetic Retinopathy

Most people with diabetic retinopathy have no symptoms until the disease is very advanced. By then, it is usually too late to do anything about vision loss. That's why it is vital to get screened for the condition as soon as you know you have diabetes. That way, doctors can take steps to protect your eyes before your vision is damaged.

I recommend having an eye examination once a year. If your eye examinations are normal for several years and your diabetes is in good control, you can decrease the frequency of eye exams to every two years.
When do symptoms occur, you may experience any of these:

» The sensation of blindness happening "like a curtain falling", even if this is transient

» Floaters in your visual field

» Blurry vision that cannot be corrected with glasses

» Floating spots or dark spots in your vision

» Trouble seeing objects that are at the center of your focus when reading or driving

» Difficulty telling colors apart

Testing For Diabetic Retinopathy

There are tests you can have with an ophthalmologist to see if you have any signs of diabetic eye disease. These tests are more commonly done:

- *Dilated eye exam:* During this exam, the eye doctor will give you eye drops to dilate your pupils. These drops allow the eye doctor to see all the different parts of the inside of your eye. After the drops have started working, the doctor looks at the back of your eye in the area called the retina. That's where blood vessel damage causes you to lose your vision.

- *Digital Retinal imaging:* For this test, a technician takes pictures of your eyes with a special camera. Then they send the images to an ophthalmologist (eye doctor). The ophthalmologist will look at those pictures to see what your retinas look like. It is a less sensitive test than the dilated eye exam but is often used if your past eye tests have all been normal. If not, you should have a regular dilated eye exam in an ophthalmologist's office.

If either the digital retinal image or the dilated eye exam shows any signs of disease, the ophthalmologist may order some other testing as well to see how much damage you have in your eyes.

Preventing Diabetic Retinopathy

The prevention of diabetic retinopathy involves managing your blood sugars, controlling high blood pressure, and reducing cholesterol. Healthy eating and exercise help you to minimize the risk of retinopathy by addressing many of the major risk factors. Avoid weight-lifting if you have known diabetic eye disease as this might cause bleeding in your retina. Talk to your ophthalmologist before choosing an activity you are unfamiliar with.

For those who have type 1 diabetes, you should start having eye exams 3 to 5 years after your initial diagnosis. We know that most people with type 1 diabetes do not have diabetic retinopathy until three to five years after their diagnosis. Unfortunately, almost all will be affected at 15 to 20 years. Type 2 diabetics should start having eye exams as soon as they are diagnosed.

Treating Diabetic Retinopathy

When mild, diabetic retinopathy does not always need treatment. Of course, you will still need medications for diabetes and should continue to monitor your blood sugar carefully. Your eye doctor must closely monitor you, even if you do not need urgent treatment. Even with mild disease, you need to keep your blood sugar and blood pressure levels as close to normal as possible. Doing so keeps the condition from getting worse.

With appropriate screening, excellent control of glucose levels and blood pressure along with early intervention with both surgical and pharmacologic therapies, you and your medical team can prevent severe vision loss.

Treatments you may need if your disease worsens include:

- *Photocoagulation:* This is laser surgery used to seal or destroy leaking or growing blood vessels in the retina. This treatment is not always the first option. Doctors typically try medicines first.

- *Medicines:* The ophthalmologist will inject medicine into the vitreous humor (the liquid in the eyeball). They sometimes use medicine alone or along with other treatments. Doctors commonly use medications such as anti-VEGF. Anti-VEGF is common for the treatment of symptomatic macular edema. Your eye doctor will let you know if medicines might help you. Anti-VEGF treatment may take months or even a few years to be helpful to you. If you cannot maintain this treatment strategy, you may want to discuss alternative options with your ophthalmologist.

- *Vitrectomy:* This is surgery to remove blood from the part of the eye called the "vitreous humor." Eye doctors do this surgery if the blood vessels in the retina leak into the vitreous humor. In diabetic patients with macular edema that is not responding to anti-VEGF treatment and photocoagulation, having a vitrectomy may be an option.

In Summary

Diabetic retinopathy is one of the more common complications of both type 1 and type 2 diabetes. Early treatment is absolutely important to prevent vision loss. Keeping the A1c below 7% and, if possible, below 6.5% is critical. Also, keep your blood pressure below 140/90 or below 130/80, if possible. This reduces one of the risks for diabetic retinopathy. Keeping your LDL cholesterol below 100 mg/dL is another way to reduce the risk of diabetic retinopathy. Exercising regularly about five times per week is also helpful.

One of the cholesterol medications, fenofibrate, can directly help reduce the risk of diabetic retinopathy, too. Your endocrinologist might prescribe fenofibrate to you if you have high triglycerides. Having diabetic retinopathy and having high triglycerides together can be a good reason to take fenofibrate.

Gastroparesis

Diabetic gastroparesis simply means "delayed gastric emptying" in the absence of mechanical obstruction. Patients feel excessive fullness, bloating, nausea, and in some cases, vomiting and abdominal pain. Longstanding diabetes, especially type 1 diabetes, is the main reason for developing gastroparesis. Diabetic gastroparesis does not often happen within the first five years of diabetes; however, after the first ten years of the diagnosis, gastroparesis tends to happen in 5% of type 1 diabetic individuals and 1% of type 2 diabetic individuals.

Patients with gastroparesis also tend to have other types of neuropathy (nervous system dysfunction) problems, such as orthostatic low blood pressure(dizziness upon standing up from a sitting position) in some cases. Some patients may also have a loss of change in their heart rhythm upon breathing during the EKG study. Normally when we inhale and exhale, our heart rate changes. In patients with autonomic neuropathy, heart rate will not change with inhalation and exhalation.

Symptoms tend to be more severe in type 1 diabetic individuals when they have gastroparesis. It also makes diabetes difficult to control because the food in the stomach might not get absorbed for a few hours and then and gets dumped suddenly after many hours of sitting in the stomach.

For insulin users, this can cause low blood sugar within the first 2 hours of insulin injection and then high blood sugars about 5 to 6 hours after food intake. This is because mealtime insulin only lasts 4 hours in your system. On the other hand, your stomach can release its content 5 hours after ingesting food. Gastroparesis typically happens among long-term diabetics; however, blood sugar spikes above 200 mg/dL (11.1 mmol/l) will also cause gastroparesis acutely. So when blood sugars are more controlled, the symptoms of gastroparesis tend to improve.

Medications That Can Cause Or Worsen Gastroparesis

Some medications can also cause delayed gastric emptying, such as narcotics (opioid drugs such as morphine), blood pressure medications such as clonidine and amlodipine, diabetes medications such as Victoza, Ozempic, Trulicity, Rybelsus, and antirejection drugs like cyclosporine. if you are on one of these medications, you may need to discuss with your physician possible alternatives.

How Do We Diagnose Diabetic Gastroparesis?

We always do upper gastrointestinal endoscopy to rule out mechanical obstruction. A barium follow-through examination can also be done. If available, CT or MRI enterography can be very helpful. If there is no evidence of obstruction, we will do a gastric emptying study. Individuals typically eat solid food, and scintigraphic imaging can detect if the emptying is slow. We diagnose gastric emptying if gastric retention of food is more than 10% at 4 hours and/or more than 60% at 2 hours when Individuals eat low-fat scrambled eggs at the start of the test. If it is more than 35% retention at 4 hours, we consider that severe gastroparesis.

How To Treat Diabetic Gastroparesis

Dietary modification is the most important initial step in managing gastroparesis. We tell our patients to avoid fatty, spicy, acidic, and high-fiber foods. Yes, high-fiber typically helps diabetics when they do not have gastroparesis. However, when someone has gastroparesis, high fiber content makes it worse and delays gastric emptying even further. One exception is well-cooked soluble fiber, which can be much easier to digest.

Liquids are much better tolerated, so if an individual cannot tolerate solid food, we generally recommend patients concentrate on liquid foods or homogenize solid foods (you can grind solid foods). If you are vomiting, we need to make sure that your hydration is adequate so enough to have enough potassium and liquid in your system.
Controlling blood sugar is extremely important. As we have discussed, sudden spikes in blood sugar will create an abrupt slowdown in gastric emptying.

Pharmacological options include metoclopramide (liquid form) 10 mg 3-4 times a day before meals. If symptoms persist, we use domperidone 10 to 20 mg 3 times a day. If symptoms continue, we will use erythromycin up to 250 mg a day 3 times a day. If everything else fails, gastric electrical stimulation can be used as a last resort.

Erectile Dysfunction

As a person ages, sexual problems such as erectile dysfunction (ED) become more common. In those with diabetes, these problems can be even more common than in the normal population. Other health problems can mean that having or enjoying sex may be difficult for you or your partner.

High blood glucose levels over time can cause blood vessels and nerves to become damaged. This damage can lead to sexual and bladder problems. One way to prevent this damage to your blood vessels and nerves is by keeping your blood glucose within the target range.

Having erectile dysfunction can be a sign that you need to manage your diabetes differently. A healthy sex life can greatly improve your quality of life. Now is the time to take action if you have any of these concerns. This is because ED is best treated shortly after you notice it.

Could Erectile Dysfunction (ED) Be A Symptom Of Diabetes?

Any change in sexual function may be an indication of diabetes. Diabetic neuropathy can happen anywhere in the body and will damage important nerves leading to your genitals or urinary tract. According to a study published in Diabetic Medicine, men with diabetes may develop erectile dysfunction (ED) 10 to 15 years earlier than men without diabetes. Approximately 50 percent of men develop ED after just ten years with diabetes.

Risk Factors For Erectile Dysfunction In Diabetics

You are more likely to develop sexual problems if you have diabetes and any of the following:

- » High blood glucose
- » Nerve damage or neuropathy
- » High blood pressure
- » High cholesterol
- » Overweight or obese
- » Not physically active
- » Taking certain medications like blood pressure or depression medications.
- » Consume too many alcoholic drinks
- » Smoke tobacco products

Other Types Of Sexual Problems Seen In Men

Diabetes can cause changes in your blood vessels, nerves, and hormones. Poor emotional health may also make it more difficult to have satisfactory sex. This can happen due to low sex desire, ejaculation problems, and/or erectile dysfunction. Diabetes and other related challenges may make it harder for you to have a child, too. These are the main issues you might face:

- *Retrograde Ejaculation:* Diabetes can rarely cause retrograde ejaculation. This happens when some or all of your semen goes into the bladder instead of leaving your penis during ejaculation. The semen mixes with urine and is later urinated out. A urine sample after ejaculation can show if you have retrograde ejaculation. In some men, ejaculation may not occur at all.

- *Penile Curvature:* Men with diabetes are more likely to have Peyronie's disease (also called penile curvature). Peyronie's disease causes the penis to curve when erect due to scar tissue on one side of the penis. These curves in the penis can cause sexual intercourse to be painful or difficult. Men with Peyronie's disease may also have ED.

- *Low Testosterone:* A man's testosterone levels naturally become lower with age. These lower testosterone levels can be the cause of some cases of ED. This is a good explanation of why some men often feel tired, depressed, or have a lower sex drive. Men who are more likely to have low testosterone include diabetic men who are older or overweight.

- *Fertility Problems:* Many studies have shown that men with diabetes may have problems with their sperm. This can make it harder to conceive. According to one study, sperm may be slow or not move very well. Sometimes sperm may not be able to fertilize a woman's egg very well. If you want to conceive, work closely with your healthcare provider as well as your partner. There are some advances in reproductive technology that might work.

In addition to increasing age, the main factors associated with ED are peripheral or autonomic neuropathy, retinopathy (diabetic eye disease), long duration of diabetes, and poor glycemic control.

The severity of ED is positively correlated with the duration of your diabetes. Moreover, poor glycemic control, diuretic (water pill) therapy, and the presence of diabetic eye disease, chronic diabetic kidney disease, or neuropathy contribute to having this sexual problem. The presence of cardiovascular disease is a huge risk factor for ED because blood vessels to the penis are blocked. If you have ED and diabetes, there is a good chance you have cardiovascular disease as well.

Types Of Sexual Problems In Women

Women with diabetes can experience low sexual desire, vaginal dryness, and painful sex. These can be caused by nerve damage, reduced blood flow to the genital area, and hormonal changes. Other conditions, such as menopause, can cause these symptoms as well. If you notice any of these changes, talk to your endocrinologist about what you can do.

Low sexual desire and responsiveness can include any of these symptoms:

- » Unable to become or stay aroused
- » Not having enough vaginal lubrication
- » Having little to no feeling in your genitals
- » Being unable to have an orgasm or rarely having one

Your body and mind go through many changes with diabetes. High and low blood glucose levels can affect your sex life if you become aroused. You may also find yourself more tired, depressed, or anxious, which can cause you to become less interested in sex. Women who keep blood glucose levels in the target range are less likely to have nerve damage, which can lead to low sexual desire and response.

These are the sexual issues that often affect a woman with diabetes:

- *Painful Sex:* Diabetes can make sexual intercourse uncomfortable or painful for some women. In women with diabetes, the nerves that signal your vagina to lubricate during stimulation can often become damaged. Prescription or over-the-counter vaginal lubricants can help with vaginal dryness. Good management of your blood glucose can help prevent this type of nerve damage.

- ***Yeast and bladder infections:*** Diabetes makes women more likely to develop yeast infections. Yeast organisms grow more easily when blood glucose levels are higher. These infections are uncomfortable or painful and can prevent the enjoyment of sex. Fungal infections are typically treated at home with prescription pills or vaginal creams. You need to discuss your symptoms with your endocrinologist.

- ***Pregnancy concerns and fertility problems:*** If you plan to become pregnant and have diabetes, it's important to get your blood glucose levels close to your target range even before you become pregnant. High blood glucose levels can harm your baby during the first weeks of pregnancy. If you are already pregnant and have diabetes, see your provider as soon as possible. This will help you make a plan to manage your diabetes.

Management And Treatment

You should see your health care provider for any problems with sex or your bladder. Problems like these could be a sign that you may need to manage your diabetes differently. You should also be able to prevent nerve damage by managing your diabetes. Better diabetic control can reduce the risk of developing sexual problems. These interventions will help the most:

> » Keeping your blood glucose, blood pressure, and cholesterol levels close to your target numbers
> » Being and staying physically active
> » Keeping and maintaining a healthy weight
> » Quitting smoking if you do smoke
> » Getting help for any emotional or psychological problems that arise

Sexual intercourse is a physical activity; therefore, be sure to check your blood glucose levels before and after sex. Both high and low blood glucose levels can cause problems during sex.

Final Thoughts

You should know that few people actually die of "diabetes"—blood sugars being too low or too high in ways that are fatal. Most people by far die of the complications of the disease; cardiovascular disease is the main fatal complication of diabetes. While things like diabetic retinopathy and peripheral vascular disease do not usually cause death, they are very disabling and can make life difficult and challenging for the diabetic for many years.

Yes, diabetes is a progressive disease with many complications. Remember the Legacy Effect, however, and make sure you do what you can to maintain normal blood sugars, manage your weight, and start adjusting your lifestyle with the idea that this is the lifestyle you will maintain for the rest of your life. This is all doable if you put your mind toward a commitment to health, even if you don't honor that commitment every single day.

CHAPTER 4 - DIABETES MANAGEMENT

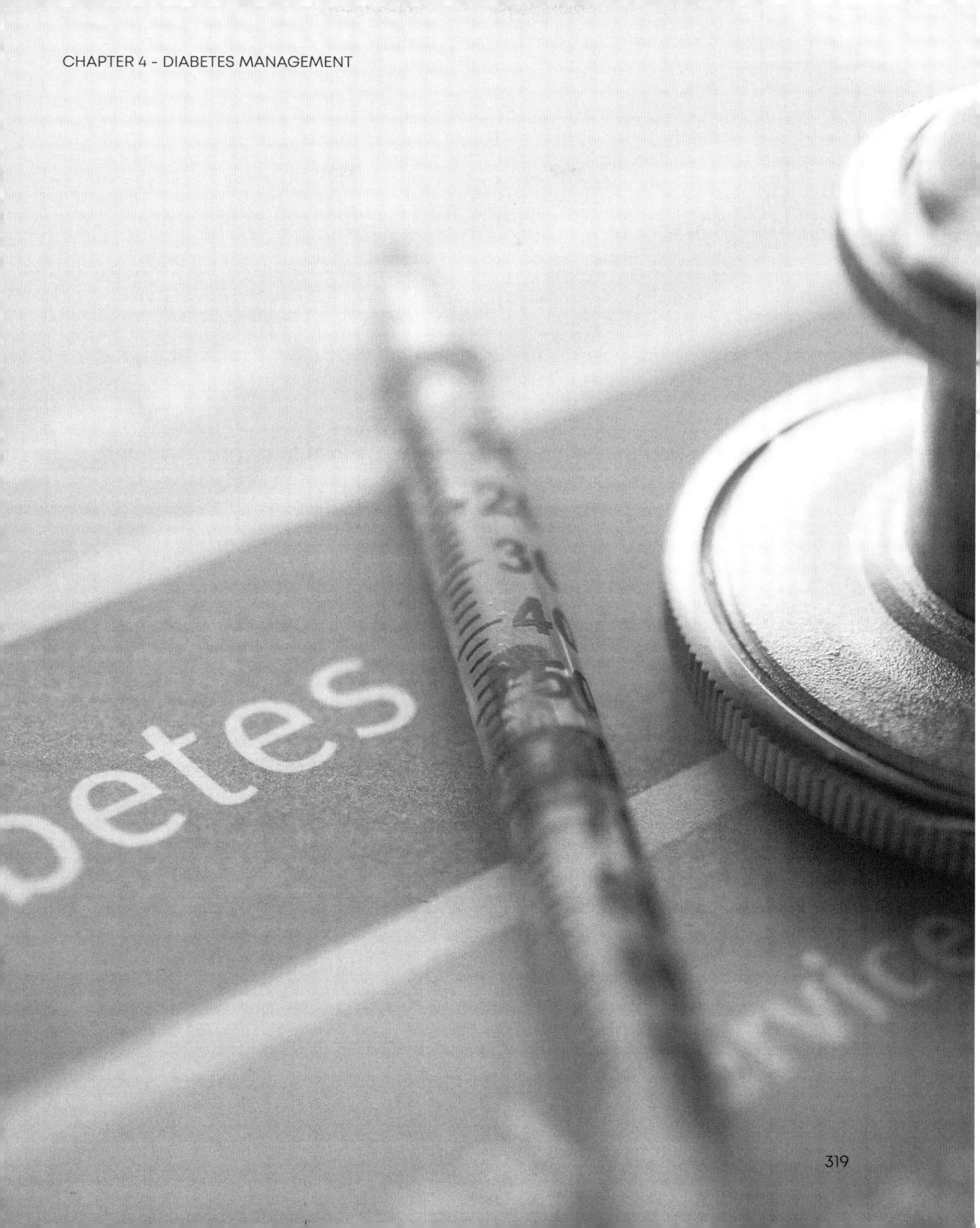

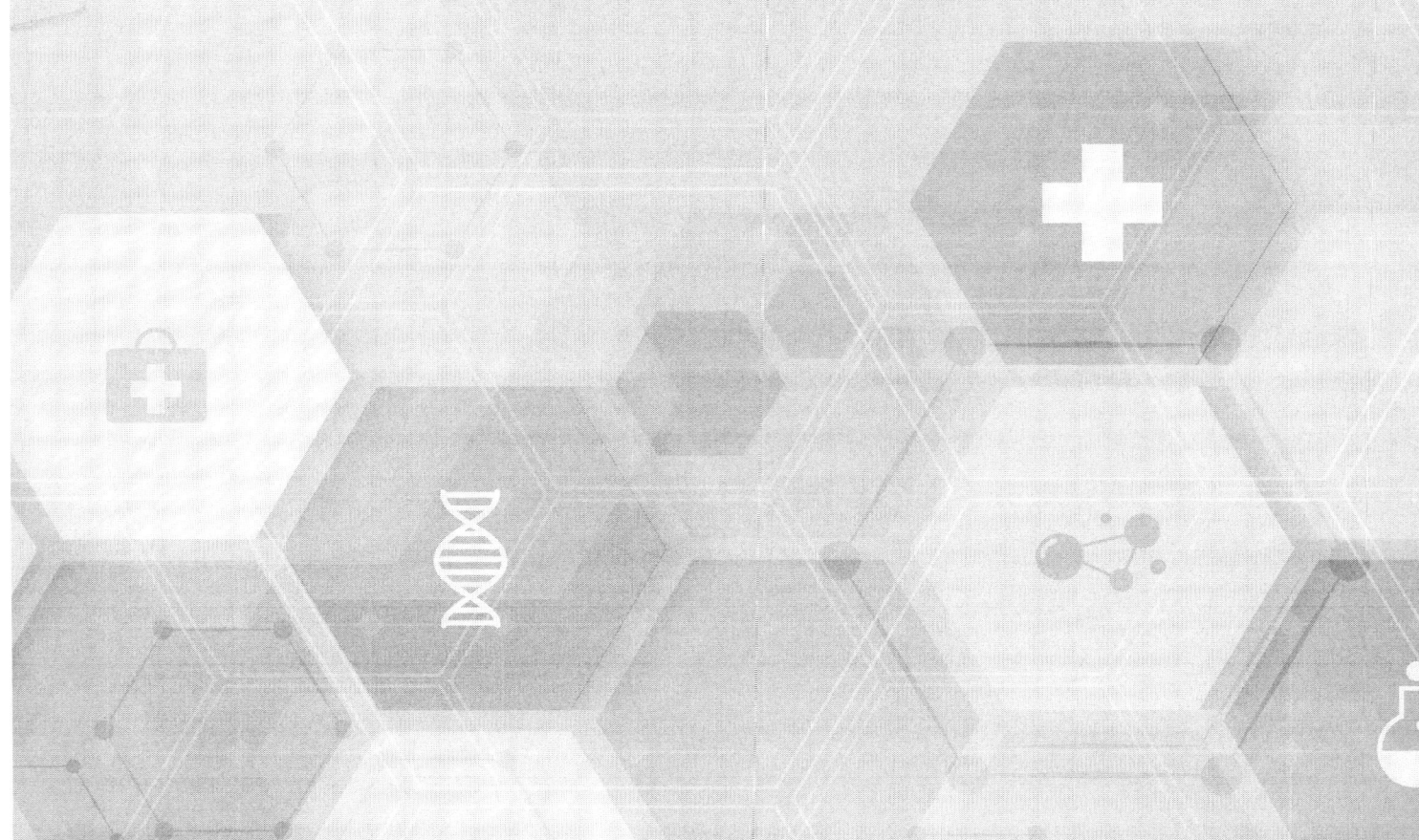

CHAPTER 5
DIABETES TECHNOLOGY

CHAPTER 5
DIABETES TECHNOLOGY

The management of diabetes has gotten to be much more high-tech than it was even 20-30 years ago. Diabetics used to guess what the effect of carbs would be on their blood sugar and take medication to account for the meal. There is a large potential for error in doing this, with equal risks for taking too much insulin or too little.

Also, what we know about diabetes is that good control makes a huge difference in the rate of adverse outcomes. Some insulin delivery systems may be complicated to manage, for example, but there is a huge payoff when it comes to reducing the chances of diabetes complications.

In this section, we will look at the different technologies you can use to help manage your diabetes in ways that were unavailable even a few years ago. These include insulin pumps, continuous glucose monitoring devices (CGMs), remote diabetes monitoring, and telemedicine.

Insulin Pumps

Diabetes, whether it is type 1 or type 2, is a serious chronic condition, but you can still manage diabetes successfully with the help of a healthy lifestyle and proper medical care. Some patients will need insulin injections at a certain point in their diabetes management. However, for those who are too busy or squeamish about dealing with an injection, a useful tool they can use is an insulin pump.

There is no such thing as the "best insulin pump." After you read this section and my recommendations, you will have a better idea of which glucose pump to choose from. There are advantages and disadvantages to each. You should also talk to your endocrinologist about which one he or she is most familiar with.

What Is An Insulin Pump And How Does It Work?

Insulin pumps are small medical devices that work by delivering insulin automatically according to your needs. It accomplishes this in a calculated, steady, and continuous fashion (referred to as the basal insulin). It also allows you to give a bolus dose close to mealtime for rapid-acting insulin delivery. So the best insulin pump or average insulin pump all do the same thing when it comes to how it works. Nowadays, pumps and CGMs work together, and knowing the nuances can improve your decision-making ability and satisfaction with your pump and the CGM.

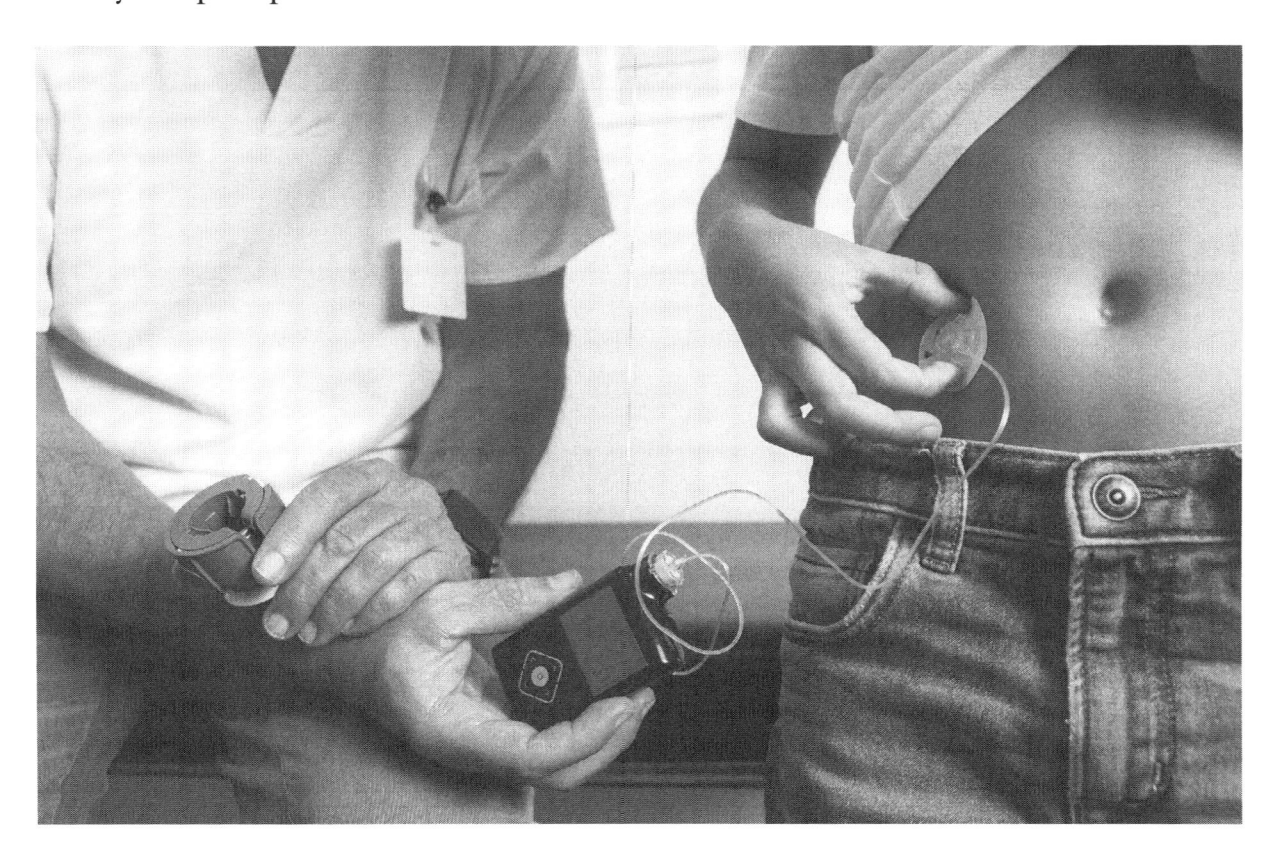

The pump is a small device, much like a pager or iPod, and is usually worn on your body. The pump has a thin catheter that is connected to a cannula. The cannula is inserted into the fatty tissue of the body to deliver insulin doses straight into the bloodstream.

The entire pump is fastened to your body with the help of an adhesive patch. This is commonly positioned around the stomach area but, based on your preferences, it can also be fastened to the thighs, upper arms, hips, or even the buttocks.

Many people love using the pump because it is small, discreet, and easy to use. You also don't have to deal with constant reminders about using it as you would with an insulin injection.

With a little education from a knowledgeable endocrinologist or diabetes educator, it is easier to understand how you can use the insulin pump, monitor blood sugar levels, and manage your condition successfully. If you've never used an insulin pump, you might want to consider one. Any type of pump can work well for you once you learn how to use it.

Who Is A Good Candidate For An Insulin Pump?

People of all ages can use an insulin pump for the management of their diabetes. Most often, insulin pumps are used in people with type 1 diabetes. Patients with type 2 diabetes who need multiple daily injections of insulin are also good candidates for the insulin pump. People who suffer from fluctuating blood sugars will benefit from insulin pumps because they can correct this problem better than the insulin you inject yourself.

Those who suffer from frequent episodes of low blood sugars will also benefit from insulin pumps. These are essentially computerized insulin delivery systems that make it a lot easier to control insulin delivery. You can avoid significant fluctuations in your sugars more easily throughout your day and prevent low blood sugars

There will be a modest improvement in your A1c as well when you use an insulin pump. The important thing to know about this is that if you have an A1c of 6.5%, you may have more noticeable blood sugar fluctuations than someone with an A1c of 9%

Is An Insulin Pump Right For Me?

Many people with diabetes use insulin pumps because they prefer a system with flexibility and a frequently adjustable insulin delivery system. Some people use pumps to avoid taking injections. Choosing between injections vs. insulin pump options usually hinges on your preferences. However, you should seriously consider an insulin pump if you:

» Frequently suffer from very low (below 70 mg/dl 3.9 mmol/l) or very high(>200) blood glucose levels.

» Have an active lifestyle and will benefit more from having changes in your basal rates. (Basal insulin need can change depending on your activity status)

» Want flexibility in your diet and like precision in insulin dosing. Using the bolus calculator in the pump helps you have better precision in your doses (allows flexibility in insulin dosing based on what you eat. It also gives you enhanced freedom regarding food choices)

» You have gastroparesis, which affects your stomach emptying. This makes it unpredictable as to when and how much sugar gets absorbed with meals.

Most people are intimidated by the words insulin pump. On the other hand, very few patients have a hard time using the insulin pump once they start. If you can use a cellphone, you can use an insulin pump. Insulin pump nurses and specially trained coaches help you a few times to get you started, and the rest is easy. Once you master it, you reap the benefits almost immediately.

Advantages Of Using An Insulin Pump

If you're still contemplating the idea of whether you should use an insulin pump or not, here are some reasons that can help you decide:

- *More Flexibility:* With an insulin pump, you can continue to live an active lifestyle without any issues. You don't have to find a special area to inject insulin into your body. Any area you normally would inject insulin will work for the pump infusion site.

- *Preventing the Risk of Low Blood Sugar:* Insulin pumps have a CGM reading system incorporated into them. Medtronic 670 G and Tandem Control IQ systems are the best examples. This CGM reading system ensures that the device monitors your blood sugar levels and automatically shuts down or injects more insulin based on your blood sugar levels. It's a safe, easy, and healthier way to consume insulin.

- *Accuracy in Insulin Delivery:* Insulin delivery can be set as needed. You have the freedom to set the dosage amount for the insulin you need. Even if you're a new diabetic, this is not a hard feature to master and will ensure that you don't accidentally have too little or too much insulin.

Disadvantages Of The Insulin Pump

The downsides of an insulin pump include the following:

- *Longer time to learn how to use it:* It may take time to learn how to program and use an insulin pump. This is honestly more of a problem for older patients or patients who are not highly motivated.

- *It can malfunction:* If the tube comes out of the skin or gets a kink, you won't get any insulin. If this happens, your blood sugar will increase unexpectedly. A CGM device will take care of this problem because it will quickly detect that a malfunction has happened. Thankfully, this problem does not happen too often with insulin pumps. There are also ways to prevent kinks if they happen too frequently.

- ***Insulin pumps usually cost more than insulin shots:*** This is a general statement. As long as pump supplies do not cost too much, most patients save money on insulin. This is because they generally use only one type of insulin. Using more than one type of insulin (long-acting plus rapid-acting, for example) can get expensive.

- ***Wearing or carrying an insulin pump all the time can be bothersome:*** Certainly, carrying an insulin pump can be an inconvenience. Yet, carrying an insulin pen, pen needles, and supplies can also be an inconvenience. Also, with an insulin pen, you will still have to expose your skin and give an injection every time. You will also have to do calculations yourself.

Components Of An Insulin Pump

Now that I've talked about what an insulin pump is, let's look closer at its components. The following are the three major components you can find in a traditional insulin pump:

The Pump

This is the main body of the insulin pump. It is computerized and battery-powered with an insulin reservoir and a built-in pumping system. Some have a touch screen, while others use buttons, which can be used to set the amount of insulin delivered into your bloodstream.

The Infusion Set

The cannula and tubing together make up the infusion set. They can either be made of steel or Teflon. The user simply fastens the infusion set to the skin with the help of adhesive tape. There are different types of infusion sets available for you to choose from. However, if you're not sure about which one is right for you, consult with an endocrinologist to see what your options are.

The Tubing

The tubing is a thin and flexible plastic funnel taped to your skin. It has a small needle inserted into the catheter, which transfers insulin to your body. Tubing lengths vary, and you can pick one according to your preferences. If you want to wear your pump at a distance from the infusion set, you can always choose longer tubing.

Various Kinds Of Infusion Sets Are Available

There are a couple of different types of infusion sets available. This makes it easy for different people and a variety of lifestyles. The following are the ones you can pick and choose from:

- *Straight Sets:* You simply insert straight sets at a 90-degree angle to the skin. They have shorter needles. They are more suitable for use on the arms or the buttocks. Additionally, you can use an insertion device with this set, which hides the needle. This is especially handy if you are afraid of needles.

- *Angled Sets:* You will be able to insert angled sets at a 30-45-degree angle into the skin. They also have longer cannulas than straight sets. This makes them more suitable for use by pregnant women, athletes, muscular people, and children. Due to the angle, you can view the needle and monitor the insertion area as well.

If you're not sure which set is right for you, ask your endocrinologist for help. They will be able to guide you when it comes to which type of set you should choose.

Various Types Of Insulin Pumps

Traditionally, insulin pumps are commonly found in two forms, such as tethered pumps and patch pumps. However, today there are more pump types available, including the closed-loop insulin pump. Let's briefly look at each of these types here.

- *Pumps that use tubing (Medtronic, Tandem):* Tethered pumps come with flexible tubing, which is tethered between the pump and the cannula. The pump also has various feature controls and is portable. Some pumps with tubing also come with a separate handset for controls. Patients can use a remote system to monitor their blood sugars.

- *Patch Pump (Omnipod):* A patch pump is a simple pump that you attach to your skin. The controls of the pump are on a separate remote control. Unlike the tubed pump, this remote can also serve as a blood glucose meter. The biggest benefit of using patch pumps is that there are no other tubes to fasten on the handles. However, you need to be very careful about accidentally knocking the pump. Also, a lot of people report sensitive skin and rashes due to the adhesive patch.

- *Closed-Loop Pumps (Medtronic 670G, Tandem Control IQ):* Also known as an artificial pancreas, closed-loop insulin pumps work completely automatically. They respond to readings the CGM device takes continuously through the glucose monitor. It's easy to wear throughout the day and is perfect when it comes to monitoring the blood sugar levels in your body. You will still have to give boluses for the food you eat; however, the pump will compensate for any calculation errors you make that can cause higher or lower blood sugars than the specified target blood sugars. Medtronic 670 G has its own CGM (guardian). Tandem Control IQ works with Dexcom.

Choosing An Insulin Pump

Now that you're ready to pick an insulin pump, we're listing down the top ones from renowned insulin pump brands. To help you make up your mind, we're sharing the pros and cons associated with these devices as well. This can allow you to choose a device that meets your needs and gives safe and continuous insulin delivery.

Tandem Pumps

Tandem insulin pump is called the T:slim X2. It relies on basal IQ technology to deliver insulin based on your glucose readings. Most recently, the company developed a control IQ system in early 2020.
The following are the pros and cons associated with their usage:

Pros

- » Recent improvements with control IQ system to prevent highs and lows. It also increases time in range (Keeps glucose as close to normal as possible).
- » They have a full-color, bright touch screen.
- » Chargeable batteries.
- » Waterproof; can be used while swimming and showering.
- » High-quality, compact design.
- » Integrates with smart devices like smartphones and CGM through Bluetooth.
- » No fingerstick blood sugar calibration is necessary. It is integrated with Dexcom G6.

Cons

- » With smaller buttons, the screen may go blank if you miss a button while indicating what you want it to do.
- » The tubing connector may snag on your clothes.
- » Unlock procedure is not simple and may cause hassle.
- » Has a weak vibration system.
- » Patients have to charge the pump 1-2 times per week.

Medtronic Insulin Pumps

These pumps use SmartGuard technology to suspend insulin delivery in case the blood sugar reaches an alarmingly low limit. They're simple to use and are available in two different types. The following are the pros and cons associated with their usage:

MiniMed 670G System

Pros

- » Great customer support. A large support team with nurses and an excellent technical team.
- » Hybrid closed-loop pumps with SmartGuard technology allow flexible levels of insulin delivery. Similar to tandem control IQ, it helps to keep blood sugar close to normal as much as possible.
- » An auto-mode feature adjusts insulin delivery according to a CGM sensor (As of 2020, it requires calibration twice a day with fingersticks).
- » A waterproof screen in full-color.
- » Choice of both fast and slow bolus delivery.
- » Patients can use the integrated meter as a remote control for insulin bolusing (contour next meter). Being able to use this meter is subject to insurance coverage, and the pump remote bolus feature has to be turned on).

Cons

- » CGM requires extra finger-sticks for safety checks and calibration.
- » Has a high learning curve to operate the pump on Auto mode.
- » Frequent alerts from auto mode can be disruptive, even after midnight!

- » If the patient does not do a calibration, the pump will take the patient off auto mode and beep annoyingly. Also, when not in auto mode, the insulin pump will not adjust your insulin delivery.

- » Staying in auto mode can be a hassle due to the need to calibrate with fingersticks multiple times a day.

- » Too many complicated menus.

MiniMed 630G System

Pros

- » Full-color screen.
- » Waterproof pump that can also sustain itself under 12ft of water for up to 24 hours.
- » Suitable for adults and children aged 16 and above.
- » A hybrid closed-loop basal adjustment that relies on predictive algorithms and CGM readings.
- » Bluetooth handset that delivers blood sugar levels to the machine.
- » Generates insulin statistics.

Cons

- » Outdated. It cannot integrate with a CGM.
- » Airplane Mode option for CGM accuracy may not be on par with other insulin pump brands.
- » You will have to pay for backup pumps.
- » Small screen and text which makes readability poor.
- » Complicated programming with lots of button pushing.

Omnipod

Omnipod insulin pumps are the only single-standing "tube-less" pumps in the market. They are pre-filled with insulin. The following are the pros and cons associated with these devices:

Pros

- » Portable and travel-friendly with no tubing required.
- » Can easily program through thick clothing a few feet away.
- » Less costly than other insulin pumps in the market.
- » Automated cannula insertion.
- » Water-tight pump.
- » Large and clear color screen with big readings.

Cons

- » It needs a separate device(called dash) to control insulin delivery. If you forget your dash device, you can not give insulin boluses for meals.
- » There is no integration with Dexcom as of 2020. They do not have their own CGM either.
- » There is no automatic adjustment of insulin, unlike the Medtronic or tandem pumps.
- » Complicated programming with lots of button pushing.
- » The hybrid closed-loop feature is still in development.
- » Pod might create a bump on the skin and stop working after 72 hours.
- » Supports only one cannula length.
- » No vibration option.

How An Insulin Pump Works

Pumps are designed to release insulin at a steady rate to provide basal insulin. Remember that basal insulin is the insulin that the body needs to keep your blood sugar at a normal rate. It is like the amount of gas your car burns in order to run at neutral/idle speed.

Pumps also give a bolus of insulin following data entered by you to account for the carbohydrates you eat with each meal. This would be like your car needing more gas when you are going up a hill. This is called your bolus insulin. The pump can do all that without an insulin needle injection since it is already connected to you under the skin.

Only short-acting (regular) or rapid-acting insulins are used with an insulin pump for diabetes. Most people use rapid-acting insulin with a pump. While they act quickly, you don't get the entire dose at once, so it acts as though you are getting long-acting insulin; it's just rapid-acting insulin given slowly over time to cover your basal insulin needs. Your doctor will help you figure out the amount of insulin that you should get in your pump to give you the basal dose you need on a regular basis. When you need bolus insulin, your pump will give a quick large dose based on the carbs you have had and your blood sugar levels.

Checking Sugars On The Insulin Pump

Checking sugars with an insulin pump is just as necessary as if you were using regular insulin shots you give yourself throughout the day. This means you will have to check your blood sugar level a few times each day.

On the other hand, if you are using Dexcom G6 or Freestyle Libre, you may not have to check your blood sugar at all (or at least only occasionally). Some insulin pumps have connections with continuous glucose monitoring systems such as the Dexcom G6 and Freestyle Libre. For example, tandem pumps work like this in what's called the Control IQ system.

With the Control IQ system, the insulin pump can adjust insulin delivery for both the basal and bolus insulin. It does not totally replace your own involvement in bolus insulin delivery. On the other hand, the system can compensate for the small mistakes you make when you miscalculate your carb intake or the effect of stress and exercise on your sugars.

Medtronic systems use their own sensors. Those CGMs are called Guardian. Guardian CGM systems can be more sensitive for picking up low or high blood sugars. Unfortunately, they are known to have many false-positive results, which can be frustrating.

The bottom line, using an insulin pump might help you keep your blood sugar levels under better control with fewer episodes of low blood sugar. This can even be more enhanced with the use of a continuous glucose monitoring system such as Dexcom G6, Freestyle Libre, or Medtronic Guardian.

Wearing An Insulin Pump

People with diabetes wear or carry their insulin pumps in different ways. They can put it in their waistband, shorts, underwear, or bra. They can also keep it in their pocket or clip it to a belt. At night, you can put your insulin pump in your pajamas or clip it to a blanket, sheet, or pillow.

Most people on an insulin pump can disconnect their pump and take it off for short periods of time—only about 1 to 2 hours. That way, you don't need to wear it when you shower, bathe, swim, or have sex.

Maintaining And Troubleshooting Your Insulin Pump

1. Change the needle and tubing every 2 to 3 days. You need to refill your insulin pump with insulin every few days.
2. Change the battery on schedule.
3. Make sure the date and time are correct on your insulin pump.

4. Keep an eye on the pump body and case for any cracks. Call the insulin pump company to get replacements if you note any structural problems. Your pump may lose water resistance with cracks.

5. Check the tubing for air bubbles occasionally and when you replace it.

6. Monitor your insertion site for infection or bleeding.

7. Discuss your rates and ratios you use for the pump with your endocrinologist to make sure they are accurate.

8. If you are changing insulin pumps or upgrading pumps for diabetes, make sure your endocrinologist knows about it and makes the transition.

9. Always have backup basal and bolus insulin in case the pump fails.

10. Try to have an online account with the manufacturer. Most diabetic insulin pump companies provide free accounts. Free accounts help you keep a record of your past settings in case you have insulin pump failure.

11. Make sure you have a glucagon injection handy. Let your family members know who to call for your diabetes-related matters when you are not able to.

12. If your blood glucose reading is abnormally high, take a corrective dose of insulin, and test again in one to two hours. If your blood sugars are remaining high or going higher, check your urine for ketones. Do a correction with fast-acting insulin to bring the blood sugar down while you also change out the tubing, reservoir, and infusion set.

13. If you are using a continuous glucose monitoring system such as Dexcom G6, pay attention to any alerts you receive. Make sure you set up the alerts correctly. Freestyle Libre does not have alerts. When your blood sugars are too high or too low from any CGM system, double-check with a glucose fingerstick.

Final Thoughts

Insulin pumps are another tool to help you achieve your diabetes goals. On the other hand, you do not have to have an insulin pump to be a successful diabetic on insulin. It is very important to discuss that with your endocrinologist to make sure the insulin pump is right for you.

Continuous Glucose Monitoring Systems

Diabetes is a chronic condition that does not have an ultimate cure; even so, it can be successfully managed with the right care and attention. Most people with diabetes use glucose meters and strips to monitor blood sugars on a day to day basis. However, another tool that is even more useful is the CGM system—a continuous glucose monitoring system. CGM devices measure your blood sugars and trends in blood sugar continuously.

There are several CGM devices available, and it can be confusing to determine which one you should use. The two most commonly used devices are the Dexcom G6 and the Freestyle Libre 2. There is another made by Medtronic called the Guardian Sensor 3. They each have advantages and disadvantages we will discuss in this section.

Dexcom G6 System- Soon To Be G7

Among the different choices, Dexcom systems have been in the market for much longer than the others. The latest version of the Dexcom CGM is called the Dexcom G6. Freestyle Libre entered the market in the last few years. Their most recent system is called the Freestyle Libre 2. There are major differences between Dexcom G6 and Freestyle Libre systems.

Whether you have type 1 or type 2 diabetes, you know how difficult it is to deal with fluctuating glucose levels in the body. Also, doing fingersticks so many times a day sucks! CGM systems continuously record your blood sugar readings every 1-5 minutes without using fingersticks.

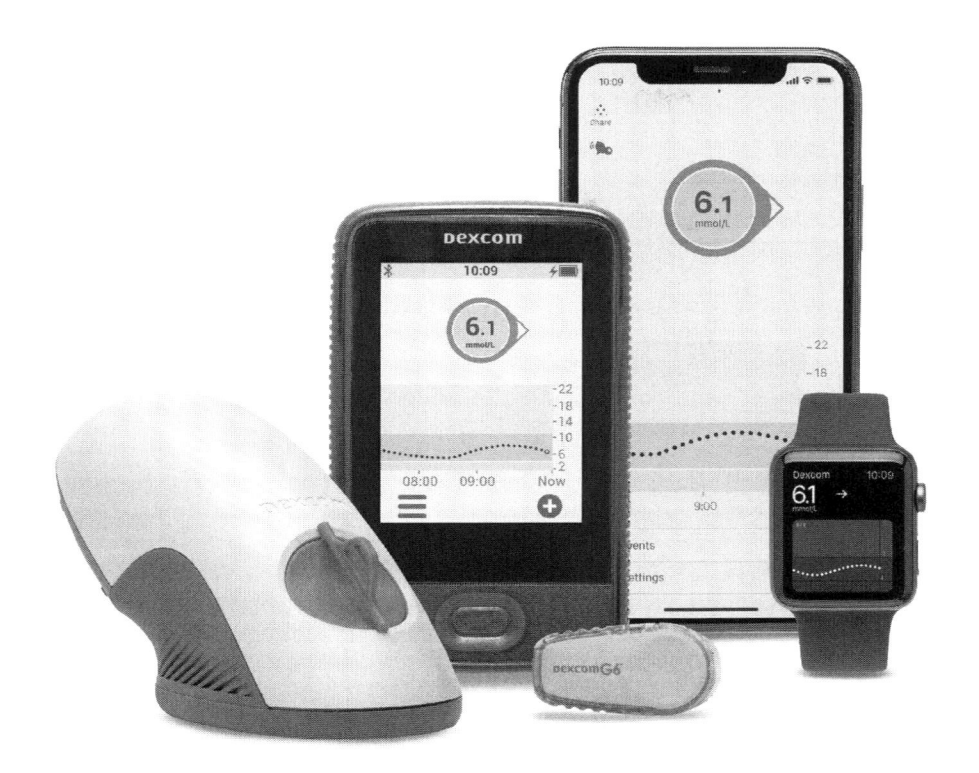

Highs and lows in glucose levels can be dangerous. With fingersticks, you can't always predict whether the sugars are rising or falling. CGM systems warn you that your blood sugars are either too high or too low and will tell you the trend it is going. They won't deliver insulin; you need to either give yourself an injection or use your insulin pump to adjust the amount of insulin you are getting.

Is CGM The Right Option For Me?

CGM systems like Dexcom G6 or Freestyle Libre are vital tools in the management of diabetes. When used along with insulin pumps or even multiple daily injections, they can improve the quality of your diabetes care and your life. Both Dexcom G6 and Freestyle Libre are approved to make treatment decisions based on the readings you receive.

If you identify with the following issues, then getting a CGM system is the best option for you:

- » If you are unable to meet and maintain the optimal levels of your A1C results
- » You frequently experience low glucose levels
- » You are mostly unaware of your blood sugar level
- » You want to lower your A1C targets safely without increasing your higher risk for hypoglycemia
- » Your blood sugar levels fluctuate frequently

Before you get a CGM system, remember to consult with your endocrinologist to see if one of the CGM systems is the right choice for you.

The Benefits Of CGM Systems

Using a CGM system can make it easier for you to manage your diabetes and to live your life with more freedom. The following are the major benefits of CGM systems:

- *Lower Your A1C Levels:* As an outpatient device, CGM systems are the most effective in helping diabetics maintain and lower their A1C levels safely. They are hailed as the best method for glycemic management in out-of-hospital settings.

- *Detect Lows and Highs:* With constant readings being offered, the CGM system can give fairly accurate readings about your glucose levels. These systems aren't perfect, as there are some problems associated with any CGM system in terms of accuracy under certain conditions. The data gathered can alert you about your highs and lows before they occur. Most importantly, your CGM system can keep you from experiencing hypoglycemia (low blood sugar) or hyperglycemia.

How To Choose The Right CGM?

Let's compare the Dexcom G6 and Freestyle Libre Systems

While there are other systems out there, these two are the most commonly used in clinical practice. Here are the general comparisons you can make between the two systems:

- » Neither the Dexcom G6 nor the Freestyle Libre requires a fingerstick (most of the time).

- » Dexcom G6 is more accurate, especially for blood sugars below 80 mg/dl (4.4 mmol/l) and above 250 mg/dL (13.9 mmol/l) than the original Freestyle Libre but new the new Freestyle Libre 2 seems to be on par with Dexcom.

- » Dexcom G6 does not require scanning the sensor via a meter or phone, while the Freestyle Libre needs scanning to find out the glucose level. The company is working on eliminating the scanning step to know the blood sugar.

- » Dexcom G6 is more expensive than the Freestyle Libre. Without insurance, forget buying the Dexcom G6. On the other hand, the Freestyle Libre can cost 120 dollars a month if you are willing to pay for it.

- » Dexcom G6 has alerts and predicts high and low glucose levels, while the old Freestyle Libre has no alerts. The new Freestyle Libre 2 now has an alert system. Unless you scan your sensor to find out your sugar level, you are still in the dark.

- » Dexcom continuously records blood sugars, while the Freestyle Libre stops recording if you have not scanned the device after 8 hours.

- » Dexcom can connect and help operate a closed-loop system with a tandem insulin pump, while the Freestyle Libre cannot be connected to any pump (and should not be used due to low accuracy).

- » Dexcom G6 has a cloud-based system and can be connected or integrated with other systems and apps.

- » The Freestyle Libre sensors tend to fail more frequently than Dexcom G6 sensors.

- » The Freestyle Libre 2 can't be used with a smartphone only, while the Dexcom and the old Freestyle Libre system can still be used with a smartphone without an actual reader.

Using CGM Systems And Troubleshooting Them

One of the biggest problems with CGM systems is inaccuracies. These can be frustrating and confusing.

These are the main reasons:

- ***The glucose level in a CGM system is that of your interstitial fluid and not your blood:*** Your interstitial fluid is the fluid your cells are bathed in. This is not the same thing as your blood. There is a delay of around 15 to 30 minutes in stable conditions when your blood sugar is not changing rapidly. If your blood sugars are rapidly changing (such as after a meal) or the blood sugars are rapidly declining (such as after a high dose of insulin), there will be a 20 to 25% or more difference between CGM readings and blood sugar levels obtained from a fingerstick.

- *The sensors are delayed:* There is also a delay because of the sensor itself. Since the sensor is not detecting the blood sugar directly, it relies on a chemical reaction to occur. The time it takes for this reaction and detection of the blood sugar is long enough to cause differences between a fingerstick meter reading and your CGM readings.

- *Fingersticks are fully not accurate either:* The fingerstick blood glucose measurement you get from your glucose meters is not 100% accurate either. If you are using the meter-obtained blood sugar as a gold standard compared to your CGM reading, you are making the wrong assumption. There are way too many meters on the market, and all have different accuracy rates, ranging from 5% to 20%. The best FDA-approved meters and strips have an accuracy level that is less than 20%. Given that there is variability in the meter-obtained blood sugar and delays in CGM systems, trying for the most accurate result is a futile attempt. Instead, you should focus on the trend, which we will talk about later in this section.

Many patients compare their fingerstick blood sugar results to their Dexcom G6 or Freestyle Libre results. Now that you know how these systems work, you should realize that this is actually a big mistake. You can't assume that the fingerstick result is accurate to begin with. Many blood sugar results from inexpensive meters can be up to plus or minus 20% of a venous blood sample. This is the blood the tech draws from your veins; it is the true gold standard test for blood sugar.

To complicate things further, your blood sugars will be different depending on the body part you take it from. A blood sugar of 100 mg/dL (5.5 mmol/l) in your fingertip may simultaneously be 120 mg/dL (6.7 mmol/l) in your toes (if you poked yourself there). The CGM systems don't even check your blood sugar levels—just the sugar levels in the fluid around your cells. This will almost always be different from your blood sugar levels, especially if they are changing; there is a delay from the time the sugar in your blood gets to the interstitial fluid. This delay will also add to the differences in sugar values you see.

<u>Focus more on the trend in blood sugar and not on the actual blood sugar level.</u> What most people do not understand is that the trend of the blood sugars is way more important than the blood sugar itself. The arrow indicators on your CGM system are more important than the exact number on the screen. So, instead of trying to do fingersticks and matching the readings with your CGM, concentrate on the direction of blood sugars.

With the readings and data gathered, your CGM system can predict the direction of your blood sugar levels. These predictions can be vital to preventing fluctuations in your blood sugar level over time. The readings also help you understand how different foods, activities, and medication can affect your diabetic condition.

Using Your CGM System To Make Treatment Decisions

No matter what system you use, you need to understand how to correctly use your CGM in your everyday life. Not all CGM systems, for example, need calibration. The manufacturer's instructions will tell you whether this is necessary. When you calibrate, the sensor understands that the electrical gradient at the time of calibration corresponds to the blood sugar that is calibrated via a fingerstick.

There are reasons why some systems must be calibrated. Remember that most CGMs have a sensor under the skin and not into the blood vessel, so the glucose readings are not true blood glucose readings. The CGM system has a chemical reaction inside the device called a glucose oxidase reaction; it estimates the blood sugar reading. The sensor detects and converts the products of the reaction into an electrical signal. If the signal observed doesn't accurately reflect the sugar level, the device will need to be recalibrated.

Interpreting Your CGM Numbers

Remember that your CGM readings are most similar to your actual blood sugar when your sugars are the most stable. This would naturally be before meals or when fasting (as long as you aren't taking insulin-secreting medications). Your screen will show a horizontal arrow next to the sugar reading:

If you see a horizontal arrow on the screen before a meal, you can be very confident and use that glucose reading as is. You do not need to make any adjustments to your mealtime treatment. We will talk about treatment decisions before meals, in between meals, or fasting.

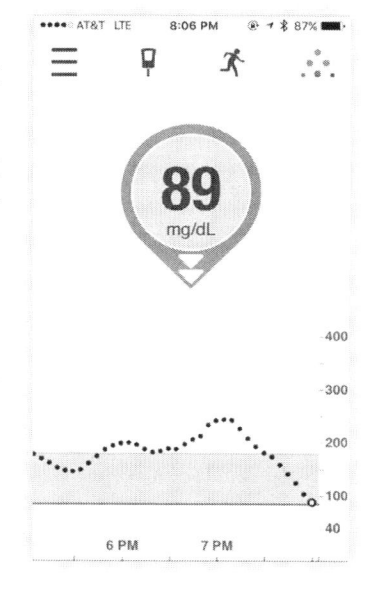

If You See An Arrow That Is Diagonal Up Or Diagonal Down:

This may indicate that your blood sugars are going up or down by about 1-2 mg/dL/min, which can lead to a 30 to 60 point change in your blood sugars over the next 30 minutes. In that case, there are a few things you can do to adjust your insulin dose.

If you are not using an insulin pump, you can add 30 points to the current blood sugar on the continuous glucose monitor screen. For example, if your blood sugar is 160, you can consider and treat it as if your blood sugar is 190. In this case, if you are using a sliding scale insulin regimen, you can determine the corrected insulin dose you need based on the adjusted blood sugar.

If you are using an insulin pump, you can enter that adjusted blood sugar into the pump, and the insulin pump will do the rest. If you are not using a pump, but you have a correction ratio for correcting high blood sugar, you can just do the math accordingly. You may also consider taking the insulin earlier than you typically take it. If you take insulin 10 minutes before a meal, you might decide to take your insulin 20 to 30 minutes before the meal when your blood sugar is already trending up.

If you see the downward diagonal arrow, the reverse is completely true. You can subtract 30 mg/dL (1.6 mmol/l) or 30 points from your current blood sugars and treat accordingly, as I just explained. In this case, you can also postpone your insulin injection until right before the meal.

If You See A Straight Up Or Straight Down Arrow On Your Dexcom G6:

This may indicate that your blood sugars are going up or down by 2-3 mg/dL/min, which can lead to a 60-90 point increase in blood sugars within the next 30 minutes. The same principle that I went through in the previous paragraph applies. In this case, you would add or subtract at least 60 points because the trend is up or down with one straight-up arrow.

For example, if your blood sugar is 160 and you see a straight-up arrow on your Dexcom G6 CGM, you should add at least 60 points, which will lead to 220 mg/dL (38.6 mmol/l) adjusted glucose levels that need to be used in a treatment decision. You would assume that your blood sugar is 220 instead of 160 mg/dL (8.9 mmol/l).

If you see a straight down arrow, you will subtract 60 points from your blood sugar on your Dexcom G6. In this case, 160 - 60 = 100 mg. This is the new adjusted blood sugar that you will use in treatment decision-making. Again, if you see a straight-up arrow, you may want to rush the insulin injection and do it earlier than scheduled. If you see a straight down arrow, you may want to wait even until after the meal to prevent a blood sugar drop.

Making Treatment Decisions Between Meals Or When Fasting Using A CGM Device

If you are not about to eat, yet you see your blood sugar is trending up with a diagonal arrow up or down, there are a few things you can consider, depending on the last time you ate and the last time you had an insulin injection or insulin bolus via an insulin pump. If you have an insulin pump, things are a lot easier as the pump will do all the math for you.

1. If your blood sugars are trending down with a diagonal arrow, one arrow down, or two arrows down, you should know by now that your blood sugars are possibly going to be at least 30 points, 60 points, or 90 points lower, respectively, based on the direction of the arrow. This gives you a heads up and gives you time to prepare for possible low blood sugars. For example, if your blood sugar is 90 and you see one straight down arrow on the Dexcom G6 screen, you know that your blood sugar may be 60 or lower within 30 minutes. It would be a wise idea to have a snack to prevent low blood sugar. If you see two straight arrows down, you should act immediately.

2. When you see a horizontal arrow indicating stable blood sugars, you will think that your blood sugars are stable. Do you have to worry about that? This depends on the situation. Exercise, for example, will reduce your blood sugars. Knowing that fact, it would be a wise idea to have a snack with a blood sugar of 90 mg/dL (5.0 mmol/l), even when you see a horizontal arrow, because your blood sugar may go low (below 70 mg/dL or 3.9 mmol/l) fairly quickly with exercise.

3. In case of upward trending blood sugars, when you see a diagonal or straight arrow up, you should know that your blood sugars will end up being at least 30 points with a ***diagonal*** up arrow, 60 points with one straight-up arrow, and 90 or more points with two straight-up arrows. For example, if your blood sugar is 180 mg/dL (10 mmol/l) 2 hours after a meal and you see two straight arrows up, you could immediately think that your blood sugar may end up at 270 mg/dL (15 mmol/l) within just 30 minutes. That means that you either did not take enough insulin or you have had too many carbs or too much fat in your meal. That can also happen if you are on steroids such as prednisone or when you are physically or mentally stressed.

If the arrow is pointing straight up and has two arrows upward, you should take immediate action to prevent severely high blood sugar. In this case, you can take a correction bolus of insulin to reduce the upward trend of blood sugars and hopefully correct it to normal levels. This can be tricky if you have had an injection within the first 2 to 3 hours, as frequent injections of insulin can lead to stacking, which later causes low blood sugars. To avoid that, you need to understand the duration of action of the insulin you are currently using.

For rapid and short-acting insulins such as Fiasp, Humalog, NovoLog, Apidra, Admelog, and insulin Lispro, the duration of action is typically 3 to 4 hours. For Novolin R or Humulin R, the duration of action can range from 5 hours to 8 hours. Typically, for rapid-acting insulin such as NovoLog or Humalog, you should know that by 2 hours after an injection, you would still have 50% of the insulin in your system. You should account for that previous insulin when you are correcting your blood sugars.

CGM Cost And Coverage Issues

Your insurance company often wants specific criteria if you can get insurance coverage for the device. These are the most common reasons why insurance companies will pay for the device:

- » Hospitalization for diabetes recently
- » Frequent low blood sugars (hypoglycemia)
- » Labile blood sugars (fluctuating blood sugars)
- » Insulin-dependent type 1 diabetes
- » Insulin-dependent type 2 diabetes

While there are reasons the insurance company thinks you need a CGM system, you might have your own reasons why you might think a CGM system is for you. A lot of my patients will want to use Dexcom G6 or Freestyle Libre just to avoid fingersticks. Unfortunately, if you are only taking metformin or only oral agents for diabetes, most insurances will not cover a CGM.

Insurance companies go by medical necessity, not necessarily patient convenience. I am all about patient convenience for my patients. On the other hand, insurance companies are there to protect their own interests. These devices are expensive and, if insurance companies start covering Dexcom for every patient with diabetes, insurance premiums will skyrocket. But do you really need Dexcom G6? Do you really need to carry a device on your body when you can check your blood sugar with a fingerstick a few times a week? And yes, some people like to see numbers and track their response to certain foods, which can help in their learning curve of how different foods affect their blood sugars.

Most of the time, individuals check their blood sugars excessively. This happens when they are newly diagnosed when they are obsessed with their blood sugars. The truth of the fact is this: if you are not on medications that cause low blood sugars and your blood sugars are typically in the same or similar range, there is no need to keep checking blood sugars every morning or every evening. Having a good idea of blood sugar levels with regular checking without being excessive is a reasonable thing to do for most patients.

Final Thoughts

Although continuous glucose monitoring systems are not perfect for exact blood sugar estimation, they are great monitoring tools showing your current glucose trends so you can make the insulin adjustments necessary. They are still fairly accurate, especially when blood sugars are stable.

When blood sugars are not stable, such as when there is a rapid increase or decrease in your blood sugars, there will be a delay in the transmission of the electrical signal that matches your actual blood sugar. Yet, they are still helpful in decision making by showing glucose trends. The CGM systems also give you high and low blood glucose alerts, giving you a heads up allowing you to act before a severe high or severe low glucose event happens.

Like everything else in life, it takes interest, persistence, and dedication to master your skills in managing your diabetes. You need to wear your CGM as much as possible and pay attention to the numbers you see on the screen, the arrow directions, and the other factors, such as diet and exercise, that affect your blood sugars. Also, a trusted endocrinologist will be your best friend in helping you have a happy and successful life with minimal influence on the quality of your life despite having diabetes.

A Modern Concept: What Are The Benefits Of Telemedicine And Remote Patient Monitoring?

There are two ways doctors can manage patients without being in the same room with them. These are called telemedicine/virtual visits and remote patient monitoring. Telemedicine is essentially a doctor's visit over the phone or on the computer. The doctor and patient get to see each other and talk to one another, but the visits are brief and may be insufficient for the diabetic patient.

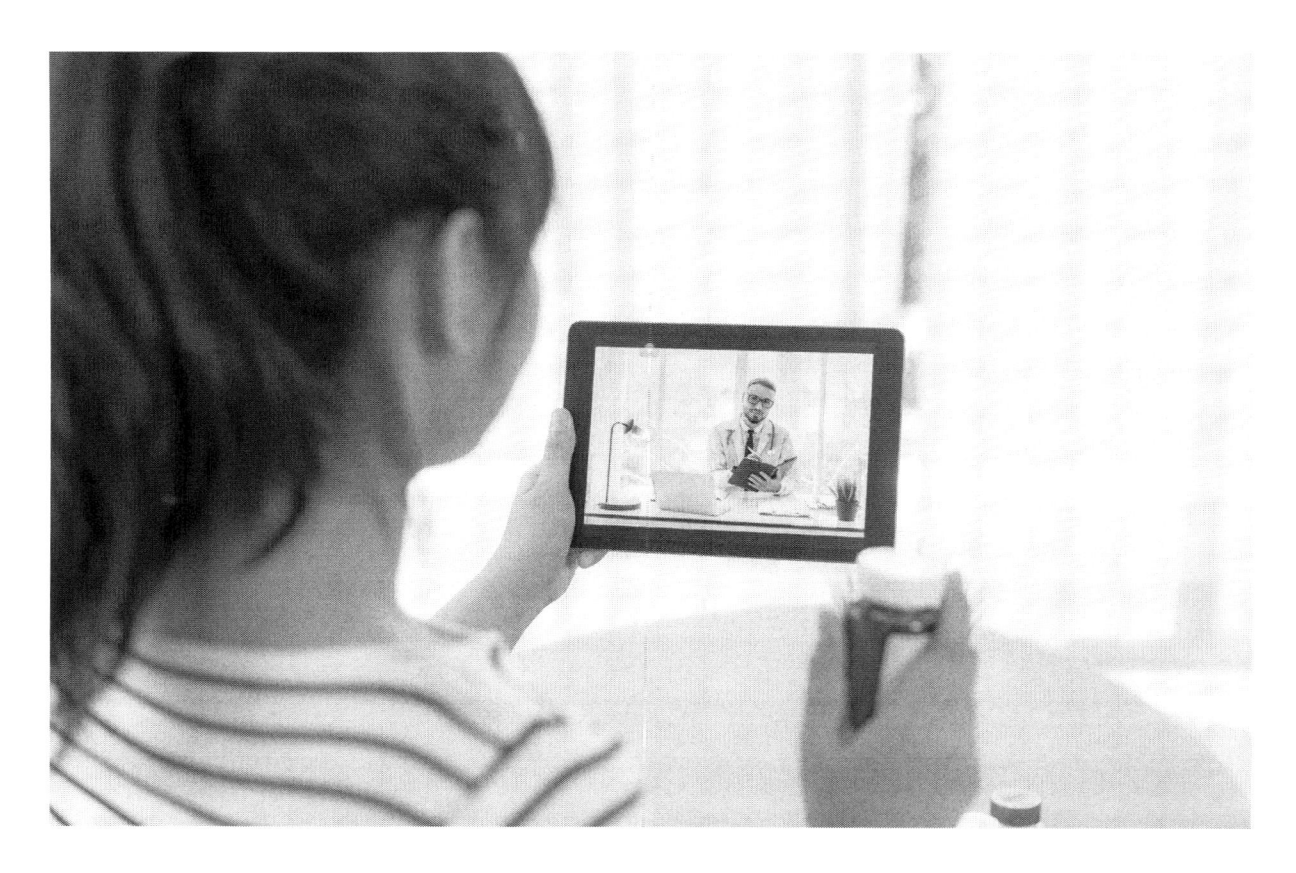

More recently, remote live glucose monitoring or remote health monitoring has become a new trend. Yet, most endocrinologists are still practicing traditional methods—reading your logs from home and trying to make sense of them. Some patients even forget to bring their logs, which cripples the doctor trying to make rational medication adjustments.

CHAPTER 5 - DIABETES TECHNOLOGY

Fortunately, there is a much more convenient option. Imagine a system where you check your glucose, and it goes to your doctor immediately, being automatically stored permanently. That would be a great idea, right? This is the basis of remote glucose monitoring. To make use of this feature, find an endocrinologist capable of doing remote medicine via remote glucose monitoring today.

Now that many diabetic patients are using CGMs, there is a lot of data that can presented on a 24/7 basis. As a patient, you have all of this information and may not know which data is important or what to do with the numbers you've gotten. Remember that CGM devices are only helpful when you make rational choices about the number you see on the device. This is where remote patient management comes in as a way to help diabetics maximize their A1c reduction with the peace of mind that they are getting quality advice about their clinical situation. ***SugarMDs is a company that delivers just that kind of service for patients who see the benefit of remote patient monitoring for their concierge members.***

How Does Remote Patient Monitoring Work?

Remote patient monitoring (RPM) can be accomplished with continuous glucose monitoring systems such as Dexcom G6 and Freestyle Libre, as well as Bluetooth or cellular meter technology. Some systems have a platform that can include all of the systems in one place. Doctors and nurses can monitor patients remotely and act instantly when the physiologic data received from a patient's device is out of range.

In this platform, patients can use their own CGM, a regular meter, or other Bluetooth or cellular meter, which transfers data automatically to the endocrinologist immediately after a blood sugar check. When patients use a special meter that has Bluetooth technology, they need a smartphone application.

Some patients do not want to use smartphones or a CGM or are not familiar with them. For those patients, cellular meter technology is the best solution.

That way, patients do not have to keep logs and do not need to use any technological device.

The bottom line is that remote patient monitoring is a subset of telehealth services. Telehealth services can still be delivered without remote patient monitoring. For example, video visits or tele-visits are examples of telehealth. Telehealth involves intermittent doctor's visits that aren't in-person. RMP is different because it is a 24/7 service that most effectively suits the problems seen in diabetes. Remote patient monitoring definitely adds a lot of value to telehealth services.

RPM doesn't replace telehealth visits. You can still see your doctor for routine visits to discuss diabetes planning and other issues or questions you might have. Every three to six months are often visits used to review your diabetes numbers and medications. By using remote patient monitoring, physicians will have a lot more information to make informed decisions regarding your diabetes. This is in addition to the day-to-day issues found during remote patient monitoring. The combination of telehealth and RPM allows for better chronic care management that becomes much more efficient and cost-effective.

How Remote Patient Monitoring And CGM Work Together In SugarMDs Center?

Remote patient monitoring or RPM works perfectly with CGM systems. Here's how it works:

- *Data is collected:* The RPM doctors collect blood sugar and blood pressure data via continuous glucose monitoring devices, Bluetooth, or cellular meters that require minimal to no involvement by the patient.

- *Data are transmitted:* Secure data transfer and correspondence occur via secure internet, phone, text, or other forms of communication.

- *Data is processed and analyzed:* The team examines the data and points out any areas of concern. The patient and the patient's healthcare team receive a report for out of range data and how this data was managed.

- ***Notification if necessary:*** Primary care doctors can see the team's remote monitoring via a secure portal or the app. They also see correspondence and reports created by the medical team. If there is an interruption in the communication or data collection, the team tries to reach the patient first. If the patient cannot be reached, local emergency medical responders are notified.

The Future Of Telemedicine

The use of telemedicine is increasing, especially since COVID 19. Recent studies have shown that telehealth interventions are effective in improving clinical outcomes and decreasing hospital admission. Telemedicine does this with excellent patient satisfaction as well. Telemedicine for diabetes specifically has also increased greatly. It shows promise in expanding access to health care, promoting disease management, and facilitating better patient health between in-person visits to their doctor.

Telemedicine for diabetes and remote glucose monitoring are particularly important in managing diabetes. Compared to other diseases, diabetes requires interpretation and responses to many types of data such as high or low blood glucose, blood pressure, and others the patient can measure in the home. These things are hard to review in a brief office or telehealth visit.

Medicare and other insurance agencies have become much more comfortable with the convenience and benefits seen with telehealth services. When it comes to RPM itself, agencies have been behind the times in seeing its benefits compared to spot virtual visits and are less comfortable with it; this is likely to change as the cost versus benefit data on this type of service becomes clearer.

CONCLUSION

Diabetes is a chronic illness that requires continual self and medical care. Self-management and education are frequently underestimated and yet, these are the most important to prevent the acute and long-term complications of this disease.

Diabetes care is complex and requires many issues beyond glucose control to be addressed. Understanding diabetes and human physiology are essential for anyone with diabetes to achieve long-standing control over their diabetes.

Diabetes is a disease, but what makes it manageable is how you deal with diabetes and adapt to it. The attitude towards your diabetes can affect your quality of life dramatically. Without the proper knowledge, most people either choose denial or ignorance due to fear. Knowledge is power, and I hope this book helped you empower yourself with the essential information you needed to have a healthy life despite having this chronic condition.

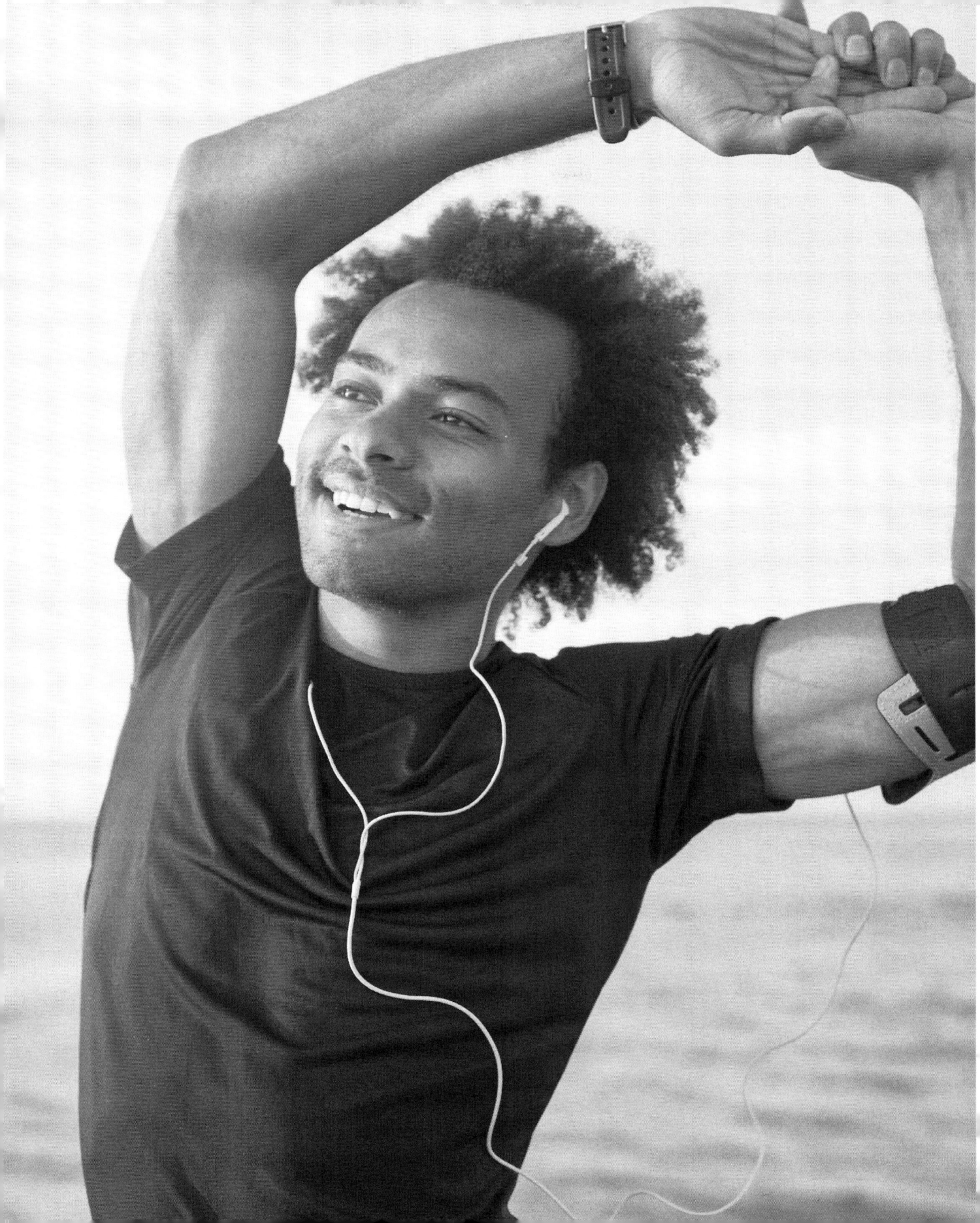

The End

Printed in Great Britain
by Amazon